SHOPPER'S GUIDE TO NATURAL FOODS

A Consumer's Guide to Buying and
Preparing Foods for Good Health

SHOPPER'S GUIDE TO NATURAL FOODS

FROM THE EDITORS OF
THE EAST WEST JOURNAL

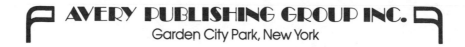

AVERY PUBLISHING GROUP INC.
Garden City Park, New York

Shopper's Guide to Natural Foods is compiled by *East West—the Journal of Natural Health and Living,* the monthly magazine that has played a pioneering role in the development of the natural foods industry for over fifteen years. Its quarter-million readers have come to rely on *East West* for in-depth articles on every facet of natural foods, as well as the latest information on holistic approaches to health and fitness. Other publications from the Editors of *East West* include *The Whole World Cookbook, Sweet and Natural Desserts, Natural Childcare,* and *Bodyhealth: A Guide to Keeping Your Body Well.*

Cover Design by Martin Hochberg and Rudy Shur
In-house Editors Diana Puglisi and Jacqueline Balla
Illustrations by Tim Peterson, Pamela Tapia, and Marilyn Cathcart
Typeset by Multifacit Graphics, Aberdeen, NJ

Library of Congress Cataloging-in-Publication Data

Shopper's guide to natural foods.

    Bibliography: p.
    Includes index.
    1. Food, Natural.   2. Marketing (Home economics)
I. East west journal (Brookline, Mass.: 1978)
TX369.S56   1987   641.3 '02   87-1098
ISBN 0-89529-233-5 (pbk.)

Printed in the United States of America

10 9 8 7 6 5 4 3 2 1

CONTENTS

ACKNOWLEDGMENT

This book has been many years in the making. In a sense it began over twenty years ago, when some of the early pioneers of natural foods first began researching whole foods, distributing them to friends and family, and organizing companies. These natural foods activists, including Herman Aihara, Paul Hawken, Michio Kushi, Robert Rodale, and Fred Rohe, along with such natural foods farmers and organic agriculture spokespersons as Frank Ford, Carl Garrich, the Lundberg brothers, and Charles Walters, Jr., planted the seeds that eventually grew into the contents of this book.

The writers and editors, the readers and friends of *East West Journal* (now simply *East West*) who have had a hand in nurturing these seeds over the past decade are also numerous. Among the most important people, certainly, are Dan Seamens and David Wollner. Their early, in-depth articles on grains, nuts, sea vegetables, and beans were the basis for a forty-page pamphlet called the *Shopper's Guide to Natural Foods* that *East West* published some five years ago. Expanding that pamphlet into the full-blown book you hold has depended upon the editorial efforts of a number of members of the *East West* staff, including Mark Mayell, Meg Seaker, Linda Roszak Elliot, Kirk Johnson, Thom Leonard, and, once again, Dan Seamens. All of these editors also contributed essential writing to the *Shopper's Guide*, rounding out the chapters with introductions, sidebars, and additional up-to-the-minute information.

Perhaps most importantly, we have to thank writers Jan Belleme, John Belleme, Ken Burns, Steve Earle, John Fogg, Barbara Jacobs, Ronald E. Kotzsch, Richard Leviton, Jacqueline Ozon, Martin Russell, Akiko Aoyagi Shurtleff, William Shurtleff, Bill Thomson, and Rebecca Theurer Wood for the insightful, well-researched articles that form the backbone of this book.

And finally, we'd like to thank managing editor Rudy Shur of Avery Publishing Group for his patience and encouragement as this project grew much beyond our initial plans in authority and scope, and Avery editor Diana Puglisi for her scrupulous attention to detail and the high editorial standards she demanded of everyone associated with putting this book together.

Leonard Jacobs
Publisher, *East West*

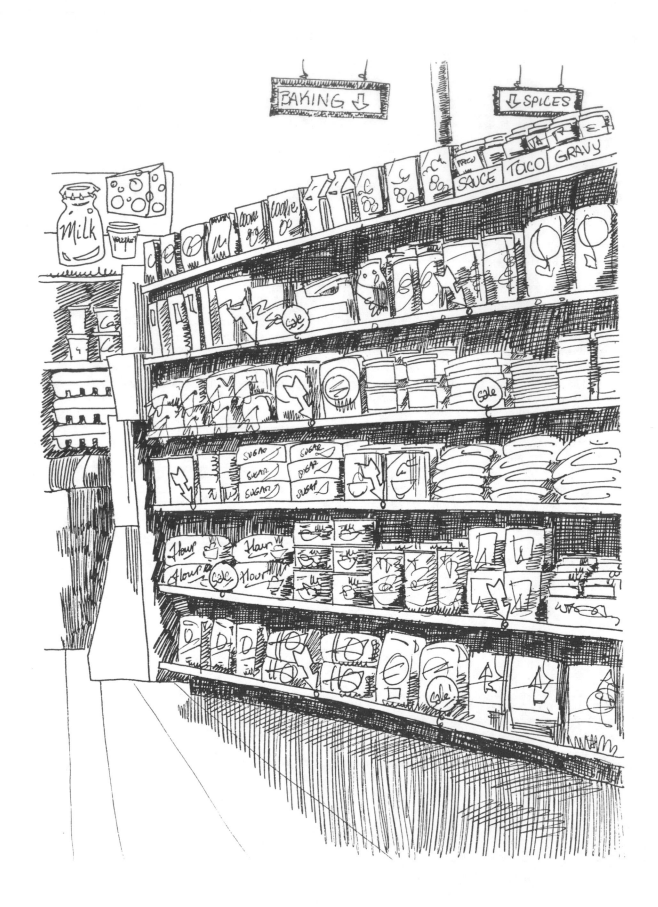

INTRODUCTION

Although the natural foods industry in the United States today represents only a small fraction of the total food market, it is an important and growing phenomenon. Even people who are still eating highly processed, chemical-laden foods are attracted to the *idea* of natural foods. Surveys have shown that, given the choice between two identical products, one labeled "natural" and the other not, most people prefer the natural. The reason why this is true is a topic unto itself, and one that this *Shopper's Guide to Natural Foods* will touch upon a number of times, but the salient point is that natural foods is a concept whose time has come.

During the rest of the 1980s and into the '90s, we can expect the increase in popularity of natural foods to accelerate, as their generally beneficial effect on health and their variety of tastes and textures attract more fans. For many people, eating natural foods will be a new and wonderful experience. It can also, however, be an intimidating experience. While some natural foods are obviously similar to their processed cousins, others are unique.

A truly natural, whole wheat loaf of bread may be the same size and shape (though a much darker color) than a loaf of commercial white bread. The whole wheat is made with different ingredients, and produced differently, in ways that many health-conscious consumers are interested in finding out about. This book is meant to be of tremendous use to such consumers.

Even for the great majority of people who are content to buy whole wheat bread simply because it is natural and therefore better than white bread, there is a need for a source of information on many other types of natural foods. Such popular natural foods as rice cakes, miso, seitan, tempeh, and umeboshi have no obvious analogues among mainstream American foods. By learning about and appreciating the broad variety of natural foods available to shoppers today, readers of this *Shopper's Guide to Natural Foods* can confidently join the millions of people worldwide who are switching to a natural foods diet—and changing their lives and their societies for the better.

What Are Natural Foods?

The beauty of natural foods often lies in the eye of the beholder. Defining natural foods is a complicated issue, and we'll go into it in more depth in Chapter 6, Labeling and Standards. Federal and state regulatory agencies have not yet agreed upon a definition for "natural," as most have for related terms such as "organic." Individual definitions of natural foods vary broadly. For many, natural foods are defined by what is missing—refined sugar and flour, chemical preservatives, artificial flavors and colors, and so forth. For others, the primary consideration is the origin of the food in nature; foods sold in as close to their fresh and natural state as possible, with minimal refining or processing. For our purposes, we can combine these two concerns and say that natural foods are recognizable as coming from nature rather than the factory, are minimally refined and processed, and have no artificial or chemical substances added to them.

Another distinction can be made between natural foods and health foods. The natural foods industry as such is really a very recent development, springing up in the late 1960s in the United States, as part of the general dissatisfaction young people of that time expressed toward other aspects of our industrial, "artificial and sterile" society. Dietary reformers such as Robert Rodale, Adelle Davis, and macrobiotic educator Michio Kushi preached the benefits of returning to a diet centered around fresh, whole foods. At the time, there was an established network of health food stores. Their main products were not foods, but rather vitamin and mineral supplements. Natural foods stores opened to provide a place where consumers could buy fresh produce, bulk grains, beans, nuts, cereals, and newly imported foods such as miso and tofu from Japan. Today, the distinction between health food and natural foods stores remains, although it is being increasingly blurred as natural foods stores broaden their offerings to include more vitamins, minerals, cosmetics, and other non-food items.

From its modest origins less than two decades ago, the natural foods industry has grown to a billion-dollar-a-year concern in 1987. This includes such pioneering companies as Eden, Westbrae, Erewhon (recently renamed U.S. Mills), Arrowhead Mills, and others with annual revenues in the tens of millions. It also includes thousands of small companies scattered throughout the U.S., Europe, the Orient, and elsewhere that are marketing natural foods products on a local or regional basis. And, especially within the past few years, the natural foods industry has grown to include well-established food manufacturing giants, as they've recognized the size and profitability of the natural foods market. Rice cake makers Chico-San and Arden Foods have been acquired by H.J. Heinz and Quaker Oats, respectively; tea maker Celestial Seasonings by Dart and Kraft, Inc.; and the natural juice company R.W. Knudsen and Sons by J.M. Smucker Company. Other food giants, such as Kellogg's with its Nutri-Grain brand cereal, are entering the natural foods market through internal product development rather than acquisitions. The wide diversity of size and expertise in the natural foods market is an indication of the vitality of the growing industry.

It is also an indication that natural foods are not a fad; they are here to stay. We might more accurately state they have returned to stay. For natural foods are what nourished the human race for over 99 percent of its existence. In the future, it may be that the past few hundred years (and especially the past fifty in the industrialized West) will be seen as a dietary aberration, a fad. As *The New York Times* nutrition columnist Jane Brody notes in *Jane Brody's Nutrition Book* (W.W. Norton and Co., 1981), "Most of the peoples of the world, including those in a number of developed countries, do not eat the way we do." Moreover, she says, "Americans didn't always eat like this"—consuming such a high percentage of foods in the form of meat, canned and frozen goods, sugary and fatty desserts, and highly processed and refined products. The natural foods alternative to the standard American diet is a logical and perhaps even inevitable choice.

Who Is This Book For?

This *Shopper's Guide to Natural Foods* is designed to be a tool for everyone interested in natural foods. If you've only recently become aware of the many advantages of eating natural foods, this book can be an introduction to a whole new world of fascinating foods, from arrowroot to wakame. Yet even veterans of the natural foods scene will find much that is new and interesting here. The natural foods industry is a young and dynamic one. New companies and product lines are introduced every year. Ancient and traditional foods, such as the grains amaranth and quinoa, are being rediscovered and offered in a variety of forms and styles. There are already some half-dozen monthly magazines, such as *Natural Foods Retailer* and *Whole Foods*, which do nothing but chronicle the comings and goings of natural foods products and companies. Most natural foods consumers have neither the time nor the inclination to become industry experts. This book offers a short course in what these natural foods are, how they are grown or produced, how they resemble or differ from commercial foods, what the best ways to use them are, and how they can improve both one's appetite and one's health.

Although you will find very few animal-based products discussed here, this book is not just for vegetarians. Many natural foods eaters are vegetarians who do not eat any red meat, fowl, or fish. Many other natural foods eaters have forsaken only red meat among these three foods. Some will eat no meat or fish, but will eat dairy products. The variations are endless. The veteran natural foods activist Fred Rohe has coined a nice word to get around this confusion. In *Nature's Kitchen: The Complete Guide to the New American Diet* (Garden Way Publishing, 1986), he offers the useful word *omnivarian*, which he defines as "a person who eats natural foods with an emphasis on plant foods, with complex carbohydrates as the principal foods, supplemented by all other types of food, including or excluding meat and animal products according to individual discretion or circumstances." Most shoppers for natural foods are probably omnivarians of this stripe, and they'll find much of value in these pages.

Only the largest of the natural foods stores generally carry meat and fish. In future editions of this book, we may well be able to include hints on what to look for in so-called "natural" or "free-range" chickens, or "organic" beef. Still, as the primary emphasis for most omnivarians is on whole grains, fresh vegetables and fruits, beans, seeds, and nuts, they are the primary emphasis in the *Shopper's Guide to Natural Foods*.

This book will be of use not only to people who shop in health food and natural foods stores, but to those who shop in supermarkets as well. Some "crossover" products, such as rice cakes and tofu, are already available in all three types of stores. Other products (such as soymilks) are on the verge of a breakthrough, while some (sea vegetables, for instance) will be found in only the natural foods store—at least for the near future. There are special considerations for shopping in these different types of stores, and we'll explore them in Chapter 1. It has been estimated that upwards of twenty million Americans buy natural foods regularly through these outlets. (A final source for natural foods is through mail order. Names and addresses can be found on page 191.)

Why Shop for Natural Foods?

Before we go any further, let's examine just what the attractions and benefits of eating natural foods are. Why do some people take extra time and make an extra effort to search out natural foods? Why do they choose from among the many natural foods that (because they are less processed than what most consumers are used to) may take more time to prepare for eating? We all lead busy lives. What makes this extra time worth it?

An important factor is the increase in nutrition and health available through natural foods. Since the beginning of the 20th century, when reliable records began to be kept, we can notice a number of distinct changes in the average American diet. These trends are, to say the least, a prescription for health disaster. Foods that have become increasingly popular include beef, cheese, processed fruit, ice cream, soft drinks, and frozen and canned vegetables. Foods that have gone down in consumption include fresh fruit, fresh vegetables, and whole grains. These are the foods that are rich in complex carbohydrates. The decrease in the consumption of complex carbohydrates has been matched by a vast increase in the consumption of sugars and sweeteners. In addition, Americans' intake of fat as a percentage of calories has probably doubled in the past 100 years, from about 20 percent to 40 percent today. When we take into consideration the vast quantities of sugars and sweeteners consumed today, we come up with the startling fact that over 50 percent of Americans' calories are ingested in the form of fat and added sweeteners.

The vast majority of nutritionists and health experts now agree with the advice of the United States Federal government, as stated in its dietary guidelines, for Americans to increase their consumption of complex carbohydrates and naturally occurring sugars (such as those found in whole grains and fresh fruits and vegetables), and decrease their consumption of refined and processed sugars, saturated fats and cholesterol, and sodium. The long-term result of such a shift in eating habits can be nothing but a reduction in debilitating, diet related conditions such as heart disease, some cancers, diabetes, and many other health problems.

Most of the natural foods that you will find described in this book are just the kind of foods now recognized as being most conducive to a long and healthful life. They are foods such as sea vegetables and whole grains, which are high in the "micronutrients" of vitamins and minerals, while being low in the harmful "macronutrients" of fat and sugar. We should note, however, that eating a natural foods diet is not a guarantee of health. There are many other factors, such as attitude and level of physical activity, that are important as well. Also, not all natural foods are equally healthful. There are on the market today natural cookies, candies, ice creams, soft drinks, and even meats. These are often qualitatively better than commercial cookies, candies, and so forth, in that the natural ones may offer more vitamins, somewhat less fat and sugar, and no harmful chemical additives, for instance. But, as we will see in Chapter 6, the difference is only one of degree. A steady diet of natural foods snacks and other high-fat, high-sugar products would not be healthful.

Health and nutrition aside, there are numerous other reasons to prefer natural foods to processed foods. One of these reasons is the greater variety of tastes and textures in natural foods. This may come as a surprise to people who think eating natural foods means "giving up and going without," but as veteran natural foods eaters will attest, it is true nonetheless. Upon consideration, its truth should be self-evident. Many people who eat a standard American diet restrict themselves to a few different meats, potatoes either French-fried or baked, and a few varieties of vegetables. The processed foods that make up the rest of the diet are limited to two main tastes—sugary sweet and overly salty. These tastes and textures are, of course, still available to natural foods eaters, but the range extends much further. The appealing taste and spaghetti-like texture of the sea vegetable hijiki, the meaty, spongy character of seitan, the chewy consistency of the hearty root vegetable burdock—these unusual culinary experiences are part of the attractiveness of natural foods.

Another advantage to natural foods that comes as a surprise to some is the opportunity to eat more economically. It cannot be denied that many items in natural foods stores are more expensive than similar products in the big supermarkets. Due to the economics of food manufacturing and retailing, small companies and small stores don't move the volume of product that industry giants do, so the markup to consumers ends up being higher. On the other hand, switching to a natural foods diet usually means buying bulk grains and beans, fresh vegetables, pastas and breads, and other nutrient-dense, relatively low-cost foods. By shopping wisely and avoiding higher-priced meats and processed foods, most people find that they can substantially reduce their food dollars.

Finally, we should not ignore the ethical or philosophical considerations of eating a natural foods diet. The foods each one of us eats affect not only the individual, but all of society. Inevitably, there are environmental, social, economic, and even political implications connected with all foods. These range from the obvious (eating lion meat may be contributing to the extinction of a species) to the more subtle (eating fast-food hamburgers may be contributing to the deforestation of the world's rain forests, since many are being cut to provide beef cattle range). Some of the common foods in the average American diet that should be carefully considered by consumers because of their broader implications include coffee, sugar, bananas, dairy foods, chicken and eggs, and chocolate. On the other hand, natural foods such as grains, seeds, nuts, beans, vegetables, and fruits carry their own set of implications. Does your purchase support an agribusiness conglomerate that is harmful to nutritional and social diversity in a region? Does your purchase reinforce a food system that wastes energy by trucking vegetables to your area from across the country or around the world? Is your food purchase a vote for natural methods of pest and weed control, or chemical poisons? By eating a natural foods diet, we do not necessarily contribute to a better environment and a more just economic and social system, but it is likely that we will have greater opportunities to do so than we would if eating a meat-based, processed food diet.

What's Here and How to Find It

This book is an anthology of articles that have appeared in *East West—The Journal of Natural Health and Living. East West* is a monthly magazine, begun in 1971 and published out of Brookline, Massachusetts, which has been in the forefront of the natural foods movement. More than a few of its writers have gained experience through working in natural foods stores, or by starting natural foods companies. Most of the articles in the *Shopper's Guide to Natural Foods* have been written within the past few years, and some specifically for this book. Older articles have been updated and revised.

The bulk of the book is made up of chapters on the broad categories of natural foods: grains and flours; breads, pastas, and seitan; produce; sea vegetables; fruits; seeds and nuts; beans; beverages; condiments; and cooking ingredients such as oils and sweeteners. There are also discussions of shopping in natural foods stores and supermarkets, labeling and standards, and the value of pressure cookers.

We have included both long, in-depth articles and short, practical sidebars. Browsing through this book, you will come upon a wealth of fascinating information, ranging from the historical origins of pasta to how cooking oils are produced. By using this book as a reference, you will also be able to find the answers to such specific questions as: How do I make a sourdough starter? What's the difference between shoyu and tamari? Is it true that heavy metals are concentrated in sea vegetables? What are the differences between the dozens of non-dairy frozen desserts on the market today?

As an area of study, natural foods is still a young and mostly unexamined field. This book falls far short of being an encyclopedia of natural foods. Yet we do think that the *Shopper's Guide to Natural Foods* is the most comprehensive and reliable report available today. We welcome our readers' comments, clarifications, and especially suggestions for other aspects of natural foods worthy of consideration in future editions of this book. The efforts of all people who are concerned about natural foods and their relation to better individual health and social health are part of the contribution toward a better world.

1. INTRODUCTION TO NATURAL FOODS

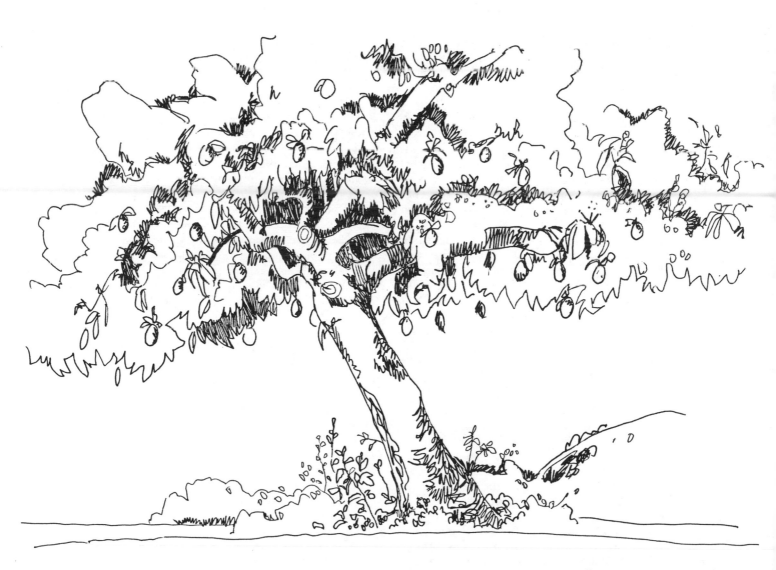

Pamela Dupie 87

A Natural Foods Store Primer

Twenty years ago, in the early stage of the natural foods movement in this country, the ''health food store'' was the principal type of alternative food outlet. This enterprise, however, actually sold very little food. Shelves were crowded with vitamins, nutritional supplements, ''natural'' medications, and various potions and elixirs. Bottles of papaya-mango juice and foil-wrapped bran biscuits added splashes of color here and there. Instead of cookbooks, the book rack offered pamphlets on such subjects as ''Vanquishing Wrinkles with Vitamin B_{17}.'' Bright fluorescent lights, vinyl floors, salespeople in medical white, and high prices all contributed to an ambience of a somewhat bizarre suburban pharmacy.

Although the health food store still exists, for the most part it has been superseded by the *natural foods store*, where the primary aim is to provide whole, unadulterated, staple foods—organically produced if possible—and sell them at competitive prices. A few natural foods stores stock only these items. Many, however, have adopted some of the characteristics of the older health food stores, selling vitamins, supplements, and other high-profit, low-bulk, nonfood items. In any case, these stores are very different from the supermarkets where Americans do most of their food buying. Shopping in such places, especially at first, can be a disorienting experience, as unfamiliar products are offered in unfamiliar ways. Let's take a tour through a typical natural foods store and see what we find.

Upon entering you will probably be struck by the size and decor. A few natural foods supermarkets boast of vast shelf space, broad aisles, and commodious shopping carts; some operate out of closets in people's homes. The typical one, however, is approximately the size of an average convenience store, featuring narrow aisles and hand-held shopping baskets. Many natural foods stores have wooden shelving and muted lighting, which create an atmosphere of rustic simplicity. But even though the natural foods store may be small and appear unsophisticated, it can meet virtually all of your food needs. And the people who work there are usually committed to and knowledgeable about the foods they sell, and are apt to be helpful and friendly.

You will probably notice that the store is dominated by barrels or bins, in which various foods are offered at ''bulk'' prices. Bulk merchandising is perhaps the most outstanding characteristic of the natural foods store, although large supermarkets now offer many items in bulk, from pasta to cookies. Eliminating unnecessary handling and packaging, bulk bins make the highest quality food staples available at competitive prices. On each bin you should find a tag identifying the contents and its price per pound. Conscientious stores will also tell you where the product comes from and whether it is organic. For example, a tag might read, ''Long Grain California Brown Rice, Organic, $.85/pound.'' Near the bins you will find a hand scoop, brown paper bags of various sizes, and a marking pencil.

Suppose that you want to buy some rice. The important thing to remember is *not* to walk up to one of the salespeople and say, ''Excuse me, would you please bag me up eleven-and-a-half ounces of brown rice?'' This is the age of self-sufficiency and self-service: courageously grab the scoop and a bag and measure out what you want—taking care not to spill the grains, beans, or nuts—and then write the price per pound on the bag. Many natural foods stores now feature plastic bins with an ingenious door spout for conveniently filling bags without the use of a scoop.

The bins contain a variety of basic foods, including whole grains such as barley, wheat, oats, different varieties of brown rice, millet, corn, buckwheat, and rolled oats. These can be cooked and eaten as bought, and any good natural foods cookbook (the store will undoubtedly carry some) will tell you how to do it. People with grain mills can also use whole grains to make fresh flour.

There will also be various kinds of flour (whole wheat, pastry wheat, and cornmeal, for instance). The flour should be ground fresh daily, or even ''on order.'' Once ground, it should be stored in a cool or refrigerated spot because as soon as the grain is broken, it begins to oxidize and loses some of its nutritional value. If the flour is simply kept in a bin, make an effort to find out when and where it was milled. The answer may convince you to purchase a home mill.

Flour products such as whole wheat noodles and macaroni, both domestic and imported, are also available. Some are made of durum wheat, and there is a line of pasta made from unenriched semolina and Jerusalem artichoke (see page 48) flour. Although only a few kinds of noodles will be sold in bulk, a much larger selection will be found in packages nearby. Observe whether the bulk noodles are protected from dust and dirt—sometimes they are just presented in open boxes.

The bins also contain a variety of beans such as lentils, soybeans, black and navy beans, azukis, black-eyed peas, chick peas, split and whole peas—the selection varies in each store but is usually diverse. In addition to being delicious and infinitely versatile, beans are a valuable source of protein. Again, if you are a neophyte, the available cookbooks will tell you how to prepare bean soups, casseroles, main dishes, salads, pates, and so forth.

Seeds and nuts are rich in protein and good-quality oil. You will find sunflower, pumpkin, and sesame seeds, almonds, filberts, walnuts, and cashews in bulk, as well as the faithful peanut (which is technically a legume, not a nut). The seeds and nuts may also be sold in the shell—they may be fresher this way. On the other hand, some may be sold roasted and salted or sprinkled with tamari, thus ready for immediate consumption. This, of course, raises the price and involves processes that are just as easily done at

home. Peanuts, soy nuts, and sunflower seeds are sometimes roasted in oil, but you will rarely see these in the natural foods store. Check to make sure the nuts and seeds are not rancid. As with any food, the closer they are to their harvested state the more fresh, economical, and healthful they will be. Ask the salesperson if you can sample them before purchasing a large amount.

Granola, which was inherited from the Swiss and German natural foods movements, has become popular throughout the United States. Granola consists of a whole grain base—usually rolled oats—and added seeds, nuts, dried fruits, sweeteners, and occasionally milk solids. Vegetable oil is mixed in, and the whole concoction is baked or roasted. You should find a wide selection of granolas in the bulk area of the store, ranging from Spartan mixtures of oats and sunflower seeds to sybaritic blends containing walnuts and Adriatic figs. Most granolas are sweetened with honey or maple syrup. Occasionally, you will come across a type that is sweetened with brown sugar. Since brown sugar is merely colored white sugar, you may want to avoid this. It is a good idea to read all ingredients care-

Ten Questions for Your Local Natural Foods Store

As the advantages of eating a natural, whole foods diet become increasingly evident, more and more stores are being opened all across the United States to cater to natural foods shoppers. Many are small "Mom-and-Pop" operations, while others are part of national or regional chains. If you are lucky enough to have a number of natural foods stores in your immediate area, your patronage at one of them is in effect a vote for its products and services. The following ten questions, which can be answered by observation or directed to a store's owner or manager, will help you to obtain a better idea of how informed the store's staff and owners are about the products they are selling, what their standards are and how they enforce them, and whether the store is the best place for you to shop for your natural foods groceries.

1. Who owns the store—a corporation, the manager, or an absentee owner? Does the store take an active part in the community, for instance, by sponsoring classes, offering food demonstrations, or donating leftover food to a local food bank?

2. Does the store have a written statement of quality standards that they post or make available to the shopper? What is the store's return policy?

3. Can the employees give you clear information about the products they carry and the standards of the manufacturers? Is the service and speed of the check-out line acceptable?

4. Are bulk food bins labeled with the source of the product and not just generically (that is, "Lundberg's Organic Brown Rice" as opposed to just "Brown Rice")?

5. Does the store sell any commercial products that you know contain refined sugar, chemical additives or preservatives, or other ingredients you wish to avoid?

6. Does the store carry organic produce and products? Are they strictly marked and separated from nonorganic food? Where does the store's nonorganic produce come from, and do they try to buy from local and regional farms?

7. Does the store sell predominantly non-food items, such as vitamins and cosmetics? Does it carry fruits, vegetables, and bulk grains, beans, nuts, and cereals?

8. Does the store buy direct from the supplier or through a distributor (and who is the distributor)? Are the store's prices in line with industry norms?

9. What day do perishables such as bread, produce, dairy, and tofu get delivered? Are they delivered more than once a week? Is the staff careful about removing out-of-date products from the shelves? Can you make special orders through the store?

10. Is the store neat, clean, and well-lit? Are the hours convenient for shopping?

No store may have the best answers to all these questions, but just the act of asking them may help to inspire a greater consciousness—on the store's part—of the importance of maintaining quality standards for products and services.

fully. Most stores list the granola's ingredients on the bin (if they don't, they should).

Peanut butter may also be sold in the bulk section of the natural foods store. If so, you will see several plastic tubs, each containing a different type: salted-chunky, unsalted-smooth, and so forth. Some stores even have a peanut grinder, allowing you to grind your own right on the spot. The store may also carry tubs of sesame butter and sesame tahini. Generally, sesame butter is ground from unhulled sesame seeds that have been roasted beforehand; it can be used like peanut butter. Sesame tahini consists of ground hulled seeds, usually unroasted, and can be used in cooking and in sauces. Other nut butters—almond, sunflower, macadamia, and cashew—are often found in jars on the shelves. Unlike commercial nut butters, these have probably not been hydrogenated, so there will be some oil separation. If there is a lot of oil, the butter may have been sitting on the shelf for too long. Because natural nut butters can go rancid, be sure to return any that have an off taste.

Save all glass jars, and use them when purchasing nut butters and other bulk products. Have them weighed by a store employee before filling them, so you will not be charged for the weight of the jars. You can usually buy jars, but they are expensive. In addition, plastic containers often cost a nickel or a dime, so why buy them when you can simply recycle a glass jar?

This recycling of glass jars will also prove useful when buying oils and sweeteners. The spigoted plastic containers in the "liquid bulk" area of the natural foods store contain sesame, corn, safflower, soybean, and sometimes olive oil, as well as maple syrup, honey, unsulfured molasses, and barley malt. Here again, a fearless and enterprising attitude is necessary. After having your jar weighed, hold it under the spout and turn the spigot. But be sure to close it before your jar is full, or some of the viscous substance will cascade over the lip and onto your hand.

Except for the consumption of dulse along the Maine coast and kelp in the Pacific Northwest, the eating of sea-weeds has never been popular in this country. In recent years, however, edible seaweeds (now frequently going under the more sophisticated name of "sea vegetables") have become increasingly popular. Some people take to them immediately. For others they are an acquired taste (but one worth acquiring) since, in terms of mineral value, they are the most nutritious vegetables around. They are also extremely versatile. Many stores offer a variety of sea vegetables, often in bulk form, including dulse, alaria, and kelps from the east and west coasts of the U.S., sea palm from the west coast, and wakame, kombu, arame, and hijiki from Japan.

All of the items that have been discussed thus far are usually available in packaged form as well as in bulk. Often, just above the appropriate bulk bin the same food will be neatly packaged and arranged on a shelf; the price, however, will be 25 to 40 percent higher. So unless you are in a terrific hurry, can't handle a scoop, or have a phobia about brown paper bags, it is most practical to purchase in bulk.

Once you have been through the bulk section, other parts of the store will resemble the corresponding sections of any food store. However, the apparent similarity belies real differences. In the produce department, in the cooler and freezer, in the bread section, among the snacks and crackers, and on the cosmetic shelves you will indeed find special quality—or at least you should. Unfortunately, placement in a natural foods store is no guarantee of the ultimate healthfulness of a product.

Thus it is important to continue reading labels. Many stores have clear, strict standards concerning the products they sell. They may refuse, for instance, to carry anything containing white sugar, white flour, synthetic preservatives, or chemical additives. Some also refuse to sell products containing fructose. Other stores, however, do not have such clear guidelines. By reading the label you will discover if there are any ingredients you would prefer not to eat.

Once I bought a pint of soy "ice cream" at a leading natural foods store in Boston and discovered that it contained fructose. I wrote to the company and learned that it has a strict ban on all products containing fructose. They were unaware, however, that this particular flavor contained it. So, as in any food store, read the label before you buy.

Vigilance is important even in the produce department. Not every natural foods store has a produce section. A good one should provide organically grown vegetables and fruits whenever possible. Out of season, the produce may come from ecologically aware growers in California and Florida. In season, it is the harvest of local growers. When this is the case, the store is doing a true service to both producer and consumer. Organic fruits and vegetables are worth the 20 to 30 percent extra cost. In addition to sparing your body some poisons, you are supporting a grower who is raising food in a way that enhances both the soil and the environment.

Often, however, shops will procure commercial-quality produce from a source used by regular food stores. If so, you are probably better off buying the same things at a produce center, where they will most likely be cheaper and fresher. Organic items are very clearly marked as such. Unless something is specifically labelled "organically grown," chances are that it is not.

The freezer and cooler sections of the typical natural foods store offer an increasingly wide variety of products. There are animal and dairy foods. Many stores carry organic meats, eggs from free-running, grain-fed hens, high-quality yogurts, and rennetless cheeses. There are also ice creams made from real cream (rather than from petroleum byproducts) and sweetened with honey or maple syrup. You can expect all of these to be more expensive, and better-tasting, than their supermarket counterparts. If you have any doubt as to whether they are worth the extra

How Much Is Enough?

When confronting an unfamiliar array of foods one must learn anew how much to buy. Several factors should be considered: how much storage space you have, how often you go shopping, how much you eat, which foods you and your family prefer and, most importantly, how strong the Sherpa is who carries home the groceries. With experience you will soon have a *modus operandi* appropriate to your household, just as you did when you were filling up the shopping cart at the supermarket.

Buy perishable items in small quantities. Flours and soy products such as tofu and tempeh should be used fairly quickly. Flours lose their freshness and nutritional value from the minute they are ground. Tofu will go bad in less than a week even in the refrigerator, although tempeh can often be kept for up to two weeks. In each case check the date of processing, choose the most recent, and buy only what you need until you go shopping again. Oils, and nut and seed butters, tend to become rancid; store them in a cool place away from light and, if possible, refrigerate them. Use them within several months' time.

You may want to buy less perishable staples in greater quantity. Grains, beans, sea vegetables, dried fruits, miso, and shoyu all keep almost indefinitely . . . with a little care. If you buy in quantity or in bulk, you may be able to get a substantial discount. A two-pound bag of dried apricots may cost only 50 percent more than a one-pound bag. If you buy a twenty-five- or fifty-pound sack of rice or

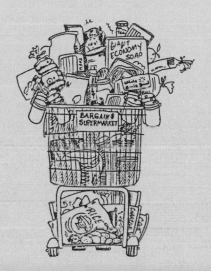

beans you will often get a substantial savings. Co-ops usually offer such possibilities; natural foods stores do so as well, to a lesser extent. If you eat rice once a day your twenty-five-pound bag will disappear at the rate of about four pounds a week. A family of four will go through the whole sack within a few weeks.

A cool, dry place in which to store these staple items is essential. Add a few bay leaves to the grains to prevent insect infestation. If you have a problem with mice, a small wooden barrel with a cover is a good investment. For smaller quantities, one-gallon glass jars with wide mouths make excellent containers.

Miso and tamari should be stored in glass or ceramic rather than in plastic or waxed-paper containers, as they contain salt and enzymes that eventually break down these materials. These salty soy products should also be kept in a cool dark place. Mellow or young misos should be refrigerated. Though these foods keep for a long time, they are more perishable than grains or beans, so plan to use them within six months. If white mold appears on the top, be sure to skim it off.

price, consider the hormones and antibiotics that are used in this country's factory farming business.

In this section you will also find some non-dairy alternatives. Tofu is a soybean product that comes in white, rectangular cakes. It is an easily digestible and excellent source of protein, long used in the Orient. Tempeh, recently introduced from Indonesia, is also made from soybeans (sometimes with added grains) which are steamed and then fermented. Tempeh comes in flat, dense cakes and, like tofu, has some of the qualities of cheese. It is a versatile product that can be prepared quickly and deliciously. Seitan, or "wheat meat," is the gluten part of the wheat (the bran and starch are removed), seasoned with shoyu. It looks and tastes similar to meat—at least to someone who has not eaten meat for a long time. There are even ice creams made from soybeans that are quite similar to the dairy product itself.

Carrot and vegetable juices, fruit juices, soymilks, non-alcoholic beers (made from water, malt, corn, hops, and yeast), and ginger and root beers are found in the cooler. Some natural soft drinks contain fructose, so if you wish to avoid this ingredient, read the labels. On juice bottles, look for labels that read "no preservatives" and "no added

sugar." Unfiltered juices show some sediment that has settled at the bottom of the bottle. Though they are less clear than filtered juices, their nutritional value is superior. Sparkling juices have had CO_2 (carbon dioxide) added. Juices made from organic fruit are rare.

Spring and mineral waters are also found in the cooler or elsewhere in the store. Some of the waters are naturally carbonated, while others have had carbon dioxide added. One company, which lists added natural carbonation in its ingredients, brings in CO_2 from a natural source and pumps it into its spring water.

Tofu, seitan, tuna, and various other sandwiches made with whole wheat breads will probably also be available in the refrigerator section. Although the ingredients will vary widely, they will be better than their supermarket counterparts—and more expensive.

An increasing number of ready-to-eat, precooked foods—such as canned or bottled soups and vegetables—have become available. There are even complete meals that you simply drop into boiling water. Frozen whole-wheat tofu pizza, frozen lentil croquettes—every day a new product appears, making the natural foods store look more and more like the local supermarket. Although the ingredients tend to generally be of a higher quality, some prepared foods are far superior to others, depending on the ingredients and the amount of processing. In a pinch or in special circumstances these foods can be quite convenient and useful. However, prepared products should always be used with discretion. In general, the more processing, packaging, traveling, and refrigeration that any food undergoes, the less fresh-tasting and healthful it becomes. In terms of taste and nutritional value, there is nothing like a home-made meal of grains, vegetables, and beans.

The same holds true for the amazing and growing variety of snack foods—cookies, chips, candies, honey ice creams, and so forth. Here, too, discretion is in order. These foods tend to be high in oils (some carob candies are almost all saturated fat!) and rich in simple sugars. A "natural" potato chip still contains about 90 percent oil, and a candy bar made with honey still gives the stomach and pancreas a sugar jolt. A bag of pretzels may contain more sodium than you probably need in a week! Such goodies are tempting (they are usually stationed near the check-out counter) and expensive. It is easy to prepare something at home that is fresh, more healthful, and just as delicious—at a fraction of the cost.

The bread and baked goods section of the natural foods store presents a wonderful and delicious array of products, including breads, rolls, bagels, cupcakes, cookies, and pastries. Three criteria are helpful in deciding what to choose among them: proximity of source, simplicity of ingredients, and density. First, the bakery should at least be regional, as baked goods shipped from afar lose their taste and quality even if they are frozen. Secondly, the ingredients should be few and wholesome. A good baker can create a masterpiece, even a delicate pastry, using elemental raw materials, while a poor baker needs all the help he or she can get. Finally, while no one is thrilled by a brick-like bread, a healthy density makes for good eating. The more air and fluff, the more likely the loaf will resemble a less nutritious "Wonder Bread" type of product. Good bread, even when past its prime and marked down in price, can be rejuvenated by steaming. The breads available in the natural foods store fall into four classifications: sourdough, yeast and quick breads, flat breads, and sprouted breads.

Sourdough bread is hearty and satisfying and will last for a long time if stored in a brown paper bag. The ingredients listed on the label will not mention yeast or baking powder but may include "sourdough starter" or "natural leavening." French, whole wheat, raisin, rye, and rice breads (made with brown rice and whole wheat flour) are all available as sourdough breads.

Yeast breads are readily available and come in many varieties. They may be made of whole wheat or unbleached white, rye, barley, oatmeal or corn flours; sweetened or unsweetened; with many ingredients or only a few. Some breads are almost cake-like; others are more plain. Quick breads are leavened with baking powder, soda, or both and include banana, date, pumpkin, and nut breads.

Flat breads include pita and whole wheat chapati. They may contain yeast or baking powder and can be sweetened. Some stores offer corn tortillas made from masa. Flat breads are usually stored in the cooler or freezer, as they go stale quickly.

Sprouted breads are on the sweet side, as the sprouting grains convert starch into maltose and other natural sweeteners. They have a sticky consistency, and taste good toasted. Flourless breads made of sprouted grains or seeds are in a class all their own. Some are leavened with yeast, but most kinds are unleavened. Nuts and dried fruits are sometimes added.

Nowadays many different kinds of crackers are available to the adventurous consumer in the natural foods store. In addition to the versatile rice cake (salted, unsalted, or low-salt; with millet, corn, buckwheat, sesame seeds, or plain), there are: Japanese potato, shrimp, sea vegetable, and vegetable crackers; Scandinavian flatbreads; and American whole wheat crackers and corn chips (salted or unsalted; baked with or without oil). Several lines of crackers based on traditional Oriental snacks have recently appeared. Some are baked without oil and salt, while others are lightly covered with tamari. Many different shapes, sizes, flavorings, and textures are available. Reading labels is a reliable way to learn not only about the ingredients, but also about the culinary tradition of the cracker and how it is made.

For spreading on your whole grain bread or crackers there are jams, jellies, conserves, spreads, and apple butters made only from fruit. The pectin, or gelling agent, comes from the fruit itself or from added fruit pectin, extracted from citrus peels or apple pomace. (Commercial pectins contain other ingredients such as dextrose or preservatives.) Spreads may be sweetened with honey or maple syrup or left unsweetened. Some are highly concentrated and are priced accordingly.

Carob is found in the natural foods store in several forms. It is available as a powder, roasted or unroasted, which is used as a flavoring ingredient in dessert recipes. Carob chips, sweetened or unsweetened, contain partially hydrogenated palm kernel oil or coconut oil, milk powder, soya lecithin, and perhaps malted corn and barley. (Some sweetened carob chips contain refined sugar. Ask if you're not sure.) Carob candies generally contain the same ingredients. Carob seeds and whole dried pods, which can be eaten as a sweet snack, are also found occasionally.

Other familiar items such as mayonnaise, salad dressings, vinegar, mustard, sauerkraut, pickles, relishes, and applesauce line the shelves of the natural foods store. These should be free of refined sugars, preservatives, and additives. Unrefrigerated pickles are usually pasteurized, which means that some of the beneficial enzymes have been destroyed by heat. However, they shouldn't contain the preservatives and other additions of commercial pickles.

Before moving on to the inevitable gauntlet of the check-out counter, we come across three more of the unique attractions of the natural foods store: teas and beverages, the Oriental specialty foods section, and toiletries.

There are many different herbal teas presently on the market. Some of these are familiar favorites, such as peppermint, chamomile, and rose hips. Others are recently developed blends with names like Pelican Punch, Enlightenment Special, and Sleepy Time. Teas are available in loose packs or in bags. These do not generally contain caffeine unless specifically noted. Those which do have caffeine usually include black tea and/or South American matte. It is difficult to find organic herbal teas.

Several excellent grain coffees are available, usually as instant powders made from roasted grains like barley, rye, or wheat and flavored with malt, beet roots, figs, chicory, or acorns. Some have a strong, bitter taste similar to that of coffee. Boiled chicory is also a good coffee substitute, and can be used to cut regular coffee. Kukicha is a twig tea from Japan that makes a delicious beverage, although it does contain a small amount of caffeine. Several companies offer organic kukicha.

Kukicha is actually one of a number of related products found in various sections of the natural foods store. These are the Oriental specialty foods developed in the Far East as part of a predominantly vegetarian diet. Most were introduced into this country through the macrobiotic movement. Many are imported from Japan although some, such as tofu and tempeh, are now produced commercially in this country.

Miso is a fermented paste made from soybeans (or another legume) and salt, and usually another grain such as rice or barley. It makes a hearty and slightly salty soup base and can also be used in spreads, dips, and to flavor beans and stews. Most miso comes from Japan, although there are now several very good domestic varieties. While most imported miso must be pasteurized, native ones do not have to be. Shoyu, or natural soy sauce, is also a fermented soybean (and wheat) product. Unlike commercial brands of soy sauce, it contains no chemical coloring and preservatives, and is naturally aged for up to three years. It is sometimes labeled as tamari, which is a similar product but, technically speaking, contains no wheat.

The umeboshi or "pickled plum" is an unripe plum pickled in salt and shiso (beefsteak) leaves. It has a puckery, sour-salty taste and is delicious in salad dressings, with grains, or in sushi. The umeboshi is said to possess medicinal qualities, and several home remedies can be made from it.

Other Oriental specialty foods that are usually available where there is a macrobiotic clientele include: *udon*, a Japanese whole wheat noodle; *soba*, a buckwheat noodle; *gomasio*, a seasoning made from roasted sesame seeds and sea salt; *tekka*, a seasoning made from finely ground root vegetables cooked for a long time in an iron pot with miso and sesame oil; *kuzu*, a vegetable thickener similar to arrowroot; and *fu*, wheat gluten in dried cake form. Amasake, a thick, sweet, milky drink made from water, koji, and brown

Cooking on a Tight Schedule

As you become familiar with new staples you will be able to choose and prepare your food according to your schedule, making your meal preparations increasingly efficient. With a little foresight, planning, and know-how, natural whole foods will gracefully incorporate themselves into your life; they do not require a great deal of preparation, as is sometimes believed.

Brown rice cooks in less than an hour, and if you wash it beforehand, all that you need to do is add water and turn on the stove when you get up in the morning or come home from work. Wheat, oats, and rye are best if soaked for a night or a day, and barley benefits from presoaking. Whole oats can be cooked overnight in a heavy pot on a very low flame: add four cups of water to every cup of oats, cover, and set the pot on two flame deflectors. Creamy whole oat cereal will be ready in the morning. Millet and buckwheat cook in fifteen to twenty minutes, so on busy days these grains are very convenient. Noodles, of course, can be prepared quickly and in an infinite number of ways. They are delightful with quick-cooking nutritious additions like tempeh, tofu, or dulse; fresh vegetables can be cooked and added or steamed on top of the noodles. Roasted nori and dried bonito flakes complement noodle dishes and add nutritional benefits.

Bean cookery requires a little thinking ahead of time, since most beans require overnight soaking (adding a piece of kombu contributes flavor, nutrients, and digestibility). Most beans are then simmered for several hours or pressure-cooked for forty-five minutes to an hour. Azuki beans do not need soaking and will cook in an hour, either boiled or in a pressure-cooker. Lentils become tender in less than an hour when simmered, and do not need to be soaked beforehand.

Tofu and tempeh are soybean products that can be prepared in many different ways. Tofu needs only to be steamed for a few minutes to be edible and tempeh can be steamed, boiled, or pan-fried in fifteen to twenty minutes. Marinated all day, both tofu and tempeh become succulent, special delicacies.

Leftover food, of course, sometimes tastes better than when it was first served, and leftover whole foods easily lend themselves to casseroles, light pan-frying, or resteaming. In short, there is no reason to spend hours in the kitchen. If you use tempeh, tofu, seitan, and all the natural, wholesome, "quick foods" available now in natural foods stores, together with foresight, planning, and the wise use of leftovers, whole foods cooking needn't take longer than any other food preparation.

or sweet brown rice, is found in the refrigerator section. Many other condiments and foods may also be available, including *wasabi* or Japanese horseradish, *kanpyo* or dried gourd strips, *daikon* that has been dried, shredded, and packaged, and watermelon concentrate, to name a few. Koji, which is grain that has been inoculated with the *Aspergillus oryzae* mold, is sometimes found. It can be used to make amasake or miso.

Finally, we come to the toiletries. Not too long ago, the natural foods store offered baking soda as its only toothpaste, and sea kelp as a shampoo. Today the natural foods store shopper is confronted with a vast display of natural shampoos and conditioners, soaps, facial and body lotions, toothpastes, shaving creams, and even deodorants and dental floss. Often these are made only with natural, vegetable-derived ingredients and are free of the harsh chemicals from coal tar and petroleum that are commonly used. Since whatever touches our skin is to some degree absorbed into the body, these toiletries present a refreshing alternative to chemical-laden commercial varieties. But read all the labels—personal care products vary widely in the quality of ingredients.

At last we approach the check-out counter. Here the basic transaction is the same as in any establishment. Your bill is tallied; you hesitatingly hand over some of your hard-earned cash, and walk out the door with the goods you have selected. One of the common objections to natural foods is the cost. How much you spend, however, depends on what you buy. If the bill seems high it may be that you have chosen a lot of prepared foods, delicacies, and meat and dairy items. The vegetarian staples—whole grains and flours, beans, and vegetables—are priced very reasonably. In fact, a family can be fed more healthfully and economically with such foods than with any other. Most importantly, you have invested in your health, and the value of that cannot be measured in dollars and cents.

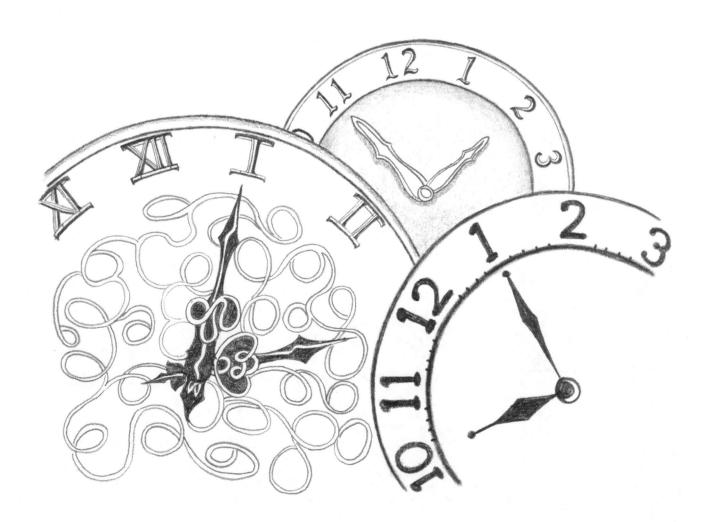

Shopping in a Supermarket

Among the "Potato Buds" & "Spaghetti-O's," Whole Foods *Can* Be Found

Visiting or living in a city without a natural foods store can be a challenge. Over 3,000 additives are permitted in foods and, unfortunately, labeling laws allow at least half of them to remain unlisted. Bread, for example, may contain over ninety "optional" ingredients that do not have to appear as ingredients. Even a food as seemingly simple as tomato sauce can contain hidden additives in the oil, salt, cheese, mushrooms, or tomatoes. Although label reading can be helpful in ferreting out better-quality foods, you cannot always tell exactly what you are getting by simply reading the label—especially in the supermarket, where there is no premium placed on natural ingredients.

Supermarkets are built for convenience—easy parking, fast service, and a selection of time-saving products. By choosing convenience, however, we increasingly lose the ability to choose healthful food. The more a food is processed, the less "real" food we are likely to get. There is one guideline, however. The "Golden Rule of Food Shopping" will steer you clear of hundreds of additives, preservatives, and chemicals, and that is: *Buy whole foods.* Buy the raw ingredients and cook them yourself.

Fortunately for supermarket shoppers, natural foods sections are starting to appear in many stores. Here you can find good-quality oils, crackers, jams, pastas, sea salt, and organic grains, the selection of which will vary from store to store. Natural foods have reached the mass marketing stage, and soon supermarkets will be moving more volume than all the other natural foods businesses combined.

In addition, some large food companies have jumped on the natural foods bandwagon and are now offering products made without chemicals, preservatives, or additives. Nowadays, a consumer can find the same items in both a supermarket *and* a natural foods store. However, it is always important to read labels and be aware of ingredients.

Most large supermarkets actually have an abundance of whole foods. Even some packaged, canned, and frozen items are acceptable, if chosen with care. However, supermarket foods that don't contain preservatives and additives are often enriched with vitamins and minerals. In addition, they may contain refined salt—something that many people are trying to avoid. You will rarely find sea salt in a supermarket. Although you may have to compromise in these and other areas, you should be able to healthfully satisfy your hunger in an emergency.

Produce

The produce department is often filled with a large variety of fresh fruits and vegetables. If that department is poor, the chances of finding anything else that is edible are slim. Perhaps it's convenience again—produce is not convenient. If the store's customers are not interested in cooking fresh vegetables, then they certainly won't be interested in cooking and preparing other whole foods. Besides the usual root vegetables, greens, and fruits, many stores now carry a variety of sprouts, specialty vegetables such as daikon and bok choy, and tofu.

Avoid produce that looks painted and waxed. When you see bushels of oranges that have the same even, bright orange color, you can be sure something was done to make them that way—they were probably treated with Citrus Red Dye #2 and mineral oil or carnauba wax. In general, buy medium-sized fruits or vegetables. Those gorgeous, giant-sized fruits are pumped with fertilizer and kept blemish-free through heavy spraying.

If it is at all possible, buy local produce. Buying locally has several advantages. For one thing, the fruits and vegetables are usually fresher, as most out-of-state produce has travel and extra storage time added to its age. In addition, many fruits are sprayed with fungicides to maintain their freshness during travel and storage. Fresh local produce doesn't need waxing, but out-of-state or out-of-country varieties of apples, citrus fruits, cucumbers, squash, turnips, and parsnips often do.

Non-local produce has another disadvantage—it is bred for its ability to travel without bruising or spoiling rather than for its taste or nutritional value. A good example is the tomato. Non-local tomatoes resemble cardboard in taste and texture. They are picked unripe, green, and rock-hard, and gassed with ethylene to make them the familiar red color we would expect. Their skin is thick and pithy, with the texture of Styrofoam.™ Local, in-season tomatoes, on the other hand, exhibit a solid, smooth, and impenetrable red color, and taste delicious.

Another good reason to buy local—or at least U.S.—produce is that many pesticides banned in this country are allowed elsewhere. Americans demand perfect specimens, and foreign growers use every chemical means available to ensure that they get it. It is tragic that American companies can produce pesticides that are banned in the U.S. and sell them to foreign markets. Pesticides such as DDT then return to us in the produce grown for American import. The use of these deadly substances is detrimental to the health of the farmers who are using them, as well as to our own.

If this makes nonorganic produce sound totally unappealing, remember that we are in a supermarket and fresh fruits and vegetables are some of the least adulterated foods available. Since many natural foods stores use nonorganic produce when organic supplies are limited or prohibitively expensive, you have probably been eating it all along.

In addition to fresh fruits and vegetables, the freezer department also has many frozen vegetables and some fruits with no added sugar or salt. Dole offers canned, unsweetened pineapple chunks and crushed pineapple, and Libby has a line of canned, unsweetened fruit.

Whole Grains

Whole grains have been the staple food of many cultures for thousands of years, and they still have a foothold in these bastions of refined food. I have been able to find four whole grains regularly in most supermarkets.

While bags of enriched white rice abound, ranging from one pound to twenty-five pounds in size, brown rice is usually found in a little eight-ounce box. It won't be organic, but then again, we *are* in a supermarket! River Rice, packaged by Riviana Foods in Houston, is simply plain brown rice. Other brands, such as Uncle Ben's, are parboiled, which means that they are precooked. Some brown rice is even cracked, parboiled, and enriched.

In addition to brown rice, another favorite grain—popcorn—is stocked in supermarkets in ample supply. Popcorn is a whole grain, retaining both bran and germ, and as such is a healthful snack.

One whole grain that is usually hidden among the dried beans is barley, which is frequently used in soups. Barley comes in a one-pound cellophane bag. Some brands package unrefined barley with the bran intact. Barley that resembles fat white rice has been ground down to remove everything but the starch. It is quicker-cooking, but is also a refined cereal. One brand, called Peak Quality, is almost identical to that found in the natural foods store. Barley is a good staple grain and can be used in soups, stews, and cereals.

Buckwheat is also commonly found in supermarkets. Wolff's, the most often-seen brand, has put more kasha on the table than anyone else in the U.S. Wolff's buckwheat comes from Birkett Mills in Penn Yan, New York, and the same brand is often sold in bulk in natural foods stores. You should buy the whole groat, either roasted or unroasted. The other types are ground and make a cereal rather than a whole grain.

Cereals

In the supermarket, other grains are usually found in a ground cereal form. Whole, unground rye, wheat, and oats are rarely seen. However, like buckwheat, these grains are available as good-quality, whole grain cereals.

The Con Agra Company of Omaha, which probably supplies most of the natural foods companies with rolled oats, also makes a rolled rye called Cream of Rye—100 percent whole rye that has been washed, cracked, and steam-rolled into flakes like rolled oats. It's delicious and an important find for people allergic to wheat or oats.

Two good-quality whole wheat cereals that are readily available are Wheatena and Maltex. Both are made by Standard Milling in Kansas City, Missouri. According to a spokesperson, Wheatena is simply cut and toasted wheat. "We just grind, toast, and package. No sugar of any type is added, nor are there any additives or preservatives." Wheatena differs from bulghur in that it is not soaked or steamed before being cut. Maltex is a creamier and fancier version of Wheatena. It is made from toasted whole wheat flakes, similar to rolled oats, and unbromated whole wheat and/or rye flour (potassium bromate is usually added to commercial flours to improve handling characteristics and rising ability). Unlike most cereals that add malt flavoring, Standard Mills adds real powdered barley malt syrup.

Beware of wheat cereals with no nutritional value. Farina, a highly refined wheat product, is delicious but not very nourishing. Pillsbury's Farina and Nabisco's Quick Cream of Wheat contain little more than farina and the few vitamins added to "enrich" them. Nabisco's Original Mix 'n Eat Cream of Wheat contains farina, guar gum, wheat germ, salt, sugar, calcium carbonate, reduced iron, partially hydrogenated soybean oil, BHA, mono- and diglycerides, and vitamins. *Always read labels carefully.*

Whole oats are difficult to find in most supermarkets, but oatmeal is readily available. Some supermarkets carry real Scotch oats, usually in cans, with tartans or Scotsmen gracing their labels. Scotch oats are steel-cut oat pieces rather than rolled oats. They make a crunchier cereal and are more expensive. The Quaker Oats Company, which has probably given most Americans their first taste of oats, produces two exceptional cereals: Quick Oats and Old Fashioned Oats. The difference between them is simply in the size of the flakes. Quick Oats are cut smaller and thinner so that they cook faster. Instant Quaker Oatmeal isn't as healthy a choice; although the label boasts that the oatmeal "prepares in your bowl instantly," it also reveals that the cereal contains salt, calcium carbonate, guar gum, caramel flavor, vitamins, and minerals along with the rolled oats. The Quaker company also has a new line called Mother's; two of its cereals are Rolled Oats and Oat Bran, both of which contain no other ingredients.

Beware also of the highly processed, cold cereals that take up a large amount of shelf space in the supermarket. Because of watchdog organizations and consumer pressure, some companies are downplaying the presence of sugar in their cereals. Even though the word "natural" appears on the front of many boxes, most of these products contain white sugar as well as other undesirable ingredients. Quaker "100% Natural" Cereal lists brown sugar as its third ingredient, while Post Fruit & Fibre lists just plain sugar as its third. Nabisco's 100% Bran, flavored with two naturally sweet fruit juices ("No Breakfast Cereal Has More Natural Fiber," and "100% Wheat Bran," the package claims), has sugar as its second ingredient. Nabisco's Shredded Wheat, containing only whole wheat, seems to be a natural product. Post Grape-Nuts, although fortified with eight vitamins, lists only wheat, malted barley, salt, and yeast in its ingredients, and the "grape-nuts flakes" contain sugar and coconut oil.

Familia, also found in natural foods stores, is a supermarket regular. The "Original Recipe" version contains turbinado sugar, but another version states, "No Added Sugar." Ralston Instant Whole Wheat Hot Cereal lists 100 percent whole wheat as its only ingredient. Kretschmer Regular Wheat Germ, packaged in a vacuum-sealed bottle, is not a whole food but does not, at least, have added ingredients.

It is especially important to read the labels of cereal boxes. Often, the vitamins are listed after the ingredients.

Beans

Supermarkets carry this staple food in great variety. In fact, the supermarket is a very good place to buy beans. It has more varieties than most natural foods stores and, unless you have an organic source, the beans are exactly the same as those sold in bulk in the natural foods store. They are often the same price. Jack Rabbit, Goya, and Peak Quality are the brands found in most stores. Some cans of beans contain only beans, but read the label carefully anyway.

Nuts and Dried Fruits

Nuts can be found in both the produce and snack sections of the supermarket. Unshelled nuts are the safest, since shelled ones are often blanched or bleached, then dipped in caustic solutions to help remove the skins. Salted and roasted nuts have hidden additives in the salt and oil, and dry-roasted varieties may contain many added ingredients. Exceptions may include unsalted roasted peanuts in the shell, raw almonds, and walnuts, but check the labels (as some of these do contain preservatives).

All supermarkets carry that most popular and natural of dried fruits, the raisin. Other dried fruits are either sulfured or contain a preservative, but not the raisin. Its package says "all natural," "no preservatives," and "nothing artificial added." A little caution is advisable, however. Golden seedless raisins have their color preserved with sulfur dioxide. And, occasionally, you will find raisins that have oil added to prevent clumping. But the regular dark, sun-ripened, sun-dried raisins seem to be fine.

So far we have covered the basic whole foods available in supermarkets—the ones that are the safest to eat. Once you have exhausted these possibilities, finding suitable food becomes very complicated. Other products, whether processed or not, are probably best purchased in a natural foods store, where you can be sure of what you are getting. But if you can't get to a natural foods store, and are willing to take a few risks, there are several other areas you can explore.

Juices

Many manufacturers are trying to make fruit juice more natural. Apple juices without sugar or preservatives are now available, although they are usually filtered. The label should read "100 percent pure juice." Avoid any product that has the words "drink," "fruit drink," "cocktail," or "punch" on its label. These contain only about 10 percent fruit juice, the rest being water, sugar, flavoring, and color.

The label of Welch's tomato juice states that it contains only tomatoes and salt, and the label of their famous grape juice boasts no preservatives, artificial flavors, or colors. Mr. Weidman, the director of Welch's Corporate Communications, affirmed that Welch's grape juice really is pure juice. "Welch's is made from the Concord grape, which is primarily a juice grape that needs no added sugar," he said. Grape juice concentrate, which has no sugar added to it either, is the other ingredient. "The color and flavor come naturally from the grape. The juice is pasteurized and bottled without a preservative, but vitamin C is added." Now that's not so bad. It's certainly more nutritious than their grape drink, which is "filtered water, sugar syrup, concentrated grape juice, corn sweeteners, grape and other natural flavors, malic acid, ascorbic acid, and artificial color." In addition, Welch's now has 100 percent White Grape Juice (vitamin C-enriched), as well as a new line of 100 percent pure fruit juices called Welch's Orchard.

Sunsweet makes a prune juice that the company claims is pure juice with no preservatives or sugar added. The Winter Hill brand offers a large selection of natural fruit juices. Apple & Eve has an apple and an apple/cranberry juice, as well as a vegetable juice made from fresh vegetables. Dole offers an unsweetened pineapple juice, not made from concentrate, with vitamin C added.

Many supermarkets—as well as natural foods stores—carry Tropicana orange juice, either freshly made or from concentrate. The freshly made juice in the carton is fine. With concentrates, you never know how much can be in them that doesn't have to appear on the label. And if you think that you can call up and ask, be forewarned: if manufacturers don't have to put it on the label, they don't have to tell you about it when you call to find out!

Supermarkets often carry spring water. But be sure that it is real and not just filtered water. The label should say "spring water," not soda. Perrier and Evian are two popular French imports; one carbonated, the other not. Poland Springs, which has natural carbonation added, is available in some east coast supermarkets. It comes plain or with lemon, lime, cherry, or orange essence added.

Oils

Finding a good vegetable oil is not too difficult if you like olive oil. One hundred percent virgin olive oil is the same in the supermarket as it is in the natural foods store. What you don't want, however, is a label that reads "pure olive oil" or "100 percent pure olive oil." Instead, it must say 100 percent *virgin* olive oil. The others are blends that contain inferior oil. All the other types of oil in the supermarket are refined to some degree. The worst ones, which say "vegetable oil" or "salad oil," are so refined that they don't even reveal what source they were made from! If you have to buy oil, get one that you can identify and that doesn't contain antioxidants or defoaming agents. Look for corn or sunflower oil. A good sesame oil will sometimes be hidden in the Oriental foods section.

Sweeteners

A supermarket is certainly the place to find sugar. In fact, most of their products contain it. But supermarkets also stock a few natural sweeteners, three of which are quite easy to find. One contains 100 percent pure maple syrup. The label should say just that and nothing else—there is no sugar, color, flavor, or water added. You can also recognize real maple syrup by its price, which is higher than that of Log Cabin or Mrs. Butterworth's. Honey is another natural sweetener that is always available in supermarkets. Try to find honey that is not sparkling clear; a cloudy or crystallized type will be less processed and thus contain more nutrients. Good quality molasses can also be found. Mott's makes an unsulfured variety, called Grandma's Molasses, which probably tastes as good as any in the natural foods store.

Odds and Ends

If you enjoy baking, or want to make your own bread, Pillsbury makes a whole wheat flour that seems to be fairly natural. Katherine Hanley, from the public relations department at Pillsbury, informed me that their whole wheat flour is neither bleached nor enriched, and does not contain a preservative. She also said that it is aged naturally and is not bromated. Some professional bakers feel that aged flour handles better than fresh, but along with aging comes a loss of nutrients and flavor through oxidation. Pillsbury also makes a white flour that is unbleached, but enriched. King Arthur stone-ground whole wheat flour, distributed in the New York/New England area, is 100 percent whole wheat; the same brand of white flour is enriched but contains no bleaching agents.

Many local companies produce natural peanut butter. The label should say simply "peanuts" or "peanuts and salt." It should be neither hydrogenized nor contain sugar, and the oil should separate and rise to the top. There are also several natural applesauces, like Seneca and Mott's Natural-Style Apple Sauce, made from only apples and water, with no added sugar or preservatives. They are not bright white in color like most applesauces, but brownish pink or slightly grey—a small price to pay for their nutritional value. Since any supermarket bread, except for an occasional hearty loaf of rye, is out of the question, you can spread your peanut butter or applesauce on crispbreads or rice cakes. Kavli Norwegian Flatbread contains whole rye, yeast, and salt; Finn Crisp is made from rye flour, yeast, and salt. There are usually several different brands of rice cakes near the crackers or at the deli counter.

You will probably want to avoid prepared deli foods. Some Italian and Greek olives in brine might be all right, but kosher pickles usually contain a preservative. The Pastene line does not contain preservatives or synthetic ingredients in its products. Some you might want to try are the clam sauce, tomato paste, green olives with pimentos, and kidney beans. DeCecco and Fara San Martino are two brands of whole wheat pasta from Italy. Although the pasta is enriched, it does not contain preservatives.

Several brands of tuna are packed only in spring water and salt, and Star-Kist offers a "diet" tuna packed in distilled water only. Some brands of canned salmon, sardines, and mackerel are water- and salt-packed, without preservatives. If there is a fresh fish counter, inspect the fish carefully for freshness. Also ask when it was caught.

A number of non-dairy ice creams (mostly based on soy products) have recently become available. Some of these are highly processed and contain artificial ingredients. In addition, they may contain only minimal amounts of the advertised soy ingredient. (For more information on these desserts, see Chapter 6.)

Supermarkets will always exist, and are an important part of the consumer's world. If you find yourself in one, remember to read the labels carefully, and make your selection wisely.

2. GRAINS

It has been said with some justification that the history of civilization is the history of grains. Certainly grains have been humanity's most important food for thousands of years. There is evidence of wheat cultivation 10,000 years ago, and rice may be an even more ancient cultivated food grain.

The attributes that attracted our ancestors to these foods are just as relevant today. Grains are relatively easy to grow, harvest, store, and transport. Almost every nutrient that our bodies need can be found in grains. High in carbohydrates, containing significant amounts of protein, and low in fat, they remain today one of the cheapest sources of nutrients in most parts of the world. Grains are also versatile and can be used in many different ways, either in their whole forms or ground into flours.

In much of the Orient, rice is still so important that it makes up 70 percent of the average person's daily diet. It has been estimated that a billion Chinese eat a pound of rice a day. Yet, sometime around the middle of this century, wheat passed rice as the most widely cultivated grain worldwide. Corn is today a close third, with oats the next most common grain.

In the United States, grains make up only about 30 percent of the average person's diet, and this figure is perhaps half of what it was a century ago. Some three-quarters of the grain consumption of Americans is represented by wheat and wheat flour. Consumption of barley, buckwheat, and corn flour is much lower in the U.S. today than it was at the turn of the century. What has increased dramatically is Americans' eating of refined grain products, such as white bread, processed cereals, pastries, and snacks.

As the first-time visitor to a natural foods store will quickly notice, this lack of respect for whole grains is changing rapidly for many health-conscious people. Most natural foods stores offer a wide variety of whole grains, including not only wheat and corn, but also rye, oats, millet, and others. And for such favorites as rice, there may be a dozen or more varieties, depending upon size of grain, color, the conditions of growing, and the extent of milling. Flours also come in an almost astonishing variety. In addition, there may be such "grain exotics" as amaranth and quinoa.

To help shoppers get a sense of the vast array of grain-eating possibilities that are open to us, the following pages offer short descriptions of various grains and flours, along with some background on how they are grown and processed. We will also briefly consider the merits of natural breakfast cereals and rice cakes; take a longer look at one of the grains, quinoa, that's recently been "rediscovered" and made available to more people; and discuss the growing organic rice movement in the United States.

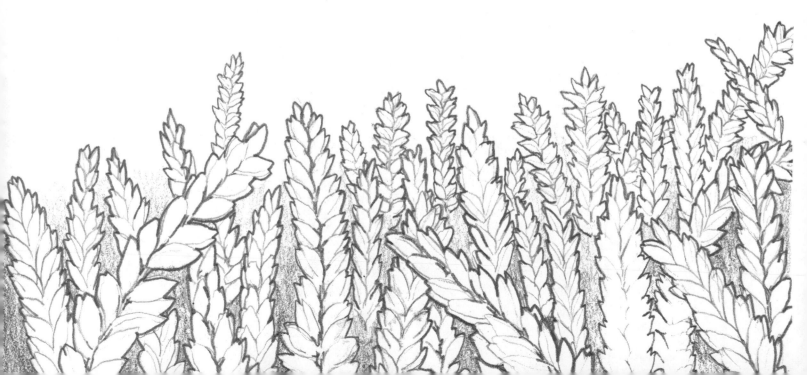

A Guide to Whole Grains & Whole Grain Flours

Grasses, the latest product of plant evolution, are the predominant species of our time. They grow everywhere on earth except in the extreme polar regions where lichens reign and in the deserts where cacti thrive. The grasses vary in form: some are petite and frail while others, such as bamboo, are tall and sturdy. Because of their adaptability and diversity, grasses are ideal companions for humans. It is only natural that we have embraced them in a multitude of ways, using them, among other things, for clothing and building materials, fuel, and food.

Cereal grains (often referred to simply as ''grains'') are grasses with edible seeds, as well as the seeds themselves. Most cereal grains are planted in the spring. Tiny green sprouts shoot skyward, grow tall through the summer, take flower as the drooping spike-like panicles develop off the stem, and become a mature golden-brown with the arrival of fall. Within the bearded faces of the mature grain are hundreds of little grain kernels. It is these kernels that are harvested, hulled, and sold in food stores as whole grains. In each kernel the fruit and seed, the beginning and end of the plant kingdom, are combined into a compact unit.

When analyzed, whole grain shows a composition of minerals, proteins, and carbohydrates in a proportion well suited for human nutrition. These elemental components are found throughout the three parts of the kernel: the bran, the germ, and the endosperm. The bran is the outermost of these three and acts as a layer of skin or peel, sealing the endosperm and the germ. Actually several layers thick, the bran varies from one type of grain to the next. Its primary component is a complex sugar called cellulose (often referred to as roughage), which gives it its hardness. One reason why whole grains should be thoroughly chewed is that cellulose is indigestible. The grinding action of teeth breaks open the bran and exposes the inner grain to diges-

tive activity. If swallowed whole or partially chewed, the grain will be only partially digested. This is also true of whole grain flours and cracked whole grains such as bulghur. After being swallowed, the bran travels the length of the digestive tract, pulling along with its bulk the other components of the grain, which are digested in different places along the way. The bran ensures that all components reach their appointed destinations without getting stuck en route.

Aside from cellulose, bran contains B vitamins, proteins, fats, and minerals. Bran, however, is only part of a greater whole and in and of itself is not a balanced food. The same is true of the germ, which has the added disadvantage of quickly going rancid unless vacuum-packed in a jar and stored in the refrigerator after opening. Grain is best eaten whole or as freshly milled whole grain flour products.

Although amounting to as little as 2.5 percent of the total kernel, the germ is a gigantic source of nourishment. The germ is to the grain as the seed is to the fruit, and it is from the germ that the new stem sprouts and the young root descends. The germ is lavishly rich, containing vitamins E, B, and A, and protein and fat that spark to life when the grain is planted. But after this primal spark, the tiny stem and root depend on stored nutriments for growing. These nutriments are in the form of complex carbohydrates contained in the third part of the grain, which is called the endosperm. The endosperm is the part of grain most familiar to the American palate for the sad reason that it alone remains after the usual milling process.

The complex carbohydrates of the endosperm reside within a sheath of intricate protein and account for 80 percent of the grain's total size. The delicious sweetness of whole grains comes from the initial breakdown of endo-

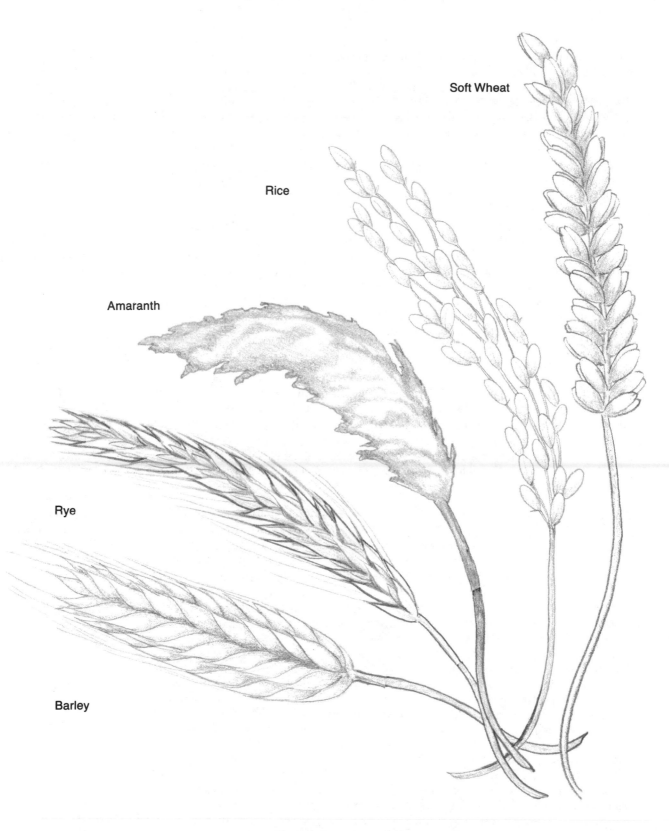

Soft Wheat

Rice

Amaranth

Rye

Barley

A Variety of Whole Grains

sperm sugars when the grains are chewed and mixed with saliva in the mouth. Most of the sugar, however, is digested and absorbed much later in the stomach and intestines, providing a continuous flow of energy. This process is what gives grain-eaters stamina, not fat. Refined grains are those that are stripped of the bran (and often the germ) and sold as is or ground into flours or cereals.

When buying grains, the shopper's first impression upon looking into the bin should be of thousands of distinct, whole individuals looking back. Closer scrutiny should reveal consistent milling. There should be no more than a scattering of grains that have passed through the milling process with their hulls intact. Nor should there be too many immature grains, which show up greenish in color. Likewise the number of broken or chipped grains should be minimal, for these have lost their potency, will not sprout, and are dead food. Stones, dirt, and nonhomogeneous-looking kernels should not be present in the bin either. The grains should not look wrinkled or withered. If they are, bring it to the attention of the store manager and ask him or her to try to find a new source for that grain.

A final test of quality—one that can be conducted at home—is to pour a cup of the grain into a pot of water. The vast majority of the grains should sink to the bottom. Those that remain at the surface, doing the dead-man's float, lack vitality. Their number should be very low, no more than one or two percent of the total.

If you are like most people, you eat the grains that taste best to you and that you can digest most easily. But when you go to the food store you may find four or five varieties of those grains to choose from and may not know what the differences are among them. Each grain and each variety of the grain has unique qualities and these qualities dictate their dietary use.

Amaranth

During pre-Columbian times, amaranth was a staple crop in areas from what is now Arizona to Argentina, rivaling corn and beans in importance in some locations. While corn and beans have become major world food crops, amaranth has persisted in its native region in only a few isolated mountain valleys in Mexico, Central America, and South America. Halfway around the world, however, amaranth has recently become an important food crop among hill tribes of Pakistan, northern India, Nepal, Tibet, and China. Now, after centuries of relative obscurity, this ancient plant is beginning to be recognized by contemporary agriculturists. A major research program at the Rodale Press experimental farm in Emmaus, Pennsylvania has already developed varieties that meet the requirements of modern growing and harvesting practices.

Amaranth is not, strictly speaking, a grain, as it is the seed of a broadleaf plant and not of a grass. But because of its high yield of nutritious edible seed, it is classified by use as a grain and amaranth species grown for their seed are referred to as "grain amaranth." These grain amaranths,

several species of the genus *Amaranthus,* are closely related to the weed commonly known as pigweed or redroot. The grain amaranths, as tall as corn, are brilliantly colored with leaves, stems, and flowers of purple, red, orange, gold, and even green. The millet-size seeds, borne in spike-like heads at the top of the plants, range in color from creamy white and golden to deep red and black, with the most common color used for food being golden.

Grain amaranth averages just over 16 percent protein, a percentage twice that of corn or rice and as high as that of either oats or the best hard spring wheat. Unlike the true cereal grains, amaranth is rich in the amino acid lysine, though low in leucine. This latter amino acid is abundant in most other plant proteins, making amaranth a good protein complement for either grain or beans.

Traditionally the seeds have been popped, milled and used to make flatbreads, prepared as a gruel, and mixed with honey to make confections. A few U.S. farmers are growing grain amaranth, and it is now available in its whole form as well as an ingredient in prepared natural breakfast cereals and crackers.

Barley

Barley originated in North Africa and Southeast Asia. Throughout its long history it was used as currency and as a standardized measure of weight, as well as for food. In Europe barley was the chief grain until displaced by wheat and rye. Barley was brought to the United States by the Dutch and English, but hardier strains were introduced later by German and Russian settlers.

Most barley has a tight hull which requires extensive milling to be removed. "Pearl" or "pearled" barley, rounded and white, has most of its vitamins and minerals removed during milling. "Hulled" barley is not as extensively milled and cooks into a chewy whole food. When combined with beans and root vegetables and seasoned with shoyu (see "The Three Flavors of Japanese Cuisine," page 165), it makes a delicious, hearty soup. Malted barley is used extensively by the brewing industry, with 10 percent of the world's crop going into the production of beer. Barley flakes, which are quicker cooking than unflaked barley, are sometimes available.

Buckwheat

Buckwheat is not truly a grain but is nutritionally on a par with grains. Botanically, buckwheat belongs to the *Polygonaceae* or buckwheat family (true cereal grains belong to the *Gramineae*), and visually it looks more like a bush than a slender-stemmed reed. The buckwheat family is generally an unsavory one which includes the notorious belladonna, of which buckwheat itself is a beneficial northern relation. Buckwheat is thought to have originated in Siberia, Manchuria, and northern India, and to have spread from there in very ancient times to the rest of Asia. In medieval times buckwheat found its way into Europe, where, possibly be-

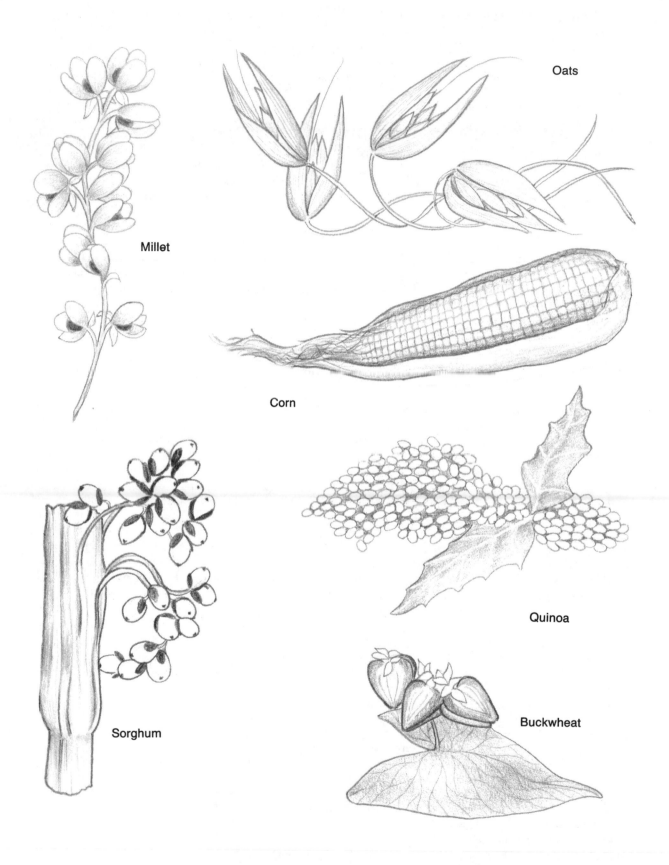

Oats

Millet

Corn

Sorghum

Quinoa

Buckwheat

A Variety of Whole Grains

cause it arrived via the Middle East, it picked up the name Saracen, the same word used to designate a Muslim person. German, Dutch, and French settlers brought this spunky plant to the United States. French Canadian loggers, known for their hearty breakfasts, ate *galettes de sarrasin*—buckwheat pancakes. Buckwheat will grow almost anywhere, with major cultivated crops in such diverse places as Minnesota and Pennsylvania.

Sold in stores as hulled whole groats, as coarse and fine grits (all of which when roasted are known as kasha), and as flour, buckwheat's hardiness makes it an ideal cold weather food. It is rich in vitamin E and is a good blood-building food as well.

Corn

Corn, known as maize to most of the world, is the only cereal grain native to the Americas. While it was grown only by Native Americans at the time of Columbus's first landing in the New World, within fifty years it was being cultivated in such faraway places as Africa and the province of Honan in China.

By 1492 corn was already being grown to its present climatic limits in the Western Hemisphere, from the Central American mountains across the Southwest deserts and into what is now Canada. The five basic types of corn developed by native farmers are still available: popcorn, sweet corn, dent corn, flint corn, and flour corn. While the selection is rather restricted today, all five of these types were once grown in varieties of four different colors: red, white, yellow, and blue. In addition to the few listed below, other varieties may be locally available.

Popcorn and *sweet corn* are the two types most familiar to the average American eater. Popcorn must have the proper percentage of moisture in each kernel if it is to pop properly. Reputable merchants will buy corn dried to this level and keep fresh stocks. After purchase, keep your popcorn in a sealed container. Sweet corn is known to most people as a delectable summer vegetable (see p. 57), but it can be dried for winter storage. Sweet corn is white or yellow or a combination of both. Many varieties are available.

Dent corn, the most widely grown corn in the U.S. today, gets its name from the dent in the crown of each mature kernel. This is the "whole yellow corn" commonly available in natural foods stores and the grain from which most store-bought yellow cornmeal is milled. It can be cooked whole, or ground into flour or meal.

Flint corn, as the name suggests, is a very hard grain. It makes a rich-tasting and sweet meal, ideal for both cornbread and cornmeal mush, and is delicious cooked whole. The flint corn commonly available is yellow or amber and is grown primarily in Ohio.

Flour corn has a soft, white, starchy endosperm and grinds to a fine flour. The only flour corn available today is "Hopi blue corn," grown in Colorado from seed derived from plantings of the Hopi Indians of New Mexico. It can also be cooked whole.

Research has shown open-pollinated varieties to be nutritionally superior to most hybrids. Ask your supplier to stock the open-pollinated, traditional varieties.

Millet

Millet's use as a food goes back farther in history than perhaps that of any other cereal grain. It is botanically a more ancient grass than rice, barley, wheat, or rye. The staple grain of the Hunza people in Asia, it is used most often in America for bird seed. Modern nutritionists claim that millet contains the most complete protein of all the grains and that it is also quite high in minerals. Millet is the only grain that is alkaline when cooked even when no salt is added.

There are many varieties of millet found around the world, but in the United States the one most frequently seen in food stores is a yellow variety called pearl millet. Millet is grown in the north-central United States and in Canada.

Oats

Oats were originally thought of as weeds that encroached on barley and wheat fields until people realized that this hearty grain could supplement the other foods in their diets. Oats are well suited to cold, damp climates, and when cultivated in their own right, they did best in Ireland, Scotland, and Northern England, where they are still the staple grain. In 1602 explorers brought them to New England, where they thrived. The largest part of the commercially grown crop in the U.S. is now located in the northern Midwest.

After oats are hulled, the inner grains are scoured, which removes some of the bran. They are then steamed at temperatures in excess of 200° F to eliminate fungus. The resulting product is the whole oat or groat.

The soft nature of oats has led to the development of unique methods of processing. "Steel-cut oats" are groats that have been coarsely cut with sharp steel blades. To make "rolled oats," the groats are flattened into flakes between rollers that resemble the wringers on top of old-fashioned washing machines.

Oats contain the highest percentage of fat of any cultivated grain. Thus they provide the populations of the cool, damp regions where they grow a staple that imparts warmth and stamina. Oats also contain an antioxidant that delays rancidity. Therefore the groats can be ground into oaten flour that is longer-lasting than whole wheat flour, in spite of its higher fat content. The flour yielded by oats is sweet and excellent for baking. It can be used as an extender for wheat flour.

Oats are a delicious replacement for people who are allergic to wheat; they also offer a feeling of satiety to those who have eaten large amounts of protein in the past.

Quinoa—Tale of a Food Survivor

Although new to North Americans, it has been cultivated in the highest continuously farmed region of the earth, the South American Andes, since at least 3,000 B.C. Compared to other grains and vegetables, it is high in protein, calcium, and iron. One researcher has said that "while no single food can supply all of the essential life-sustaining nutrients, it comes as close as any other in the vegetable or animal kingdoms."

This amazing ancient food now in the process of being rediscovered by modern eaters is quinoa (pronounced keen-wa). In South America, a renewed respect for indigenous crops and traditional foods has reversed a 400-year decline in quinoa production that began with the Spanish conquest. And within the past few years, quinoa has begun to be grown for the first time outside South America, in Colorado's Rockies.

The late scientist David Cusack, an early proponent of quinoa and at one time a partner of Quinoa Corporation founders Steve Gorad and Don McKinley, said that his and others' efforts in promoting the grain were aimed at making the ancient grain of the Incas better known, helping its revival in the Andes, and making it a viable alternative crop for farmers in the Rockies and other mountainous, cool, and semi-arid regions. And, as Cusack stated, "The shortest marketing route for quinoa from Cuzco (the former capital of the Inca Empire) to Lima (the modern capital of Peru) may be through the U.S. health food market."

What is this strange grain that holds so much promise? Quinoa is a small seed that in size, shape, and color looks like a cross between sesame seed and millet. It is a disk-shaped seed with a band around its middle, and is usually a pale yellow in color. Some species, however, may be white, pink, orange, red, purple, or black.

Quinoa is not a true cereal grain but is botanically a fruit in the *Chenopodium* genus, which also includes the common lamb's-quarters. *Chenopodia* characteristically have leaves shaped like a goose's foot. Quinoa is an annual that grows from three to six feet high, and like millet, has seeds that form large clusters at the end of the stalk.

The seeds are covered with saponin, an extremely bitter resin-like substance that makes a soapy solution in water. For the seeds to be edible, the saponin must be removed. This has been accomplished traditionally by hand-scrubbing the quinoa in alkaline water.

Some agriculturists maintain that a saponin-free strain of quinoa should be developed. Many ecologists, on the other hand, observe that the bitter-tasting saponin probably prevents insect and bird predation and that it is better to wash away the saponin than to have to rely on insecticides.

Because quinoa has been grown for centuries under varied ecological conditions, there is no "pure" strain. Quinoa is predominantly an inbreeder and any given crop is composed of a mixture of inbred lines. Thus, quinoa varies greatly within a given region and from region to region.

Some wheats approach quinoa's protein content, but other cereal grains, including barley, corn, and rice, generally have less than half the protein of quinoa. In addition, quinoa has a good balance of the various amino acids that make up protein. Like soybeans, it is exceptionally high in lysine, an amino acid not overly abundant in the vegetable kingdom.

Quinoa also supplies methionine and cysteine, and is thus a good complement for legumes, which are often low in these amino acids. Moreover, quinoa is a relatively good source of phosphorus, calcium, iron, vitamin E, and several of the B vitamins.

As important as quinoa's nutritional benefits are its hardiness and flexibility. Unlike most other food crops, quinoa thrives in areas with high altitudes and low rainfall, and can grow in poor, sandy, alkaline soil.

This flexibility has allowed quinoa to remain the staple of millions of descendants of the Inca Empire. The Aymara and Quechua Indians who live in the high mountains of Ecuador, Peru, Bolivia, southern Colombia, and northern Argentina and Chile grow most of the world's quinoa. In the Altiplano region of Peru and Bolivia, where annual rainfall may be as low as four inches, quinoa is the principal food crop. It is prepared whole, cooked in soup, or made into flour for bread and biscuits; its leaves are eaten as a vegetable or used for animal fodder; the stalks are burned for fuel; and saponin-filled water from rinsing the quinoa is reserved for use as shampoo.

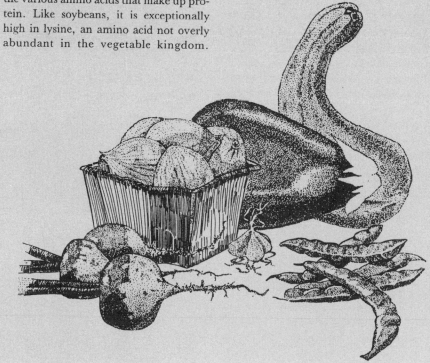

Quinoa would still be appreciated only by native South Americans if it weren't for the dedication and foresight of Cusack, Gorad, and McKinley. They knew of quinoa from their travels in South America, and in early 1982 managed to bring fifteen pounds of quinoa seed into the United States. The quinoa was planted in the spring and harvested that fall.

"We harvested it by hand," recalls Gorad, "threshed and winnowed it by hand, and washed the saponin off. Then we cooked it and ate it and it was delicious."

In 1983, they tested forty-eight varieties of quinoa on some fifty acres in Colorado, and only six varieties grew. In 1984, 100 varieties were planted on over 125 acres and a few more grew successfully. These figures may sound inconsequential, but the corporation is most optimistic about quinoa's progress in Colorado. The introduction of a grain into a new environment is a lengthy process, and according to the experts, quinoa is right on target.

"That our first seed even grew," Gorad commented, "was pure grace. It has now grown in Colorado for four summers and it's still working well."

After it's been cooked (see the following recipes for suggestions), the grain seems to melt in your mouth. But the tiny bands offer just enough tooth resistance to create a minute crunch, affording a varied and pleasant sensation. Eating quinoa is an experience to be savored, and one that deserves more popularity.

COOKING WITH QUINOA

Satisfying yet light, quinoa is so delicious that you may prepare the following simple recipes either for everyday fare or for entertaining. Cooked quinoa lends itself to numerous dishes that will save you meal preparation time the next day. This grain may be cooked as is or toasted. Toasted quinoa is light with a full-bodied and rich flavor. Quinoa is not enhanced when pressure cooked or cooked starting with cold water.

Basic Quinoa Recipe

Makes 4 cups

>   1 cup quinoa
>   2 cups water
>   1 pinch sea salt

Rinse quinoa several times by running fresh water over it in a pot and then pouring it through a strainer. Place water and salt in a saucepan and bring to a rapid boil. Add quinoa, reduce heat, cover, and simmer until all of the water is absorbed (15–25 minutes).

Variations: For a rich, nutty flavor toast quinoa (with or without oil) in a skillet, stirring constantly, before adding it to the water.

Shrimp Fried Quinoa

Serves 4

>   2 tablespoons unrefined oil
>   1 teaspoon grated fresh ginger
>   1 onion, minced
>   3 stalks celery and leaves, chopped
>   4 cups cooked quinoa
>   2 tablespoons shoyu
>   1 cup green peas
>   1 cup cooked shrimp, chopped
>   1 tablespoon sake or dry white wine
>   (optional)

Heat a wok or a large, heavy skillet. Add oil and ginger. Over medium to high heat, saute onion briefly. Add celery, sauteing until it is partially cooked. Add quinoa and shoyu, stir once, cover, and cook for 5 minutes. Add peas, shrimp, and sake. Cook for 2 minutes, covered, or just until the peas are tender.

Quinoa, Leek, and Tofu Casserole

Serves 5

>   1¹/₂ cups tofu
>   2 teaspoons sesame oil
>   1 clove garlic, pressed
>   1 leek, chopped
>   2 cups cooked quinoa
>   1 teaspoon sea salt, or 2 teaspoons
>   shoyu
>   dash black pepper
>   1 cup bread crumbs
>   1 cup soymilk (see page 148)
>   ¹/₂ cup cheese, grated (optional)

Preheat oven to 350 °F. Working with ¹/₂ cup tofu at a time, squeeze out water with hands. Set aside. Heat a large skillet or wok and add oil. Add garlic and then leek. Saute until lightly browned. Add quinoa, then tofu, sauteing for 2 minutes after each addition. Add seasonings.

Oil casserole. Add ¹/₂ cup bread crumbs and rotate casserole to coat evenly. Gently add the quinoa mixture. Press a well in the center of the quinoa and pour in soymilk. Cover with remaining bread crumbs and cheese. Cover, and bake for 20 minutes. Remove cover and continue to bake until cheese is nicely browned.

Almond Quinoa Cookies

Makes 1¹/₂ dozen

>   1 cup almond butter (or tahini or
>   peanut butter)
>   ¹/₂ cup maple syrup or honey
>   ¹/₄ cup unrefined sunflower or
>   safflower oil
>   1 tablespoon vanilla
>   ¹/₃ cup water
>   1 cup whole wheat pastry flour
>   1 cup quinoa flour
>   ¹/₂ cup toasted almonds, chopped
>   9 whole almonds
>   pinch of sea salt

Preheat oven to 375 °F. In a mixing bowl, blend almond butter, sweetener, oil, vanilla, and water. Sift together flours and salt, add chopped almonds, and combine with wet mixture.

Using hands, form dough into small balls and place on an oiled cookie sheet. Press each cookie gently with the tines of a fork. Cut whole almonds in half and press one piece, cut side up, into each cookie. Bake for 12 to 15 minutes or just until golden.

If your local natural foods store does not carry quinoa, or to obtain more recipes or information about this grain, you can write to the Quinoa Corporation, P.O. Box 7114, Boulder, CO 80306.

Quinoa

Quinoa (pronounced keen-wa), like amaranth, is a grain that has been grown by traditional peoples for thousands of years and is just now being rediscovered by a wider population. "The mother grain of the Incas," quinoa survived only in small pockets of the South American Andes until the early 1980s, when entrepreneurs Steve Gorad and Don McKinley formed the Quinoa Corporation in Boulder, Colorado and decided to grow quinoa in the Rockies and market it to natural foods stores. It is a hardy, nutritious grain, with a unique texture and taste, and shows early signs of catching on in the United States. See the sidebar "Quinoa—Tale of a Food Survivor," on pages 19–20.

Rice

Rice, presently the staple crop for over one-half the world's population, was originally grown in India and Southeast Asia. Alexander the Great brought it to Europe, and Europeans brought it to North America. The first attempt to grow it here, in Virginia in the mid-17th century, failed because the variety selected did not suit the climate. At the end of the 17th century, farmers in South Carolina had better success and rice began to catch on as a cash crop.

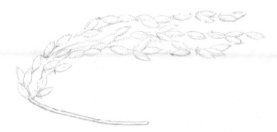

Worldwide, about 90 percent of the rice crop is grown in continuously flooded fields. Rice plants have the unique ability to transport oxygen from their leaves to their submerged roots. Flooding rice fields during most or all of the growing season helps to minimize weed competition and tends to increase yields.

Rice is commonly thought to be a tropical crop but it also grows in temperate regions. In the United States, rice is now grown primarily in Louisiana, Arkansas, California, and Texas. California grows mainly short grain rice, while the southern states raise mostly long grain. Even within states, different growing regions contribute different characteristics to the rice and veteran rice-eaters often have their preferences. Each variety lends itself to different uses, seasons, and tastes, and calls for different methods of cooking.

The sizes rice is available in include medium grain in addition to long and short grain. The short grain is the hardest variety, and contains less protein but more minerals than the others. Americans are more familiar with long grain rice, usually sold milled white and packaged in the supermarkets. It is available in its whole form in natural foods stores, and increasingly in supermarkets. Long grain rice is lighter than short grain; medium grain, as the name implies, falls somewhere between the two.

Rice is often parboiled to improve its milling, nutritional, and keeping qualities. This process—soaking, steaming, and drying the grain—drives the water-soluble nutrients of the bran into the endosperm where they are preserved during milling. "Converted rice" is the modern term for rice that has been processed in this manner, which has been used in the United States since 1942. Parboiling, however, has been practiced for generations in Asia.

White Rice

In the United States, more than 98 percent of the rice sold for direct consumption is milled and thus white. Throughout the rest of the world the percentage appears to be just as high, although exact figures are not available. Rice has been milled and polished into white rice in India and China since ancient times. Up until the 19th century, white rice was obtained through hand-milling with pestles, a very labor-intensive process.

In rice milling, the grain is identified at three major stages of the process—rough, brown, and white. Rough or paddy rice is the whole grain with the inedible outer hull intact. Following removal of the hull, the remaining kernel is called brown rice. This consists, in most varieties, of seven outer bran layers that encase the starchy endosperm and the small germ or embryo resting at the base of the endosperm. Brown rice is milled into white rice by a gradual abrasive action that strips away all the bran layers and some of the endosperm, including all the germ. This milling process, according to one study, denudes rice of 2 percent of its protein, 83 percent of its fat, 66 percent of its fiber, 17 percent of its calcium, 60 percent of its phosphorus, iron, and potassium, and much of its thiamine, niacin, and riboflavin. The bran and germ byproduct, a nutritional gold mine, is sold for cattle feed and the manufacture of vitamin concentrates.

Brown Rice

All whole grain rice is called "brown" though the grains may actually be gold, cream-colored, or even red. Only the hull of brown rice has been removed. All types of brown rice—short, medium, or long grain—can be purchased organically grown, and will be clearly labeled as such. Nutritionally, brown rice is a good source of vitamins, minerals, carbohydrates, and fiber. Traditionally, rice is eaten with a complementary legume and thus can be a reliable source of protein.

Organic Rice in the U.S.

Rice is so important in the Far East that the word for it in some languages is the same as the word for "meal." Confucius considered it "a necessary and appropriate food for the virtuous and graceful life." In the United States today it is, to most people, a somewhat insignificant supermarket item that rouses the memory of an avuncular character named Ben and that is eaten now and then to break the monotony of potatoes.

It is difficult for the average American—who eats an average of twelve pounds of rice a year and whose diet consists of a spectacular assortment of grains, vegetables, fruits, fishes, meats and dairy products—to fully grasp what this small seed means to the average Asian. Many Asians eat two to four hundred pounds of rice a year and derive between 30 and 70 percent of their total calories from it. Quite simply, the rice paddy is all that stands between them and starvation.

Rice doesn't have a 5,000-year history in the United States as it does in the Orient—it was first introduced into South Carolina in 1694. But it is in the United States, one of the largest exporters of rice in a world where 50 percent of all rice is consumed within eight miles of where it is grown, that efforts to return to organic farming and consumption of brown rice show the most promise.

The growth of the natural foods movement in the United States over the past fifteen years has given birth to a new class of rice eaters in America who are unwilling to settle for converted rice or artificially seasoned rice mixes. And the persistent call from an increasingly health-conscious public for an uncompromised grain of rice has also helped to create a market for organic rice. Hardly a dominant force in the rice market, the country's several farmers of organic rice nonetheless guard against a monopoly of chemically farmed rice.

Our country's 30,000 rice farmers presently harvest around 7 million tons, and usually two-thirds of the production is exported. What we keep is mostly packaged into white rice of one form or another, although smaller portions are processed into baby or cereal foods or used in brewing beer. Of all the rice we eat, only 1.6 percent is brown and, by rough estimate, just .3 percent is organically farmed. In other words, organic brown rice has not yet found its way into mainstream America.

If you are one of the few who pays two or sometimes three times as much for organic rice, you are most likely eating the rice of one of five established organic growers and/or distributors in the U.S.— the Lundberg brothers of California, Carl Garrich in Arkansas, the Vincent family of Texas, Louisiana's John Baker, or the Chico-San Company of Chico, California.

As these organic rice growers earnestly aim to restore agricultural sanity to an industry that has gone chemical-crazy, they cannot escape the inevitable profit-and-loss pressures that squeeze any business. Their major hurdle is price, which depends on many ever-changing factors. Naturally, a farmer's yields will affect the price, weather often being the crucial determinant. The overseas harvest also affects price: if exports are low, domestic stored supplies will mushroom, forcing the mills to dump as much rice as possible onto the domestic market at lower prices.

This may not seem to affect the organic farmers who sell a specialty product ostensibly far removed from the exported white rice. However, when an abundance of rice lies in storage, millers strive to move it in all forms, one of which is brown rice—

which can be sold as "natural" to people who identify any brown rice as a health food, regardless of the toxic chemicals that may have been used to grow it. Much of it will end up in the brown rice bin at the natural foods store at, say, $.39 a pound, right next to Lundberg's or Garrich's Arkansas organic rice, selling for $.89. Cost-conscious buyers, though they may suspect the organic is a better product, will choose the cheaper grain if the price disparity is great enough.

For most people it's impossible to see, smell, or even taste any difference between $.39 and $.89 rice. Barry Stice led me on a tour of the Lundberg Farms in August last year before the harvest and showed me what the customer is getting for the added cost. Since Lundberg raises both a minimally sprayed and an organic rice, it's possible to see immediately in the sprayed fields a weed-free environment, while on the organic fields a battle ensues between the watergrass weed and rice. The watergrass weed is a major reason why Lundberg's organic rice yields hover around twenty to thirty (100-pound) sacks per acre while commercial growers can get one hundred or more sacks per acre.

Sometimes, Stice says, when the weeds take over, they have to plow the whole field under, rice and all, and take a loss. In addition, the Lundberg brothers leave all of the organic fields fallow every other year, and they grow a humus-enriching cover on the fields in the winter. And, of course, they don't spray the bugs.

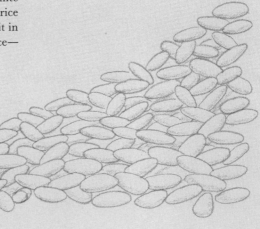

Sweet Rice

Sweet rice, which is usually a short-grained variety, contains slightly more protein than other types of rice, and is very sticky when cooked. It is often used for puddings, and such specialty foods as mochi, a pounded rice product sold in shrink-wrapped squares in many natural foods stores. Mochi is a traditional Japanese food, and is one of a number of special foods made out of sweet rice in the Orient.

Aromatic Rices

Basmati rice is an especially flavorful and light long grain rice grown primarily in Punjab in central Pakistan. Although imported Basmati rice is generally polished white rice, domestically grown, unpolished Basmati brown rice has recently been introduced to the United States natural foods market. Because of its unique aroma, Basmati rice is sometimes called "scented" or "aromatic" rice. *Wehani* rice, a specially developed aromatic rice grown in California is, like Basmati, a long grain variety and is said to have an aroma like "hot buttered peanuts" when cooked. Wehani is unique among commercially available rice in that it has a red bran layer.

Wild Rice

Wild rice is not actually a rice, but is the seed of a wild aquatic grass that grows in the shallow moving waters at the inlets and outlets of lakes in central North America, primarily the lake regions of western Ontario, eastern Manitoba, Wisconsin, and Minnesota. The traditional staple of the Native Americans in this area, wild rice is high in protein (14 percent) and relatively low in oil. Much of the commercially available wild rice is actually harvested from cultivated paddies, rather than from the wild.

One of the major suppliers of rice to the natural foods market, Lundberg Foods of Richvale, California, has introduced what they call "Country Wild" rice. This is not actually a wild rice but a mixture of three different domesticated varieties of rice: red Wehani, a black strain, and a standard long grain brown rice.

Quick Brown Rice Products

A relatively new product available in some natural foods stores is rice flakes. To make their "Tasty Flakes," Lundberg Foods starts with long grain brown rice, which is then steamed, flattened by steel rollers, and dried in an oven. Because more surface area of the grain is exposed, the preparation time is reduced from the 45 minutes usually needed to cook brown rice to five minutes. Lundberg claims that very few nutrients of the whole grain are lost in the process.

Another version, "Quick Brown Rice," is made by Arrowhead Mills of Hereford, Texas. The company uses a brief blast of dry heat to drive out the moisture in each kernel of rice. (Grains may seem dry, but most, including wheat and rye, contain about ten percent water by weight; it's this life-preserving moisture that enables the kernel to sprout when growing conditions are favorable.) As the moisture escapes, it creates microscopic fissures in the grain. The cracks allow hot water to penetrate as it cooks, so that cooking time is shortened to twelve minutes.

These products are more expensive than run-of-the-mill brown rice. In Boston, they typically sell for around thirty cents per 2 oz. serving, three times the price of bulk brown rice. They do have a long shelf life, though. The processing heat stabilizes the oils in the rice bran so that they resist deterioration. While regular brown rice begins to show faint signs of rancidity after sixty days with no refrigeration, these packaged products have a normal shelf life of three to six months. Those of us who scrutinize food labels will also be pleased to know that this durable grain suffers negligible nutrient losses in processing.

A new approach to convenient brown rice is being taken by Whole Earth, Inc. of London, England. They combine organic northern Italian and Indian basmati brown rice with vegetables in a 10.5 oz. enamel-lined can, seal it shut, and bake it slowly so that none of the flavor or nutrients escape. The rice is cooked "al dente" and ready to heat and serve. It is slightly more expensive at around forty cents per 2 oz. serving. Whole Earth products are now distributed nationally in the United States.

A Shopper's Guide to Rice Cakes

They sure don't make rice cakes like they used to—at least not here in the production-minded West. In Japan, where the snack originated, one can still find street vendors who produce rice cakes the traditional way, pouring moist grains of rice into a mold that has been heated over a bed of coals. The kernels expand as they cook, and after a short while, out pops a single crunchy disk. Different cooks will add their own signatures; one man habitually places a single soybean in the center of the mold to be puffed along with the rice kernels.

On this side of the Pacific, old-fashioned rice-cake cookery defers to mass production, a move that has changed the way these snacks look and taste. Here gigantic machines spew out thousands of rice cakes each hour, each one emerging from a pressurized cylindrical chamber where blazing heat induces the kernels to puff up and stick together like intertwined popcorn.

The most prominent difference is consistency. Because American cakes contain less rice and more air than the originals, they are lighter and not nearly as filling. An hour after you eat one, you might say, you're hungry again.

Another key difference: flavor. American companies, particularly the larger ones, are fond of sprinkling in assorted grains or a pinch of seasoning. It distinguishes their product from other rice cakes and has the potential to build a loyal base of customers who have grown enamored of a particular flavor. There are rice cakes flavored with buckwheat, barley, corn, even Italian spices and apple-cinnamon. To the pizza and the oatmeal bowl the rice cake moguls have turned for their modern-day signatures.

Nutritionally, all rice cakes are pretty similar. They bring the quality nutrition of brown rice but in a less concentrated form bite for bite, since a typical cake contains just over a tablespoon of rice. Most cakes carry about 35 calories. Even salted varieties often weigh in at around 30 milligrams of sodium per half-ounce serving, low enough to be legally labeled "very low sodium." The cost comparisons given here are based on manufacturers' suggested retail prices (as of October 1986) for basic rice cakes. Prices for flavored varieties may be higher.

The California-based natural foods company **Chico-San** first introduced the rice cake to America back in 1967 and went on to become the industry leader. In November 1984 the company was acquired by H.J. Heinz Co., of Pittsburgh, which continues to market the rice cakes under the labels Chico-San and Spiral. The latter is available in the delicatessen sections of food stores. Shortly after the purchase, the president of Heinz remarked to the *Wall Street Journal* that rice cakes "are almost inedible and have the consistency of wallboard." His, evidently, was a minority view.

Chico-San cakes come in seven varieties: Rice (only), Organic Rice, Sesame, Buckwheat, Millet, Corn, and Rye. Each is available sodium-free or (sea) salted. We like how they resist crumbling despite their thinness.

The rice itself is produced by California farmers according to Heinz's specifications. The company says its organic rice is grown to standards more stringent than California's organic produce law. *Price:* moderate ($.99 for a 5¼ oz bag, or $.19/oz).

From a small operation in rural Asheville, North Carolina, **Arden** grew to be the second-largest rice cake producer in the country before it, too, was approached by a food giant with an offer too good to refuse. Quaker Oats of Chicago bought the company in 1985 and promptly pumped in $10 million of advertising that produced the country's first television commercials for rice cakes.

Except for one organic version, which is available only in the Eastern U.S., Arden cakes are made with commercial long grain brown rice. Six other varieties are available nationwide: Plain, Sesame, Multigrain, Buckwheat (unsalted), Corn (salted), and Barley-Oat (salted). Arden's rice cakes are thick, but to us they seem airy and overpuffed, which makes them fragile and not as richly flavored as other brands. *Price:* moderate ($.99 for a 4¼ oz bag, or $.22/oz).

The natural foods giant **Hain** of Los Angeles puts out a line of miniature rice cakes about the size of a silver dollar and half the thickness of full-size cakes. They are densely textured and flavorful, and the smaller size makes them good for spreadables and dips. The company uses commercial short grain brown rice in all its rice cakes.

Mini Rice Cakes come two ways: Plain (regular and no salt) and Teriyaki, an innovative if salty (80 milligrams of sodium per ½ oz) blend of rice, soy sauce, honey, and dried bonito. *Price:* expensive ($1.39 per 4 oz package, $.35/oz).

For less adventurous souls, the company also manufactures standard-size cakes. They come in five varieties (Plain, Regular No-Salt, Sesame, Sesame No-Salt, and Five Grain). *Price:* moderate ($1.04 for a 5 oz package, or $.22/oz).

True to its name, **Lundberg Family Farms** of Richvale, CA, remains a family-owned and operated company. Eldon, Wendell, Homer, and Harlan Lundberg grow their own rice, mill it on the property, and hand-select a fresh batch each day to be made into rice cakes. Because the Lundbergs pack twice as much rice in their cakes as their competitors, the end product is heavier, chewier, and more substantial. They are also the least expensive of any rice cake we surveyed.

Lundberg's cakes come in five varieties: Brown Rice, Organic Brown Rice, Wild Rice, Wehani (an aromatic specialty rice native to India), and Sweet Mochi (cooked sweet rice). All varieties come in unsalted and lightly salted versions. Lundberg aficionados say the Wehani and the Mochi are sweeter than the other

three. *Price:* inexpensive ($1.09 for an 8 oz bag, or $.14/oz).

Pacific Rice Products of Berkeley, CA, entered the market in 1984 with Crispy Cakes, a product that brought several innovations to the genre. The company uses rice flour, not kernels, cooked with water and sesame seeds. The resulting slurry goes into something called an extruder, which steam-heats the mixture under pressure and squirts it into a continuous ribbon that is cut into three-inch squares and oven-toasted. The result is a thin, delicately textured, cracker-like product that resists crumbling. Sales have been brisk enough to quickly move the cakes from natural foods stores to supermarkets such as Safeway.

Crispy Cakes are labeled a "good source of fiber," a claim more accurately applied to brown rice than to rice cakes, which contain a fairly small amount of actual grain. You would have to eat forty Crispy Cakes to match the fiber in a single slice of whole wheat bread.

The rice for Crispy Cakes comes from individual farmers and from a rice co-op that pools commercial rice harvests from a number of California growers. The cakes come in three varieties: Natural, Apple-Cinnamon, and Italian Spices. The Apple-Cinnamon is sweet with apples, and the Italian is piquant, spicy, and salty (135 milligrams of sodium per half-ounce) with tomato powder and soy sauce powder. The company is also introducing three new flavors: Honey Raisin Spice, Sourdough, and Onion Herb. *Price:* moderate ($1.19 for a 5¾ oz bag, or $.22/oz).

The latest entry to the market travels the greatest distance to get there. In October 1986, **Westbrae Natural Foods** of Emeryville, CA, introduced American shoppers to a first: rice cakes made from rice grown on Japanese soil. The cakes are square and thin, much more like even-textured crackers than the traditional round disks, and are made with commercial Japanese brown rice.

Westbrae's cakes come in three Asian-inspired flavors: Double Sesame, Teriyaki, and Sesame Garlic, each of which starts with a tasty coating of shoyu, brown rice malt, and umeboshi plum. Three Western-style flavors—Plain, Buckwheat, and Organic Sesame—are due to be released soon. These will be made domestically with California-grown organic brown rice. *Price:* moderate ($1.39 for a 5¾ oz bag, or $.24/oz).

Rye

The first recorded mention of rye as a cultivated crop was made by Pliny the Elder, a Roman who lived in the first century A.D. During medieval times rye flour was an ingredient in bread recipes throughout Europe. Able to thrive in severe climates, rye is still consumed in much of Eastern Europe and Russia. Cultivated rye was brought to North America by Dutch settlers, although wild varieties are found here. Rye cultivation today is sporadic and does not constitute a major cash crop. Like wheat, rye is threshed clean and does not need to undergo further hulling.

Rye may be cooked whole and is delicious mixed with other grains. It may also be cracked like wheat and prepared as a breakfast cereal or side dish. Many natural foods stores carry rye flakes that may be toasted and added to a homemade granola recipe.

Of all the grains rye has the highest percentage of the essential amino acid lysine. As proportionally high as rye is in lysine, however, it is as low in gluten. Rye flour is better used in unleavened baked goods or mixed with wheat flour if leavening is used. In this century, scientists have crossed rye with wheat to produce a grain, called triticale (tri-ti-kay-lee), that is high in both lysine and gluten.

Sorghum

Although most Western cooks may not even know what it is, a recent United Nations survey on food consumption ranked sorghum as the third most important cereal in the world (after wheat and rice). It is an extremely hardy grain capable of withstanding drought and high temperatures. As the staple grain of Africa, sorghum is freshly ground and cooked as a porridge. Sorghum is usually available only as the unrefined cooked syrup made from the sweet juice, squeezed from the stalks.

Wheat

Wheat is the world's most widely distributed grain. Because of the popularity of bread, wheat has been carried into the home territories of the other grains, so that now it is grown in nearly every country. Not native to the United States, it has become a major cash crop, along with soybeans and corn. Columbus brought wheat seeds with him to the West Indies in 1493. Cortez took seeds to Mexico in 1519, and missionaries traveling up the Pacific Coast carried wheat to what is now California. Presently, the major producing areas are the Great Plains and the Pacific Northwest. Like rye, wheat is threshed clean—it does not have to undergo extensive hulling.

Wheat is available in hard and soft varieties. The hard wheats contain higher levels of protein than the soft wheats, and the soft wheats contain higher levels of carbohydrates. Both hard and soft wheats are further classified as being spring or winter varieties. This refers to the season in which they are planted. Spring wheat is planted in the spring and harvested in the fall; winter wheat is planted in the fall and is harvested in late spring or early summer when the warm weather allows it to grow and mature. Spring varieties are planted farther north and winter varieties farther south where the milder winters allow for their cultivation. Wheat is further classified by color — usually as red or white.

The hard wheats, because of their higher gluten (protein) content, are the basic bread wheats. It is the gluten that reacts favorably with a leavening agent and turns out a light, evenly textured loaf. Generally the hard spring wheats tend to have a bit more gluten than the hard winter wheats, but both may be used for baking bread and for making seitan (seasoned wheat gluten; see pages 40–44). Semolina is a granular flour obtained from the endosperm of durum wheat, a hard variety. Semolina contains a large amount of protein and is used in the production of pastas.

Because they do not rise as well as the hard wheats, soft wheat varieties are used in making pastries or blended with the harder varieties for bread baking. Pastry wheat, a white spring variety that is very low in gluten content, is used for crackers or pastry dough. Some of this is exported to Japan for making udon noodles.

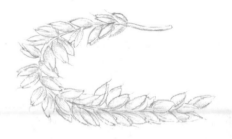

Do not think that baking with wheat flour is the only way to make use of wheat. The whole grains of any variety (sometimes called "berries") can be cooked, either alone or mixed with other grains to make a main dish. When cracked or coarsely ground, wheat makes a nutty-tasting breakfast porridge or side dish. Bulghur is cracked wheat that has been lightly cooked and parched (dried or roasted) prior to being cracked. It is the staple grain in southeastern Europe and the Middle East. A related product is couscous, which starts as durum wheat, a grain whose hardness and high gluten content makes it ideal for pasta. Semolina, the heart of the durum kernel, is extracted and ground into flour. Then it is mixed with water and formed into spaghetti-like strands, which are broken into tiny uniform pieces, steamed, and dried. The pale yellow granules that result are couscous.

Couscous has 100 percent of its bran and germ removed and differs in this regard from its whole wheat counterpart, bulghur. Couscous cannot be considered a whole grain. As an occasional change of pace to complement a natural foods meal, it can be delightful, but nutritionally it is a washout.

A Guide to Whole Grain Flours

The first flour was made by crushing grass seeds on a flat stone with a second, handheld stone. Virtually all flour produced up until the 19th century was ground in stone mills of various sorts, ranging from simple mortars and pestles through hand-turned querns to massive burrstones turned by falling water or blowing wind. Although high-speed steel rollers have replaced the old millstones for most commercial flour production, the best flour is still ground between slow-moving natural stones. Stone-ground flour retains more of the nutty flavor of the whole grain, maintains its electromagnetic charge, and has the unique texture necessary for making naturally leavened bread.

Even though most commercial bakers and millers will insist that flour must be aged (usually artificially with chemicals instead of precious time) for better handling, the best flour is that which is milled immediately before use. As soon as grain is crushed, oxidation starts and nutrition and flavor begin to decline. Obviously it is best to have your own stone mill if you use much flour. Alternatively, you could purchase a good mill with a group of people, so that all might share in the cost and benefits. A third option is to locate a natural foods store that carries freshly stone-ground flours and meals.

While whole wheat flour is the most commonly used of the following varieties of whole grain flour, the others can make delicious additions to your regular baking or serve as the basis for unique, special breads.

Whole wheat bread flour: Milled from either hard red spring or hard red winter wheat, whole wheat bread flour is high in gluten and ideal for bread and seitan (see page 41).

Whole wheat pastry flour: Pastry wheat is often not stone-ground, but rather milled in a hammer mill that reduces the soft white or soft red wheat to small, uniform particles. This flour is used for pie crusts, crackers, and cookies, and in any pastry recipe. Very finely milled stone-ground pastry flour is sometimes available.

Cornmeal: Usually milled from yellow dent corn, but occasionally from flint or flour corn, cornmeal is used for cornbread and cornmeal mush. Combined with wheat flour in your favorite bread recipe it will produce a slightly crumbly, crunchy, sweet loaf. The corn flour sold in some stores is simply finely ground cornmeal. (In English-speaking Europe the term "corn flour" is used to refer to a highly refined product similar to our cornstarch, used as an inexpensive thickener for sauces and gravy.)

Barley flour: If you're milling your own flour, lightly roast the barley (preferably hull-less) before grinding. If you buy barley flour, roast it lightly before using. Roasting greatly improves flavor. Barley flour gives bread a rich, cake-like quality.

Brown rice flour and *sweet brown rice flour* are both used in the preparation of Japanese-style pastries and can be added sparingly to wheat flour to give breads a moist, smooth texture.

Millet meal must be freshly ground or it has a bitter taste. A cup or two in a batch of bread dough imparts a unique dry and crunchy texture and a richness of flavor.

Oat flour, rarely available, was once common throughout Scotland, Wales, and Ireland, for use in the preparation of various forms of oatcakes. You'll probably have to grind your own oat flour, but if you use it either as the primary ingredient in traditional oatcakes or as an ingredient in moist, chewy wheaten bread, you'll be well rewarded for the extra effort.

Buckwheat flour: The best buckwheat flour is stone-ground from unhulled buckwheat, and contains small dark flecks. These are small bits of the hull that remain after the coarser hulls are removed when the milled flour is sifted. Buckwheat pancakes with maple syrup—what could be better on a cold winter morning?

Rye flour: Used alone, rye flour makes a very sticky dough and a heavy, moist bread. Combined with wheat it results in a delicious bread that is less likely to mold in warm weather than all-wheat bread.

Unbleached white flour: Although certainly not a whole grain flour, good-quality unbleached white flour, milled from organically grown wheat, is available in many natural foods stores. When used occasionally, it is ideal for imparting a lightness to baked goods. Since this flour is neither stone-ground nor fresh, you may find it worthwhile to make your own from stone-ground whole wheat flour by sifting it through a very fine screen. The bran remaining in the screen can be used as a pickling agent.

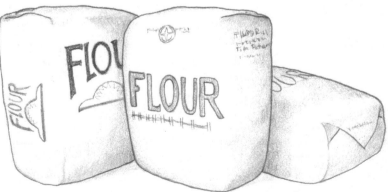

Breakfast Cereals Go Natural

Fifteen years ago, the natural breakfast cereal market consisted of some bulk granolas that could have passed for horse feed, and Nabisco's Shredded Wheat. Today, ready-to-eat breakfast cereals are one of the most innovative, profitable, and hotly contested segments of the natural foods market. Sales are estimated to be over $10 million and rising. That old mainstay, granola, is still popular, but increasingly it is losing out to natural foods versions of favorites from the baby boomers' childhood. Cereals styled after such favorites as Cheerios, Rice Krispies, and Raisin Bran are now available devoid of artificial ingredients, preservatives, colorings, synthetic vitamins, and in many cases, salt and sugar.

Although organically grown grains are a rarity in ingredients, a wide range of whole grains (rice, corn, millet, oats) prepared in various tasty ways is available. At the huge Bread & Circus natural foods supermarket in Hadley, MA, over thirty varieties of ready-to-eat cereals are sold, and that represents only a portion of all the natural cereals on the market. Most are minimally sweetened, often with barley malt and occasionally with fruit juices.

In the following review of various natural foods companies' cereals, we're looking mainly at ready-to-eat, non-granola cereals that don't need to be cooked.

An original industry leader, **Arrowhead Mills, Inc.** of Hereford, Texas, has been growing and selling whole grains and whole grain products for over two decades. One of their latest offerings, Grainstay, made of five grains and raisins, is an ambitious attempt to concoct the nutritional wonder cereal, the natural version of Grape-Nuts. Two kinds of wheat, oats, yellow corn, oat bran, raisin paste, honey, barley malt, and baking powder are mechanically blended and extruded into crunchy, dark brown bits. The result is a pleasant, nutty taste. Arrowhead Mills also offers Nature-O's, which are Cheerios look-alikes made from oats, rice, and defatted wheat germ. Additionally, they market several puffed whole cereals: Puffed Rice, Millet, Corn, and Wheat. For these cereals the whole grains (not organically grown) are mechanically cleaned, steamed, then pressurized in air-

tight containers where they puff up like cumulus clouds to several times their original size.

NEOPC, Inc. of Leominster, MA, first began as an organic produce distributor, but got into product development with their highly successful Pickle Eater's pickles. Equally promising are their **New Morning** cereals. These are among the most impressive lines of natural boxed cereals at present, both for ingredients, nutritional strengths, taste, and packaging. The grains are sufficiently toasted, flaked, baked, or puffed to make them light and crunchy and are sensitively blended with barley malt. New Morning Oatios is a snappy new cereal that is confidently hailed as "America's Favorite Breakfast

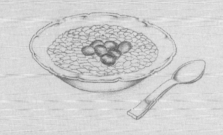

Cereal in its natural form." They are offering an alternative to Cheerios, of course, but without the additives. Oatios are bigger, more free-form puffs than the General Mills cereal, but arrive with a fresh, delicate aroma, and go well with either soymilk or fruit juice. New Morning makes six other boxed cereals, including Maple Nut Muesli, Cornflakes, Crispy Brown Rice, Super Raisin Bran, and—their newest—Fruit-e-O's. These are "loops of real fruit-flavored whole grains," meant as the natural replacement for sugar-laden Fruit-Loops.

This year **Erewhon, Inc.,** based in Wilmington, MA, celebrates its twentieth anniversary as a distributor and producer of natural foods. One of the most recent additions to its line of natural breakfast cereals is Crispy Brown Rice Cereal, a ready-to-eat puffed whole rice cereal that is probably the best of the many available. Erewhon's distinction is twofold. First, they use organically grown medium grain brown rice. Second, after puffing the grains, they blend them with barley malt

and a touch of unrefined sea salt, and roast them for a nutty, rich, but light flavor. The oven-toasting accentuates the delicious grain flavor, while the use of the medium grain rice keeps the puffed cereal looking small, tidy, and like its less natural forebears. New Morning's Crispy Rice, by comparison, is much larger, the puffed grains more sprawling and airy and less flavorful. Possibly the Erewhon brand's only drawback is its relatively high sodium content (185 mg/oz.). But fear not—Erewhon also boxes a low-sodium version with only 15 mg/oz.

Erewhon's recent acquisition of the cereal manufacturer U.S. Mills of Omaha, NB, has enabled them to expand their ready-to-eat cereal line. In 1987, they plan to introduce three new cereals made from rolled whole wheat flakes sweetened with barley malt: Fruit 'n Wheat (with dates, raisins, and walnuts), Raisin Bran, and Wheat Flakes.

Grainfields is a division of the British mainstream cereal maker Weetabix, and their fivefold natural breakfast offerings are reminiscent of Kellogg's earlier Nutri-Grain attempt at looking like one of the natural selections on the shelf. Distributed out of their Clinton, MA, location, Grainfields makes Cornflakes, Wheat Flakes, Crispy Rice, Crispy Brown Rice, and Raisin Bran, in identically styled, somewhat uninspired boxes. The cereals are solid, if unspectacular. The Cornflakes, for instance, are paperthin, almost airy, and are made simply from milled corn and barley malt. Kellogg's Cornflakes, by comparison, have three sweeteners (sugar, barley malt, corn syrup) plus synthetic nutrients. Grainfields doesn't explicitly state "whole" corn, which is possibly why the product is relatively inexpensive. But the nutritional profile is similar to the other brands.

Health Valley Foods of Montebello, CA, has over 300 products ranging from peanut butter to frozen dinners, including a line of popular boxed cereals, such as Sprouts-7, Orangeola, Amaranth (with raisins or bananas), and Bran. Some of these are innovative and tasty, while others are pale imitations of popular favorites. For instance, their version of the classic Raisin Bran will never outpace Post's

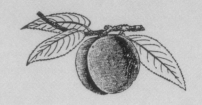

standard, nor does it hold its own against Grainfield's and New Morning's contributions, despite the high quality ingredients and well-intentioned recipe. They make the mistake of using roller-flattened roasted whole wheat kernels (too chewy and raw-tasting) and sweetening it with a heavy hand on the barley malt. They are generous with the plump, sugary raisins,

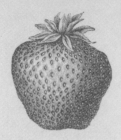

which contribute to their "old-fashioned flavor reminiscent of pioneer days," but the overall taste and texture is disappointing.

From **Perky Foods** in Newport Beach, CA, comes a light and refreshing new line of breakfast cereals. They take their name from Henry Perky, who invented shredded wheat in 1893. Following in his spirit of innovation, Perky Foods has created three breakfast varieties: Perky's Apple and Cinnamon Crispy Brown Rice, Carob Crispy Brown Rice, and Nutty Rice. The crispy rice styles are tasty little squares of crunchy toasted rice puffs. You wouldn't think of a breakfast cereal as being refreshing, but these really are. The Nutty Rice is a granulated, toasty, nut-flavored cereal much like Grape-Nuts but without the tooth-jarring texture.

The natural cookie mogul of the West Coast, **Barbara's Bakery** in Novato, CA, has joined the boxed breakfast cereal market with four offerings distinguished by their triple-play use of fruit sweeteners in place of barley malt. Their Breakfast O's, for example, another variation on the popular Cheerios, is made from whole grain oat flour, brown rice flour, concentrated juice of pineapple, pear, and peach, oat bran, and salt. Other favorites include Corn Flakes, Raisin Bran, and Brown Rice Crisps, all handsomely boxed. While being delicious, crunchy, and gaining points for their innovative use of fruit sweeteners, Barbara's cereals lose out when it comes to sodium content. Their Corn Flakes have a whopping 310 mg/oz.—almost twice the sodium of popular salty snacks such as Fritos corn chips.

Composition of Whole Grains and Whole Grain Flours (by percent)

Type of Grain or Flour	Water	Protein	Fat	Carb.	Fiber	Ash
Amaranth	8.0	14.5	5.7	66.0	4.5	3.1
Barley, pearled	11.1	8.2	1.0	78.8	0.5	0.9
Buckwheat, whole grain	11.0	11.7	2.4	72.9	9.9	2.0
Corn, white or yellow	72.7	3.5	1.0	22.1	0.7	0.7
Cornmeal, whole ground white or yellow	12.0	9.2	3.9	73.7	1.6	1.2
Millet	11.8	9.9	2.9	72.9	3.2	2.5
Oatmeal or rolled oats (dried form)	8.3	14.2	7.4	68.2	1.2	1.9
Oats	12.5	13.0	5.4	66.1	10.6	3.0
Quinoa	11.4	16.2	6.9	63.9	3.5	3.3
Rice, brown	12.0	7.5	1.9	77.4	0.9	1.2
Rye	11.0	9.4	1.0	77.9	0.4	0.7
Wheat, whole grain (hard, red spring)	13.0	14.0	2.2	69.1	2.3	1.7
Wheat flour, whole grain (from hard wheat)	12.0	13.3	2.0	71.0	2.3	1.7

As these values are averages, they do not add up to 100.

3. BREADS, PASTAS & SEITAN

Not the least of various grains' attractions is their versatility. Though usually most nutritious in their whole form, there are myriad ways to process grains without sacrificing too much of their nutrition. The combining of flour with water to form dough—and then breads, pastas, pastries, and so forth—is only the most obvious of grains' many applications.

"Wheat meat," which is becoming more commonly known by its Japanese name of seitan, is a high-protein flour product that has the potential to become "the tofu of the '90s." Barbara and Leonard Jacobs' tips on how to shop for it, make it, and cook with it provide a valuable introduction to this promising food. In addition to the discussion of seitan, this section features several articles about natural breads and pastas—Martin Russell's "A Guide to Leavening Agents," Ron Kotzsch's "A Return to Real Bread," and Thom Leonard's "The Twists and Turns of Pasta." In the following pages, we will offer a new perspective on these familiar foods, as well as take a look at the ways in which seitan can greatly expand the natural foods consumer's diet. The result hopefully will be a renewed appreciation of grains' many faces.

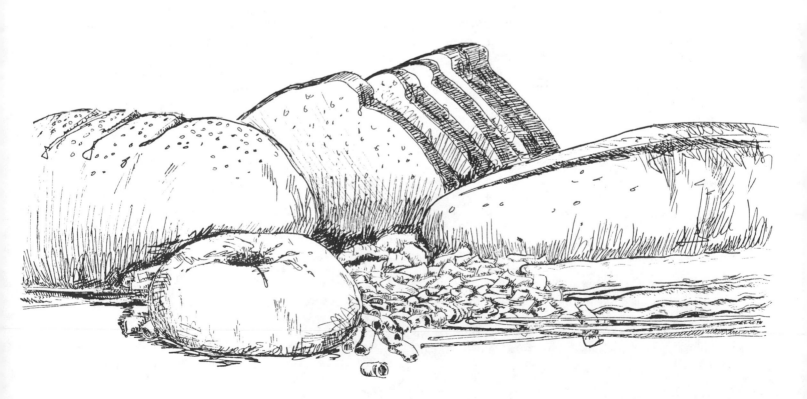

A Guide to Leavening Agents

The last of the restaurant customers had long since departed and I was doing my best to get the kitchen back into shape. At the same time, Evan Root, head chef of Sanae (a Boston whole foods restaurant that was founded in the late 1960s), was slowly kneading the dough for the next day's rice bread, which had become a Sanae staple.

Whole wheat flour, corn oil, water, sea salt, and the brown rice left over from the day's cooking were the bread's only ingredients. Instead of yeast, lactic and acetic acid bacteria and wild yeasts inherent in the flour and air would be the leavening agents.

The first step in making the bread was the mixing of the preliminary or sponge dough (which consisted of whole wheat flour, water, and cooked rice) in a huge metal bowl. After he had kneaded it sufficiently, Evan placed the dough on top of the oven (kept warm by a pilot light), covered it with a wet apron, and left it overnight to slowly produce and nourish the necessary colonies of bacteria and yeast. Evan had, in fact, made his own leavening factory.

Early the next morning, Evan would make the final dough by adding oil, sea salt, and additional flour and water to the sponge and kneading it again. Then, after the dough had received a second, much briefer, rising period, he set it on the table. By now it was fermenting and had become warm, soft, and light. He cut it into equal pieces, tightly formed them into loaves, and placed them in the waiting bread pans, seasoned from years of use. There they would rest on top of the oven while the leaven did its work of breaking down the carbohydrates and exchanging them for alcohol and carbon dioxide.

When sufficiently risen, the loaves were slid carefully into the oven and slowly baked. By the time I arrived at the restaurant that afternoon, the bread, cooled and spilling its aroma throughout the kitchen, beckoned me for a taste. It was always moist, cakelike, and sweet. Yet with each day's batch, there were subtle changes in texture and taste. The signature of each individual dough was uniquely set down through variations in time, temperature, humidity, ingredients, and kneading time and intensity.

Sourdough and Desem

Traditionally, throughout the ages, bread was made without the help of today's modern, commercial yeast, with few but wholesome ingredients, and in small batches. Today, as an alternative to the white factory-produced bread that is commonly available, people are seeking a denser loaf with a rich, satisfying taste, like the bread that is made from natural leaven. As a result, the traditional art of making sourdough bread is being resurrected in both Europe and the United States. Sourdough bread can be made from a sponge of whole wheat flour, water, and other, optional ingredients, mixed together the night before, as in Evan's bread. Or it can be made from a sponge that has as its foundation a starter—a mixture of flour and water that already contains certain microorganisms. A small quantity of starter is saved from the sponge each time to be used for the next batch. (See the sidebar ''Making Your Own Sourdough Starter,'' page 37.)

Desem—Flemish for ''starter''—is a unique starter dough made from organic wheat and pure water. The particular microorganisms that live in the desem leaven the bread and are responsible for its slightly sour, delicious flavor. Hy Lerner and Paul Petrofsky brought the desem method from the Lima Bakery in Belgium to the United States. It is practiced at the Baldwin Hill Bakery in Phillipston, Massachusetts, as well as by other traditional bakeries.

The term ''free leaven'' indicates any organisms, used as leavening agents, that live freely in the environment, not being commercially produced or added by the baker. Since desem is a free leaven, it is susceptible to contamination by other bacteria and yeast and must be kept refrigerated at around 55° F so that the lactobacilli (lactic acid bacteria), which are able to grow and reproduce in the colder environment, are most active. Unlike yeast, which digests only starch, desem works on all the flour's component parts (carbohydrates, proteins, fats, and cellulose). It breaks them down to create a more digestible, chewy loaf of bread,

A Comparison of Various Leavening Agents

Leavening Agent	Description	Use(s)
Sourdough		
sponge	is made from whole wheat flour and water; should be mixed together the night before; add other ingredients for variety	breads, sweet breads, pancakes, muffins
starter	some should be saved each time you bake; resulting breads are dense and richly textured	breads, sweet breads, pancakes, muffins
desem	is starter dough made from organic wheat and pure water; gives slightly sour flavor	breads
Yeast		
fresh	commercial yeast is a single, isolated strain that yields uniform, predictable results	breads, sweet breads
active dry	easy to store; stays fresh a long time; has great rising power	breads, refrigerated doughs for sweet breads
quick-acting	exhibits best qualities of fresh and dry yeasts; acts quickly	breads, sweet breads
Baking Soda		
(bicarbonate of soda)	a refined product; use with acidic ingredients or cream of tartar; gives light, smooth texture	quick (unyeasted) breads, muffins, cookies, cakes, pastries, pancakes
Potassium Bicarbonate	low-sodium alternative to baking soda	same uses as baking soda
Baking Powder	is baking soda plus acid; also contains cornstarch and sometimes other ingredients; gives fine texture	same uses as baking soda; baking powders containing aluminum should be avoided
Ammonium Bicarbonate	suitable only for porous doughs	used commercially for cookies and crackers
Eggs	enhance taste, texture and keeping quality; for best results, beat egg whites and yolks separately	cakes, batter breads, muffins, pancakes

made from a basic dough composed only of whole wheat flour, water, and sea salt. I have been making desem bread on and off for several years, and I like to add whole cooked grains and barley malt to the dough, which results in a chewier, denser loaf.

As my diet and moods change, I alter the type of leaven. Today a chewy rice bread, next week sour rye rolls—leavened with a sourdough starter that is constantly replenished with whole rye flour and prevented from going rank by the addition of fresh chopped onion. When I crave a sweet and lighter bread, I just go with yeast and unbleached white flour.

Yeast

In 1867 Louis Pasteur published the results of his studies into yeast fermentation. Before Pasteur's work, yeast cells were thought to be inanimate objects that at some point were spontaneously transformed into living organisms. Starting with a colony of yeast cells that could sit on the head of a pin, Pasteur produced more than two pounds of yeast, thus invalidating the theory of spontaneous generation in fermentation and proving yeasts to be living, growing, and eating organisms that transfer their life via reproduction before the mother organisms die.

Pasteur's experiment led to yeast factories like the one I toured recently in Baltimore. Today's modern production technology is quite different from the methods used at the time (beginning in about 1819 in Vienna, Austria and soon spreading to other parts of Europe) when bakers relied on breweries for their yeast, which was skimmed off the top of large beer-brewing vats, then dried and compressed. Today—from the beginning of a batch production when a single yeast cell is inoculated into a nutrient medium; to the regular feeding of the batch with molasses, phosphoric acid (chemically leached from rock phosphate), and ammonia (obtained from distillates of the coking process of coal); to the drying of the yeast via centrifuge—the entire process at the yeast plant is precisely orchestrated. Most impressive is the huge scale on which everything is done. From a catwalk in the Maryland factory I visited, I looked down into mammoth cauldrons over twenty feet high. Their yeasty contents were constantly aerated like an aquarium to provide a rich oxygen supply for the many trillions of yeast cells. Yet the yeast, batch after batch, came out uniformly.

Since World War II, when a need developed for a yeast low in moisture that stayed fresh longer and required no refrigeration, we have had active dry yeast. Many bakers, both home and commercial, prefer active dry yeast for its ease of storage and long-lasting freshness. As for performance, it is noted for its superiority in producing a greater volume in some sweet doughs. It also retains its rising power after sitting in a refrigerated dough for many hours prior to baking.

The strains of dry yeast, however, are unable to match the strength and speed of fresh yeast in raising bread dough. Contemporary yeast researchers have come up with quick-acting yeast that exhibits the best qualities of both fresh and dried yeast, and in addition acts much more quickly on the dough to provide for shorter rising times. Quick-acting yeast can now be purchased by home bakers in vacuum-packed jars or nitrogen-flushed packets.

No matter which of these commercial yeasts you use, they will all give you good results in bread and sweet doughs. I would suggest, however, that if you plan to refrigerate a sweet dough before baking, use dry yeast for its better tolerance to the cold.

Although yeast is convenient and yields predictable, consistent results, there may be good reason to use a free leaven instead. Commercial yeast is an isolated, single strain of yeast, *Saccharomyces cerevisiae*; the bread that is leavened with it doesn't have the richness, complexity, or digestibility of a loaf that contains many different strains of bacteria, wild yeasts, and other elements existing in the immediate environment. (See "A Return To Real Bread," page 35.)

The Leavening Process

The purpose of both commercial and free leavens in the dough is the same: to produce carbon dioxide gas through metabolic action on the various simple and complex sugars in the dough and to condition the dough and make it more elastic, so that it will yield readily to the pressure exerted on it by the carbon dioxide gas. The transformation of these sugars by the leaven gives us the familiar, delicious aroma and taste of risen bread.

The leavening process involves complex biochemical actions and reactions. On a molecular level, two proteins in the flour, glutenin and giladin, are arranged in long chains. Kneading breaks down these protein chains and interconnects the glutenin and giladin. When the proteins are bonded in the shearing action of the kneading, they create an elastic matrix throughout the dough, which is the gluten. The dough becomes capable of stretching like a rubber band, but it is actually tighter due to the initial physical bonding of the proteins.

When the dough is resting, the leavening, whether it is yeast, desem, or sourdough, effects a complex interaction of enzymes, both in flour and in the leavening, which solidifies the gluten bonds. At the same time the interaction mellows both the gluten and the starch in the dough (which has become interwoven with the gluten), so that the dough loses some of its tightness. This enables the dough to stretch when the pressure of the carbon dioxide, which is formed as a result of the leavening's fermentation activity, builds up.

Baking Soda

Yeast has its limitations as a leavening agent. In the mid-19th century, an alkaline salt developed from carbon-dioxide-treated soda ash revolutionized the baking industry. In 1846 John Dwight and his brother-in-law Dr. Austin Church started to produce baking soda (bicarbonate of soda) in the kitchen of Dwight's Massachusetts home. It was called Dwight's Saleratus (aerated salts). A cow was adopted as its trademark because the soda could be used with sour milk to produce a leavening action. This opened the door to a new level of cake and pastry making, and soda—used either with an acidic food or as a basic component of baking powder—has become one of the basic ingredients in the modern baking era.

Today baking soda is produced by the Solvay method, in which a brine solution is run into saturation tanks where it mixes with ammonia gas. Then this ammonia brine combination is injected with carbon dioxide and voila—bicarbonate of soda. Since the newly formed soda is insoluble in its briny ammonia bath, it is precipitated (separated out), drawn off, filtered, washed in cold water, dried, and milled into the refined white powder we know as baking soda.

If you choose baking soda as your leavening agent, you must use it in conjunction with an acid. When these two ingredients are mixed in the correct proportions with a liquid, they almost completely neutralize each other, forming water and carbon dioxide gas, which literally lifts the batter or dough and creates a light, smooth-textured goody; a few blandly flavored salts remain as end products.

The acid used with baking soda can be of several types. Acidic foods that are in the recipe, cream of tartar, or the more powerful chemicals used in today's commercial baking powders are all effective. Though baking soda is a refined substance that you wouldn't want to use frequently, it should be avoided altogether when other chemical ingredients are added to its simple acid/alkaline foundation.

If you want to use the natural acids in foods to react with baking soda, make sure that barley malt, honey, lemon juice, chocolate, cocoa, spices, or other acidic foods are in the recipe. When using soda in this manner, start off conservatively as far as the amount of soda is concerned, because if it is not completely neutralized by the acid, it leaves a terrible aftertaste. I would suggest not more than $1/2$ to $3/4$ teaspoon of soda per 2 cups of flour, depending on the amount of acid present. Also, the soda reacts with the acid as soon as the liquid is mixed into the dry ingredients, so whatever you are making has to get into the oven quickly.

Baking Powder

Cream of tartar, a byproduct of the wine making industry, was the acid companion to baking soda in the early formulas for baking powder. The sediment on the sides of wine barrels (called crystals of argolis) contain tartaric acid. These crystals are ground, purified, dried, and reground to produce cream of tartar. This acid, like others, reacts with soda in the presence of water to create a gas. The reason, however, that bakers today prefer modern compounds to cream of tartar is that tartar reacts with soda quickly once exposed to water. As a result, a large percentage of the leavening power is dispersed before the mix is panned and placed in the oven. In the old days, items produced in bakeries, as in the home, were placed in the oven soon after preparation, and enough power was left in the mix to sufficiently raise it and create a fine-textured, airy baked good. In today's bakeries, with their intense schedules, things don't always go straight into the oven, but may be refrigerated or "retarded" to be baked later. With the demand for lighter, finer-textured cakes and cookies, bakers have opted for more complex and powerful baking powder formulas that produce "double-acting" reactions.

Approximately 400 million pounds of baking soda are used each year worldwide in all its various applications, but as far as I know, a cream of tartar-based baking powder is no longer made nowadays. It is, however, easy enough to make at home. Cream of tartar can be purchased in any supermarket. Mix together two parts cream of tartar, one part baking soda, and two parts arrowroot. If you don't want to use baking soda, potassium bicarbonate is an alternative. Because potassium bicarbonate is not sodium-based, those concerned with their salt intake may prefer it to baking soda (sodium bicarbonate). Potassium bicarbonate is available over-the-counter in pharmacies, and potassium-based baking powder is now available in some natural foods stores.

The widely available Rumford brand of baking powder is a simple acid powder using only calcium phosphate (extracted from phosphate rock via an evaporation process), bicarbonate of soda, and cornstarch. It is labeled "double-acting" since it reacts both in the mixing bowl and in the oven.

This brand exemplifies what commercial bakers are looking for to produce a light dough on a baker's schedule. They want a double-acting leavening agent in which the initial action takes place when the powder is mixed with a liquid and, in conjunction with the mixing process itself, air cells are created. The second chemical action takes place when the batter is exposed to the heat of the oven chamber and the air cells expand during baking like thousands of tiny balloons being blown up simultaneously.

Other brands of baking soda used by commercial bakers also have double-acting power. The ingredient list of some, however, contains not only sodium bicarbonate, cornstarch, calcium phosphate, calcium sulfate, and often calcium silicate (to keep it free-flowing), but also sodium aluminum sulfate. Aluminum is a metal extracted from bauxite ore. Studies have shown that aluminum salts can be absorbed from the intestines and concentrated in various human tissues, and that high aluminum levels are found in the brains of patients with Alzheimer's and Parkinson's diseases. In addition, aluminum is linked to bone degeneration and kidney dysfunction.

So although this type of double-acting baking powder is convenient, saving most of its strength for the oven, and has great leavening ability, is it worth it? One piece of cake made with aluminum baking powder has 5 to 15 mg of aluminum. Chances are favorable that, if you eat a commercially baked sweet that contains baking powder, it has aluminum in every bite.

Sodium acid pyrophosphate, another acid often used in commercial baking powder, is also chosen for the convenience of its slow reaction rate until it reaches the oven. However, this chemical compound has a dark side: according to Bernard Oser, an FDA researcher, studies into its use in the food industry show a risk of possible fetal harm in pregnant women who regularly ingest it.

Sometimes it is necessary to make an adjustment in the amount of baking powder used in home baking. Since the atmospheric pressure is lower at high altitudes, less leavening is required to raise whatever you are baking. If you live at an altitude over 5,000 feet, try using only three-quarters as much chemical leavening and raise the oven temperature by about 30° F.

Ammonium Bicarbonate

There is one odd leavener—ammonium bicarbonate—that acts independently. It needs no chemical mate to create carbon dioxide, just heat and water. When it encounters them, it decomposes and releases carbon dioxide and ammonia. Ammonium bicarbonate is used mainly in the cookie and cracker industries, since these types of porous dough allow for the eventual escape of ammonia gases, which, if retained, would leave an ammonia odor. This leavener also alters the protein structure of the dough, helping it to spread as it bakes.

Eggs

If you desire to avoid chemical leavening agents altogether, yet still would like to get a rise out of baking, try the incredible egg. Not only will it act as a leavener, but it will contribute greatly to taste, richness, texture, aroma, and keeping quality. Sponge and angel food cakes rely on whole eggs or whites for their leavening. A baker I once worked with told me that the trick to using eggs effectively is to separate yolks and whites and to beat them separately. (Yolks should be at room temperature and whites should be cool and the bowl very clean.) After all other ingredients have been incorporated into the batter, stir in the yolks, then gently fold the whites into the mix. When beaten, the eggs trap air and encase it in the form of tiny cells which, when baked, expand, raising the batter. This method works best in cakes, batter breads, muffins, and pancakes.

As a commercial baker over the last fifteen years, I owed my livelihood in part to yeast and baking powder. I'm currently just baking at home when time allows and getting used to baking more and more with desem, sourdough, and eggs as leavening. I feel safer and it is more challenging to bake this way.

Frank Kern, director of the Tidewater Detention Home in Chesapeake, Virginia, is doing pioneer work in the field of diet and behavior within this institution. He recently told me that, along with other substances, he has almost totally eliminated baking powder from the inmates' diets because of its adverse effects—both physically and psychologically—on their health.

So to leaven or not to leaven, that is the question, and if so what kind, how much, and how often? If you love to bake as I do, these questions are the starting point for meditation, observation, and endless experimentation.

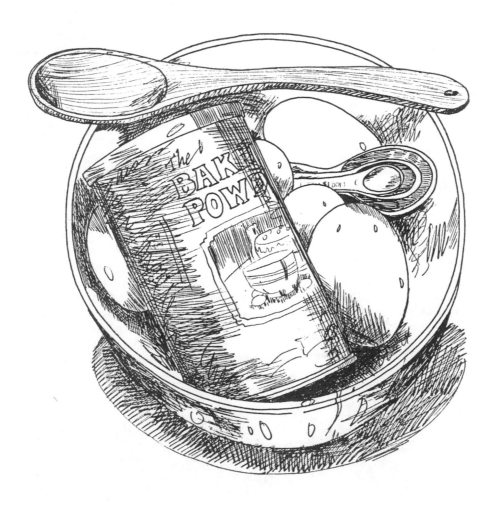

A Return to Real Bread

Let's suppose we want to bake a loaf of real "traditional" bread, the same as that which nourished our European ancestors. We gather the simplest and best ingredients: whole grain wheat and rye, pure water, sea salt, and the finest cake yeast available. We grind the grain into flour. We dissolve the yeast in warm water, and then blend that frothy mix with flour, making a dough. Dressed in medieval peasant garb and reciting our favorite Chaucerian verse, we knead the dough, let it rise, then knead it again. After allowing a final proofing, or rise, in baking pans, we bake it slowly in a wood-fired brick oven. The bread emerges golden brown, filling the house with its earthy and sweet aroma. Our ancestors smile benignly from their celestial posts, fluttering angelic wings in approval. We have faithfully recreated the staff of life, the nutritional cornerstone of Western civilization for centuries.

Right? Wrong! Despite our consummate care we have not made traditional bread at all. Rather we have produced something which, until the late 19th century, was completely unknown, which for years afterwards was outlawed by the French government, and which has been linked by modern researchers to anemia, rickets, intestinal problems, and even cancer. We have made only one error, but it is a crucial one. We have used the wrong leavening agent: baker's yeast.

The baking of bread goes back to the dawn of Western civilization. Archeological remains indicate that Stone Age residents of Europe were mixing crushed grains with water and cooking them on flat stones. These cakes were the forerunners of the unleavened flat breads still popular in northern Europe, and of the late but unlamented macrobiotic Ohsawa loaves of the 1960s.

The development of leavened bread is usually attributed to the Egyptians of around 2,300 B.C. They discovered that a mixture of flour and water, if left uncovered for several days, begins to bubble and swell, and that if this is mixed with fresh dough and allowed to stand for a few hours before baking it yields a light and sweet bread. The Egyptians learned also that a small quantity of raised dough removed before baking can replicate the process a few days later.

The phenomenon of leavening is based on several facts. One is that the air contains a variety of microorganisms, such as fungi and molds. Another is that when these alight on a proper host, and conditions of moisture and humidity are correct, they will initiate fermentation, the breaking down of complex carbohydrate molecules into simpler sugars or monosaccharides. This process, employing a "starter" culture and a sponge (see page 37), is the method of making traditional sourdough bread—light, sweet and sour, and totally digestible.

Natural leavening remained the basis of Western bread baking for 4,200 years, and bread remained the basis of the Western diet. In the Rome of the 2nd century B.C. there were large public bakeries, equipped with mechanical mixers and kneaders driven by animal power. Although much of the art of baking was lost during Europe's "Dark Ages" (5th through 13th centuries), by late medieval times, the baker was once again a highly trained and skilled craftsman. Before being admitted to the baker's guild he had to master the subtleties of the art during a long apprenticeship. This training was essential. Naturally leavened dough is a living thing, and to control it under varying conditions, to turn out a consistent product day after day, is a fine art.

In the middle of the last century a major change occurred. The work of scientists like Justus von Liebig (the founder of modern nutritional science) and Louis Pasteur led to the discovery and identification of the microorganisms that are responsible for the fermentation process. One of these, the single-celled yeast species *Saccharomyces cerevisiae*, was isolated and cultured. Used by itself it was found to cause a very rapid, uniform, and predictable raising of dough. Yeasted bread was born.

The initial advantage of this type of bread was mainly to the baker. Its proofing time was several hours shorter, which meant several hours more sleep. It was more predictable in its behavior and easier to work with.

Gradually, steadily, it displaced traditional, naturally leavened bread so that today, even in France, "the nation of bread," it is very difficult to find even white-flour naturally leavened bread. We have come to think of yeasted bread as the true bread of history. But no civilization has been nourished on it.

There are good reasons for considering a return to traditional bread. The most basic perhaps relates to taste. To the

The Back-to-Basics Goodness of Sprouted Breads

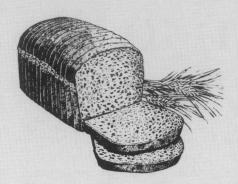

Sprouted breads take the back-to-basics philosophy of whole grain loaves one step further. In their most basic form, their principal—and only—ingredient is grain, usually wheat, sometimes rye. No added yeast, no salt, no fat, no dairy, no sweetener. This is a loaf of simplicity.

The bread is made by soaking whole kernels of grain in water until they sprout, usually within two to three days. The sprouted grain is ground and formed by hand into a round loaf. After a couple of hours of slow baking, the loaf emerges from the oven heavy, moist, chewy, thick crusted, and densely textured.

Germination sets off changes in the grain that give it several advantages over standard whole grain breads. Some of the starch in the kernel gets converted to sugars such as maltose; this eliminates the need for honey or refined sweeteners. Sprouting increases the grain's store of vitamins, minerals, and fiber. It also prolongs the bread's shelf life.

The absence of added ingredients makes sprouted loaves a natural for people who are sensitive to or would rather not eat yeast, dairy products, or other common bread constituents. Sprouted wheat bread is even enjoyed by some people who cannot otherwise tolerate wheat, according to Lifestream Natural Foods of Richmond, B.C., Canada, the company responsible for Essene, one of the most widely distributed sprouted breads.

Variations on the sprouted bread theme abound. Some bakers use yeast and add a little honey to create a lighter loaf, some add a variety of nuts, others toss in dried fruits. For home bakers intrepid enough to try their hand at a loaf, *The Laurel's Kitchen Bread Book* (Random House, 1984) offers easy-to-follow baking recipes and several baking tips, for example, the addition of 1/2 cup of dates to each pound of sprouted wheat.

---

lover of good bread there is nothing as delicious and satisfying as a piece of well-made, naturally leavened bread. It is moist and rich, with many layers of sweetness. Taken alone it is a meal in itself. Taken with soup, salad, and a good dark beer it is the substance of a wholesome feast.

According to a small group of anti-yeast activists here and in Europe, recent scientific research has uncovered other, health-related reasons for preferring the genuine bread of the past. Jacques de Langre of Magalia, California, who's been active in the natural foods movement for over twenty-five years, has been deeply interested in bread as the basis of a healthful diet for Western people. De Langre, citing many other researchers in his book, *Bread's Biological Transmutations* (Happiness Press, Magalia, CA), claims that naturally leavened bread is superior to yeasted bread. In his book he makes the following assertions regarding naturally leavened bread:

•It is more nutritious. The long proofing allows the fermenting agents to break down the cellulosic bran of the grain. This releases valuable minerals, which are dissolved into the rich, dark soup of the dough.

•It is easier to digest. The bread itself contains the lactobacillus, which is essential to the proper digestion of complex carbohydrates. This helps restore the functioning of the digestive tract, including the peristaltic action of the intestines, resulting in proper elimination.

•It is believed to be a cancer inhibitor. In yeast fermentation the starch cells of the bread actually explode. The patterns they form are identical to those of cancer cells. According to French researcher Jean Claude Vincent, the bioelectrical energy of the dough also is identical to that of cancer cells. In contrast, the starch cells of naturally leavened bread expand and swell like ripe fruit. In his book *Checkmate to Cancer*, the German researcher Dr. Johannes Kuhle asserts that yeasted bread is a cause of cancer and that naturally leavened bread is an inhibitor. Kuhle's work has been carried on by Dr. Max Wahren, of the Swiss Association of Master Bakers. Author of over thirty books on the subject, Wahren is a leader in the movement to promote traditional bread.

•Naturally leavened bread contains no deleterious phytic acid. This acid, known also as phytin, is a natural ingredient of wheat, and has been tied to anemia, rickets, and nervous disorders. According to the experiments of R. Hauspy of the Lima Factory in St. Maartens, Belgium, phytin can be neutralized by baking or by natural bacterial action. In naturally leavened bread the combination eliminates all phytin, while in yeasted bread about 90 percent remains.

•Finally, it remains fresh and edible much longer. Yeasted bread may lose its moisture within hours, becoming dry and stale. Sourdough bread holds its moisture tenaciously, and a well-formed loaf with a continuous crust will remain moist and impervious to mold for days, even weeks. According to Kuhle, the healthful properties of the bread reach their peak in five to ten days.

Many of de Langre's assertions are controversial and remain unproven. Nevertheless, it is a happy fact that in America as well as in Europe naturally leavened bread is indeed making a comeback.

Making Your Own Sourdough Starter

A number of "Alaskan" and "San Francisco style" sourdough starters are commercially available. Buy one once, give it loving care, and you'll always have it. If you can't find one of these, and your friends don't have family heirlooms they'll pass on to you, this recipe should get you—and your starter—started.

2 cups stone-ground whole wheat flour
2 cups spring water

It's important to start with whole wheat flour and, if at all possible, to grind your own. The extra freshness will produce a much better rising quality and flavor and will also have a bearing on the types of wild yeast spores attracted to the flour.

Place flour and water in a ceramic or glass bowl and stir with a wooden spoon to form a thick yet pourable batter. If necessary, add more flour and/or water to achieve this consistency.

Scrape down the sides of the bowl and cover with a clean dishtowel. Let the mixture sit at room temperature for two to five days, or until it smells slightly sour. Stir daily with a wooden spoon. Stir back in any liquid that forms on the top.

Transfer the mixture to a small crock or jar. Leave it uncovered at room temperature for one to three days, until a sweet flavor develops (during this time, skim off any dark or grey liquid that might form on top). Then cover the starter loosely and store it in the refrigerator. If the starter becomes thick, adjust it to the original consistency by adding a little flour and water.

Use your starter according to the directions of the sourdough recipe you are fol-

lowing. Many recipes call for a "sponge" to be made the night before. This is usually done by pouring the starter into a bowl, adding spring water and flour to it, and leaving it overnight. Clean the starter jar with hot water only and then refill it the next morning from the sponge, before you add salt or other ingredients to the sponge.

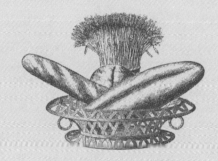

For pancakes, waffles, or quick breads, you can add about one-and-a-half teaspoons of finely sifted wood ash to the sponge before adding other ingredients. Besides providing valuable nutritional benefits, this alkaline ash neutralizes the acid formed by the sourdough fermentation: the gases given off by this reaction help to leaven the pancakes. Only clean, completely burned ash from vegetable

matter is satisfactory; make certain you don't use ash from burnt newspaper or trash. Sift the ash well to remove any lumps, foreign matter, and unburned charcoal.

If you do not use your starter very often, feed it with a little flour and spring water about once a week. If it becomes too sour, remove some from the jar and discard, then add fresh flour and water to the remaining starter. Allow to sit at room temperature for several hours before refrigerating. With a little care and regular use your starter can be kept going indefinitely—just like the precious, generations-old starters the early European settlers carried with them across the Atlantic and then across the continent. If your starter doesn't at first have as strong a leavening action as you would like, be patient. It will get better with continued use.

Another type of traditional leavening—known as *desem* in Belgium and *levain au naturel* in France—can be made by a more complex method with rewards well worth the effort. The method differs from the above "sourdough starter" in several ways: (1) the desem is a dough, not a batter; (2) it doesn't rely on the airborne yeasts and bacteria in your kitchen but on organisms and enzymes that naturally occur on and in organically grown wheat; (3) it is nursed to life not at room temperature, but between 50° and 65° F. Detailed instructions for making and using this traditional European leaven can be found in *The Laurel's Kitchen Bread Book* by Laurel Robertson with Carol Flinders and Bronwen Godfrey (Random House, 1984).

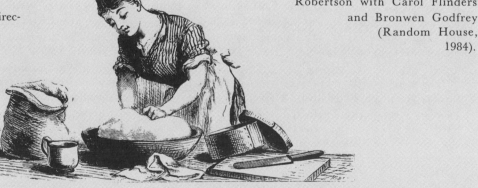

The Twists & Turns of Pasta

No doubt you've heard the story about Marco Polo introducing pasta to Italy upon returning from his expedition to China in the 13th century. This story, implying that spaghetti belongs more to Chinatown than to Little Italy, has had vermicelli scholars poring over the literature for years. The earliest reference to support this theory is an article entitled "A Saga of Cathay," which appeared in the October 1929 edition of the *Macaroni Journal*, an American pasta-industry trade publication. The anonymous article tells how Polo sent a sailor ashore in search of fresh water, and how, while on land, the sailor observed natives preparing long strands of dough. He brought some back to the ship, and Polo named them after the sailor, one Signor Spaghetti.

Considerably earlier evidence supports the theory that pasta in the Mediterranean region predated Polo's trip. Etruscan murals, circa 400 B.C., depict a floured table with rolling pins, knives, and a lasagna-cutting roller, all tools still found in Italian kitchens today, and used for the preparation of *pasta casalinga*, homemade pasta.

Marco Polo did convey in 1298 that he had observed Orientals eating "lasagne" made from breadfruit flour and that this flour was "used to make other things, just as we use wheat flour." Twenty years earlier a Genoese notary listed a chest of macaroni among the items of a soldier's estate. Flat pasta, now called *tagliatelle* by the Italians, has been known since the earliest centuries of the Christian era by various names deriving from the Latin *nodellus* (little knot, describing how the long strands get tangled up in little knots on the plate). These names include the French *nouilles*, the German *nudelin*, and of course the English *noodles*.

The evidence supports the existence of pasta, both in Cathay and in Italy, well before Marco Polo's time. Independent invention and subsequent dispersal seem more likely than that either culture learned to make noodles from the other. And it is also likely, in both China and Italy, that steamed and boiled dumplings preceded the more modern-style pasta.

The pasta available in natural foods stores today reflects both of these centers of development. Whole grain spaghetti, linguini, tagliatelle, lasagna, rotini (spirals), shells, cannelloni, elbows, and alphabets are all derived from Italian forebears. In the U.S. today, they are made primarily in factories established by Italian immigrants. In the Far East, noodle-making spread to Japan where, like many other transplants from the mainland, it has been further developed and uniquely adapted. Today's imported Japanese *soba, udon, somen,* and *ramen* are the culmination of centuries of adaptation.

There are two basic methods of making pasta: the extrusion method and the roll-and-cut method. Although some small, local pasta makers use rollers and cutters to make their fresh fettucine and tagliatelle, most domestic and imported European pasta is made by the extrusion process. Flour and water are mixed and continuously fed into the extruder, a machine that has a long "tunnel" with an auger running through it. The extruder resembles, in both form and function, a small meat grinder of the type used to make hash. As the auger turns, it kneads the flour and water into a dough and then forces the dough through a die plate at the end of the tunnel. The shapes of the holes in this plate determine the shape of the pasta. Pasta is formed into ribbons, cords, tubes, or special shapes, all originally developed for specific characteristics, such as the ability to retain heat, absorb liquid, or hold sauces. A rotating knife cuts the shaped pasta to the appropriate length. This moist pasta is hung on racks or spread on trays and transferred to a drying room before being packed for distribution.

Most commercial pasta is made from enriched semolina, a refined flour that is derived from the endosperm of durum wheat. Nevertheless, many natural foods stores offer a complete line of whole grain pasta, both domestic and Italian. The best is made from fresh, 100 percent whole wheat flour, milled from organically grown, hard amber durum wheat. Durum wheat contains a large proportion of gluten, which holds the dough together. Because type and quality of wheat, freshness of flour, handling during manufacture, and method of drying all affect the taste and texture of the finished product, different brands of whole wheat pasta may vary significantly. If what you've tried tasted bland or felt like strands of wet sawdust in your mouth, try another brand. Some are quite smooth, and, because they are made with freshly milled flour, can have a delicious, nutty taste.

The Japanese pasta sold in natural foods stores is, for the most part, made by the roll-and-cut method. First, a dough is made from flour, water, and (for most varieties) salt. This dough is kneaded in a machine that is very much like the ones used in American bakeries to make bread dough. The dough is allowed to sit or "rest" for several hours before being rolled into a long, thin, continuous sheet. This is done by passing it through a series of rollers (like those on an old-fashioned wringer washer) which gradually make it thinner and thinner. When the desired thinness is reached, the sheet of dough passes through a set of knives that cuts it into the proper width. The noodles are then hung on racks, dried, cut to length, and packed.

While Italian and domestic pasta is generally made from very hard durum wheat, most of the wheat flour in the best Japanese pasta is milled from varieties of soft white wheat. Because of the lower gluten content of soft white varieties, the more gentle rolling and cutting method is required to make good noodles. The addition of a small proportion (approximately one percent) of salt helps to strengthen the gluten and bind the dough. The soft white wheat also accounts for the lighter (as compared to domestic whole wheat pasta) color and the smooth, soft texture of many of the Japanese varieties.

The varieties of domestic and Italian whole grain pasta differ primarily from each other in shape, as virtually all of them are made from 100 percent whole wheat flour. Some specialty products may contain small amounts of rice, soy, or sesame flour, and even vegetable powder; but for the most part the ingredients remain the same for different varieties, whether they be tubes, elbows, spirals, shells, or letters.

Japanese noodles, on the other hand, vary little in form, but may be made from several combinations of ingredients. Varieties sold in natural foods stores fall into three general categories: those made primarily with wheat flour, those that include a portion of buckwheat flour, and precooked instant ramen, which are also called "Chinese-style" noodles.

Udon are thick, flat, wheat noodles, available in several combinations of whole wheat and sifted wheat flour. The label should state that the product is made from 100 percent whole wheat flour, 100 percent wheat sifted flour, or a combination of the two. *Tsuru udon* is made from 60 percent whole wheat flour and 40 percent sifted wheat flour. Brown rice udon is made from a combination of whole and sifted wheat flour with 25 percent brown rice flour added. *Somen* noodles are cut thinner than udon and cook more quickly. *Tsuru somen* is made with all sifted flour; whole wheat somen (sometimes called *hiya-mugi*, because it is a wheat—*mugi*—noodle that is usually served cold—*hiya*) is made entirely from unsifted whole wheat flour.

Soba, noodles made with buckwheat flour, are somewhat thinner than udon and square in cross-section. While some varieties are made entirely of buckwheat flour, those made with various combinations of buckwheat and sifted wheat flour are lighter and more popular. Soba in natural foods stores may contain as little as 40 percent buckwheat flour. *Ito soba* is a very thin variety made with 40 percent buckwheat flour and 60 percent sifted wheat. *Jinenjo soba* combines flour from the root of a Japanese mountain yam with buckwheat and wheat flours. *Yomogi soba* includes green mugwort powder for color, flavor, and nutritional enrichment. *Cha soba* contains green tea powder.

Ramen are the curly, precooked noodles that come packed in cellophane wraps, often accompanied by an envelope of instant soup base. The noodles themselves can be made from combinations of whole and sifted wheat flours, buckwheat flour, and brown rice flour. Ramen are made by a process similar to the one used for other Japanese pasta, except that before they are dried, the noodles are precooked with steam. The less expensive, mass-market versions are precooked by frying in oil.

Three other types of oriental noodles, all transparent, are sometimes available. *Seifun* or *bifun* are made from mung bean starch and are sometimes called "cellophane noodles" or "bean threads." *Maifun* are similar in appearance, and are made from rice. *Kuzu kiri* are made from kuzu powder (processed from the root of the wild kuzu, or "kudzu," plant) and potato starch.

Worth mentioning are two other rather unusual pasta products. One of these is made from 100 percent corn, containing no wheat at all. This pasta has an attractive yellow color, and requires careful cooking to prevent it from becoming too soft. If overcooked the pasta more closely resembles cornmeal mush than macaroni. The other product is made from a combination of refined durum wheat flour (semolina) and flour from the tubers of the Jerusalem artichoke.

Technically speaking, "noodles" must include eggs, "macaroni products" are made without eggs, and "pasta" and "alimentary paste" are all-inclusive terms. Virtually all commercially available egg noodles are made with whole egg powder, and certainly not the dark-yolked, fresh eggs you would choose if making noodles at home. In common usage, "noodles" and "pasta" are interchangeable words, and there is no need for us to change our vernacular to accommodate FDA labeling requirements.

Freshly made pasta should be refrigerated and used as soon as possible. Dry pasta can be stored indefinitely if kept in a cool, dry place.

Although pasta has long been unjustly maligned as a starchy, fattening food, it is now being recognized as a good source of complex carbohydrates. Whole grain pasta is a nourishing and wholesome food, as nutritious as the grains it is made from— high in fiber, rich in B vitamins, and a major source of complex carbohydrates. As the primary ingredient in a main course, or included in soup or salad, the variety of pastas available today in many natural foods stores offers real versatility for the cook. With cooking times from three to fifteen minutes, noodles lend convenience for those who want to eat a whole foods diet but find times when they're too busy to cook a pot of brown rice. But you don't have to be in a hurry to enjoy whole wheat-sesame spirals made into a pasta primavera or soba swimming in a steaming shoyu broth, topped with sizzling fried tofu and scallions.

Flour Power!

Cooking with seitan, a nutritious and low-fat food made from wheat, is an excellent way to reduce cholesterol, fat, and calories in your daily diet. Its full-bodied, hearty flavor and familiar texture remind many people of meat and thus it is also a very good food to use when making the transition to a meatless or less-meat diet. For the same reasons, seitan makes an exciting introduction or a satisfying addition to any natural foods diet.

Seitan has a relatively long history. Although not widely known in the West, it was traditionally eaten in China, Korea, Russia, and the Middle East. The name seitan, which means "gluten that has been cooked in soy sauce," comes to us from the Japanese, who have prepared it for several thousand years. However, only during the past ten to fifteen years has this method of preparing whole wheat been discovered by the natural foods movement in the U.S.

To make seitan, water is added to wheat flour. The mixture is then kneaded to a consistency similar to that of bread dough. The bran and starch are then repeatedly rinsed out of the dough, until only the gluten remains. Next, the gluten is simmered in a broth of natural soy sauce and water, with the addition of a few optional ingredients such as kombu sea vegetable or ginger root. Even though seitan is easy to prepare and highly nutritious, some people are reluctant to use it because it is a partially refined food. However, if it is made at home (see pages 41–43), the starch can be used in other recipes, and even the bran need not be thrown away.

Seitan was introduced to the U.S. natural foods industry about sixteen years ago when a Japanese variety, shrink-wrapped and dry and salty, was first imported. Nevertheless, there had been several other varieties of wheat gluten available from vegetarian groups, primarily the Seventh-day Adventists and the Mormons. In addition, Chinese restaurants in this country have been preparing wheat gluten for many years. The Chinese call it *mien ching*, or *yu mien ching*. (Chinese restaurants often refer to it as "Buddha food," claiming that it was developed by Buddhist monks as a meat substitute.) Dried wheat gluten, called *fu* by the Japanese and *k'ao fu* or *kofu* by the Chinese, is also available in Oriental food markets.

Within the past several years, there has been some success in getting seitan distributed to supermarkets, but the vast majority of all seitan commercially prepared is sold through natural foods stores and restaurants. Upcountry Seitan, a company in Lenox, Massachusetts, is the largest manufacturer we located in a recent survey of the industry. It makes 600 pounds each week and distributes through six states. The smallest enterprise we came across makes approximately 10 pounds and sells to only one store. Extrapolating from these figures, it appears that in the U.S. about 2,500 pounds of seitan are made commercially each week, or about 125,000 pounds per year. Although the seitan industry is still in its infancy, there may be more companies in the natural foods industry making seitan now than there were companies making tofu ten years ago, when *The Book of Tofu* by Bill Shurtleff and Akiko Aoyagi was published.

All the companies we contacted (with one exception) make their seitan from 100 percent organic whole wheat flour. There is some debate whether hard red winter or spring wheat is the best. The taste and texture of seitan depends upon such factors as well as upon the flour's freshness, how finely ground it is, the farm it comes from, and so forth. Nutrition will also be affected somewhat by these factors. However, the biggest difference among seitan makers that we discovered seems to be in the percentage of cooked gluten derived from the flour, which ranges from a low of 50 percent to a high of about 110 percent. (Absorption of water and soy sauce accounts for the possibility of getting more gluten than the original amount of flour.)

Shelf life for commercially prepared seitan ranges from two to three weeks, depending on the temperature and amount of salt used in the cooking. Among the makers we contacted, retail prices ranged from a low of $1.69 per half-pound to a high of $3.50 per half-pound. Although each company noted a dramatic increase in their sales over the past several years, it is unclear whether this is due more to an increased number of outlets for their product or to an increased demand in each outlet.

In addition to being an excellent source of protein, seitan is also relatively low in fat and calories and supplies some vitamins and minerals. The single potential nutritional drawback is the amount of sodium (from the soy sauce used to flavor and preserve it). Very few of the current seitan makers list any nutritional information at all on their packages, so sodium figures are hard to come by. Still, common sense says that if you're on a sodium-restricted diet, you should not eat seitan at every meal.

How to Make Seitan

When I first tasted seitan (pronounced say-tan), about sixteen years ago, I was fascinated by its flavor and texture. I had stopped eating meat for intellectual rather than sensory reasons, so the idea of using a grain-based product which had the texture of animal food was an appealing one. There were a few problems, however. The only seitan available at that time was expensive, and salty. And the pieces of seitan, as they came out of their jar from Japan, were tiny and hard. Perfect for beer-snacks, but not really useful for other purposes.

Some years later, a Japanese woman working at a natural foods restaurant in Boston taught me how to make seitan. That knowledge became a wonderful gift that has benefited many people, including my family. Consuming seitan as a regular staple has given us great varieties in taste as well as nutritional advantages.

CHOOSING THE FLOUR

Seitan is always, by definition, made from a high-gluten wheat flour, whether it be in the form of whole wheat flour, unbleached white flour, or extracted gluten flour (available in natural foods stores). These flours may be used alone or in combination, but seitan preparation follows the same general process regardless of the flour used.

The correct flour is essential to the success of your seitan-making experience. I have found that hard red winter wheat flour works well, but other cooks will recommend spring wheat flour. Whole wheat flours that are available in supermarkets are generally adequate. If you prefer an organic flour, request it from your natural foods store manager. Some stores stock a bulk "bread flour," which may be good for bread but for various reasons may not be appropriate for seitan.

I have had many experiences in which an entire batch of seitan has gone down the drain because the flour was not right. The safest thing to do is to buy one or two cups of many types of wheat flour (but don't bother with pastry flour—it has hardly any gluten at all), labeling each one to identify its type and place of purchase, and then try to make a sample batch of seitan

from each. The purpose of the experiment is to determine how well each one "sticks together" when cooked, and which will give you the smoothest texture. When you have determined which flour will yield the most firm and fine-grained gluten, as well as which gives you the largest quantity of gluten for the amount of flour used, make a note of it. This is an important preliminary for creating great seitan.

Preparation of the gluten for making seitan occurs in four phases: mixing the flour with water, kneading the flour and water into a dough similar to bread dough, resting the dough, and rinsing it to separate the starch and bran from the gluten. Most commonly, the gluten is cooked soon after its preparation, and this is what we call "seitan." I usually refer to the uncooked gluten as "uncooked seitan," to simplify things.

MAKING THE DOUGH BY HAND

When making the dough by hand, it is helpful to use a mixing bowl that is at least four inches taller than the size of the dough it is to contain, although it should fit into your kitchen sink for most efficient processing. I usually make double the amount of seitan listed below, and use a 12-quart stainless steel mixing bowl. This is adequate for a dough of 16 cups of flour and very comfortable for smaller amounts, but of course smaller bowls may be used. Do not use a wooden bowl as it could be damaged by the time it spends in the water.

To Make 2–2¹/₂ Cups Uncooked Seitan

4 cups whole wheat flour
4 cups unbleached white flour
3¹/₂–4 cups water

Mixing

1. Put all the flour for the batch of dough into the bowl, blending well with a fork prior to adding the water. Add the water one to two cups at a time, and mix well with a spoon after each addition. When all the water has been added, begin to mix the dough with one hand while holding the bowl steady with the other. If

you do this while the bowl is in the sink, additional water will be accessible (you can operate the faucet with your dry hand) in case you need to wet the mixing hand to prevent the sticky dough from accumulating on it.

Kneading

2. Knead with the "mixing" hand for 50 or 60 strokes with a motion which scoops up a generous handful of the dough from the bottom of the bowl and deposits it on top, so that it can then be pushed down firmly with the heel of the mixing hand or the backs of the fingers. Rotate the bowl a few inches between kneading strokes to achieve thorough mixing.

Resting

3. Let the dough rest for 20–30 minutes. If you have to leave for a more extended period of time, cover the dough with a damp cloth, as if leaving bread to rise. It is during this time that the gluten develops, so be sure to allow *at least 20 minutes*. If the gluten does not develop well, much of the dough will simply turn into batter and wash away in the next phase.

Rinsing

4. After the resting period, knead the dough again, with damp hands, for 20 or so strokes. You should be able to notice that the consistency of the dough, while still fairly soft, is much more dense than before.

5. It is during the rinsing that you will actually separate the gluten from the starch and bran. With the bowl containing the dough placed in the sink, run lukewarm water into the bowl at the edge of the mass of dough. Fill the bowl with water. Begin to manipulate the dough by lifting a section of it in both hands and compressing it gently but firmly between the palms of your hands. Repeat this about 15 times, then run more water slowly into the bowl. Repeat this squeezing motion under the stream of water, picking up a new double handful of dough every so often and compressing it under the running water. Turn off the water and continue to pick up

dough from the bottom of the bowl, squeezing it a few times between the palms. The water should now be very thick and white.

6.   Pour off water into a large measuring cup (the easiest way I know of to transfer it), and pour it from the measuring cup into a large glass jar (one gallon is good). Repeat the steps of filling the bowl with water, squeezing the dough thoroughly, and pouring off the milky "starch water." If you have extra jars, you can save up to 3–4 gallons of this starch water, which will, in about 2 hours' time, separate into layers (see note below). You may want to save only the starchy water from the first one or two bowlfuls. I recommend using a glass jar so you will be able to see the separation of the starch and bran from the main body of starch water.

Note: It will be useful to save at least half of the starch you have separated. Pour off the top clear liquid and refrigerate the thicker starch and bran that has settled to the bottom of the jar. Use the starch as a thickener for stews, soups, sauces, and desserts. This is referred to in the recipes as "Thick wheat starch from preparing seitan." (You can also save some of the top liquid to use as a base for the same dishes.)

7.   After two complete cycles of step 6, the dough should be treated much more vigorously. Continue to squeeze the dough under gently running water, but as you observe the developing gluten, which you can recognize by its stringy, elastic qualities, you can increase the strength of the water stream and the vigor of your squeezing, until you are really stretching and pulling the gluten in all possible directions. You may alternate water temperatures, as warmer water makes the gluten softer, more easily releasing the starch and bran. Cold water makes the gluten more dense and firm.

8.   When the gluten has formed a fairly solid mass, is all quite elastic and holding together well, and there are no longer any small loose pieces floating about, put it into a colander with large holes (not a mesh strainer) to finish the rinsing process. By this time, most of the saveable starch and bran have already been either saved or discarded. The final kneading is to remove any traces of starch that are still evident. Any remaining bran need not concern you, as it will not impair either the final taste or texture of the cooked seitan. Squeeze the seitan firmly,

Making Seitan Step by Step

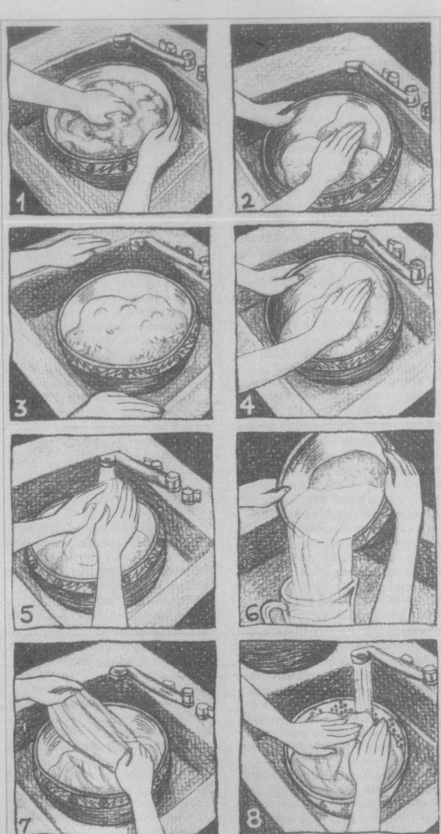

Illustration by Marilyn Cathcart

away from running water. Any water that comes out of it should be almost clear. If there is too much starch present in the finished seitan, it will have a sticky consistency when it is cooked.

When the rinsing has been completed, place the uncooked seitan in a bowl of cold water for 15 minutes to rest.

In spite of the length of these instructions, the total time for rinsing need not be more than 20 minutes for a double batch (5 cups of seitan), and possibly less for the amounts specified above, after you have practiced it once or twice. With good ingredients, a little patience, and a hearty spirit of adventure, you should have great success!

USING A FOOD PROCESSOR TO MAKE THE DOUGH

Some people prefer to prepare seitan dough in a food processor or another type of kneading machine rather than by hand. This is fine, and in fact will give excellent results. I have done both, but I find that it takes almost as long to clean the machine afterwards as it does to knead the dough by hand. If you do use a food processor, make the batch of seitan in two parts. Follow this recipe twice to make 2 cups of uncooked seitan.

To Make 1–1¼ Cups Uncooked Seitan

2 cups whole wheat flour
2 cups unbleached white flour
1¾–2 cups water

Put the flours into the bowl of the machine and turn it on and off once to mix them before adding the water. Add 1¾ cups of water and mix for about 1½ minutes. Stop the machine and push the dough down if needed. Add water up to 2 cups total (including what is already in the dough) and process for about 30 seconds more. Remove the dough from the processor and place it in a bowl, then proceed to step 3 (page 41).

Note: Amounts of water will vary according to the machines and flours used. The end result should be a smooth, elastic dough, not too firm and not too soft.

SEITAN RECIPES

Simmered Seitan Cutlets and Cubes

The most frequently used method for cooking seitan cutlets and cubes is to simmer the uncooked seitan slowly, in a broth flavored with natural soy sauce, kombu sea vegetable, and a variety of other seasonings which can be anything from fresh ginger root to an elaborate combination of spices.

The flavorings you choose will be determined by the effect you want to create. Although I am only presenting the most basic cooking method here, there is an extensive range of effects that can be created by various methods of cooking the "uncooked seitan." This is really the fun part of the cooking, where each cook can let his or her own personality and creativity shine.

2 cups uncooked seitan
4 cups water
3-inch strip kombu (for young children and others with salt and oil restrictions, prepare the seitan using only kombu as seasoning)
¼–½ cup natural soy sauce (in recipes calling for "mild natural soy sauce broth," use ¼ cup or less)
1 tablespoon sesame oil (omit oil if seitan is to be pan- or deep-fried)
4–6 ⅛-inch slices fresh ginger root (use ginger only if seitan will not be cooked with any other seasoning mix)

Place the water and kombu in a pot and bring to a boil. Remove the pot from the heat and add the natural soy sauce, oil, and ginger (or other specific seasonings required by the recipe). Allow the broth to stand for five minutes before adding seitan. During this rest period for the broth, prepare the seitan for cooking.

First, remove it from the water you have kept it in and place it on a slightly wet cutting surface. Roll it into a cylinder and let it rest for a moment. The shape will relax somewhat, but don't let it lose shape completely. If you are called away, put the seitan back into the water and when you return, squeeze it and begin again.

Slice the cylinder into 6 slices about ½ inch thick, or 10–12 slices ¼ inch thick. When cooked, these will almost double in thickness. Uncooked seitan may also be cubed before cooking, to be used in stews or skewered dishes, or other recipes calling for cubes. Pieces that are cut into cubes before cooking will have quite a different appearance than those cut into cubes afterwards.

Bring the broth to a boil, then reduce the heat and add the slices or cubes of seitan one by one, keeping them separated in the broth so they don't stick together. Partially cover the pot and simmer gently for one-half hour to 2 hours. The length of time required for cooking will depend upon the thickness and overall size of the pieces being cooked. Some very tiny pieces may only need to be simmered for 15 to 20 minutes. Make sure that the broth does not begin to boil; very few bubbles should be evident. Boiling the cutlets or cubes will result in a texture that is too spongy.

Stir the pieces occasionally by lifting and repositioning them to minimize breakage. After about 2 hours, most or all of the broth will be absorbed into the cutlet pieces. Save any remaining broth for flavoring gravies or other sauces or soups. Even when the pieces are well cooked, they may be fairly soft and tender; they are still fragile, so handle them carefully. They will become firmer as they cool. Cooling is best done by uncovering the pot and allowing the seitan pieces to remain in the broth until they cool to room temperature. In this way, they will be less delicate when removed.

Cover the cooked seitan and broth and store them in the refrigerator until you are ready to use them in a further recipe. If you can't wait, use the seitan in a sandwich with mustard and pickles or serve it plain as a side dish.

Watercress Salad with Crispy Seitan and White Mushrooms

Serves 6

This is one of my daughters' favorites—if you love watercress as much as we do, maybe you should double it.

½ cup uncooked seitan
oil for deep-frying
2 large or 3 small bunches watercress
½ pound white mushrooms, cut in ⅛-inch vertical slices
¼ cup creamy umeboshi dressing (below)

Cut the seitan into ¼-inch slices. Cut each of these slices into long, very thin strips. Deep-fry them until they are golden and crispy (they will puff up). Turn the strips to the other side as soon as the first side looks golden. Deep-fry three or four strips at a time.

Blot the strips on layers of paper towels. Then transfer them to a colander and pour boiling water over them to remove excess oil. Squeeze, and cut into 2-inch lengths.

Immerse the watercress in boiling water, one bunch at a time, for half a minute each. Remove and plunge into cold water. Squeeze firmly and cut each tightly packed bunch into 2-inch pieces.

Place the sliced mushrooms in a colander and pour boiling water over them. Wait half a minute, then pour cold water over them. Drain well.

Combine the vegetables and seitan, cover with dressing, and toss lightly. Both dressing and vegetables should be at room temperature for best results.

This salad may be prepared ahead of time. Do not add the dressing to the vegetables until just before serving.

Creamy Umeboshi Dressing

Makes 1 cup

2¹/2 tablespoons umeboshi paste
1 cup plain soymilk (see page 148)
4 teaspoons sesame or safflower oil
1 teaspoon brown rice vinegar

Thin the umeboshi paste by adding the soymilk to it, little by little. Mix well. Add the oil a little at a time while mixing with a fork or whisk. Add the rice vinegar and mix well. Refrigerate, and shake well before using.

Banana Dream Pudding

Makes 6¹/2 cups

Close your eyes and let yourself be transported to a tropical isle. . . .

4 cups boiling water
¹/3 cup unroasted almonds
3¹/2 cups clear starch water (top water from making seitan)
2–3 bananas
³/4 cup plain soymilk
pinch sea salt
1 teaspoon vanilla
¹/2 cup maple syrup
1 cup thick wheat starch from preparing seitan
¹/2 cup unsweetened shredded coconut

Blanch the almonds by parboiling them for 2 minutes in the boiling water, then drain them in a colander. Remove the skins by squeezing the wide end of each almond; the nut should slide through the skin at the pointed end. Put the almonds in a blender or food processor with 2¹/2 cups of the clear starch water and process until creamy. Place this mixture in a saucepan.

Note: The almonds may be prepared ahead of time. After blanching, place them on a screen, pastry-cooling rack, or other well-ventilated surface. Leave them in the open for one to four days, depending on the temperature and humidity. I put mine in the oven with only a pilot light on. They may be stored in a paper bag for future use.

Process the bananas and the soymilk in the blender together with the remaining cup of clear starch water. Add this mixture to the almond mixture in the saucepan.

Heat to medium, and add the salt, vanilla, and maple syrup. Mix the thick starch well so it is homogeneous and add it to the rest of the ingredients in the pot. Keep stirring until the entire sauce is thick and creamy. Simmer for 20 minutes, stirring frequently.

In a dry, heavy frying pan, toast the coconut until it is golden and very fragrant, stirring constantly and shaking the pan back and forth periodically. Use a low to medium heat.

Pour the pudding into individual serving bowls or cups, and sprinkle the toasted coconut over the top. Chill.

Banana Dream Pudding may also be used as a pie filling for individual single-shell pies.

Note: With exposure to air, the banana pudding may change color and become darker. This affects its appearance only and luckily the taste is as good as ever. Banana Dream Pudding will keep well when refrigerated, up to 3 days or more depending on the temperature of your refrigerator.

Cheap Eats

A cost analysis shows that 1¹/2 pounds of cooked seitan cost $1.28. This analysis comes from the following:

Cost of flour at $.48 per pound winter wheat

3 cups flour in one pound
$.16 per cup of flour
8 cups whole wheat flour costs $1.28
8 cups flour yields 2-2¹/2 cups gluten
2 cups gluten equals one pound

After cooking, this increases to approx. 1¹/2-1³/4 pounds seitan

For a total cost of $1.28, this cooked seitan (along with other dishes) can serve 4 to 6 people, each person getting a little over ¹/4 pound of seitan.

4. VEGETABLES

The word vegetable comes from the Latin *vegetare,* which means "to enliven"—the opposite of our modern connotations for "vegetating" as "a sinking into inanimate stupor." The ancient Romans knew that vegetables aren't dull, and the current interest in eating a wider variety of fresh vegetables indicates that we moderns are becoming aware of vegetables' attractions, too. With the federal government and virtually every nutritional expert recommending greater consumption of fresh vegetables for their high levels of vitamins, fiber, and other nutrients, and their low levels of calories, sugar, and fat, it is obvious that this is a food category of almost limitless appeal.

Our hesitation is giving vegetables their due often stems from a lack of familiarity with the different varieties. We rely on a very few to satisfy our needs, and too often these are canned or frozen. Yet the fresh vegetable display is the most beautiful in the store, combining many of the colors, shapes, textures, and tastes of nature. Cooking with fresh vegetables provides endless opportunities for creativity and satisfaction as each season offers its specialties to be prepared in countless ways.

To help you get to know a wider variety of nature's offerings, we have included a capsule summary of some fifty different vegetables, discussing their origin, season, selection, and nutritional value. We've provided a sidebar with general tips on selecting and storing vegetables. Finally, we discuss the many advantages, to both the individual consumer and the wider society, that come with supporting local, regional agriculture instead of agribusiness. We hope that as you learn to shop for vegetables with a more knowledgeable and discerning eye, you'll find that the closer you look, the more you will grow to love these gentle pillars of our daily lives.

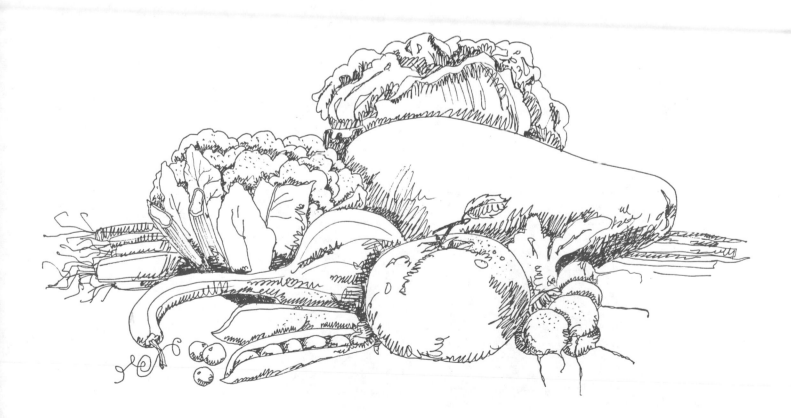

A Guide to Fresh Vegetables

The information in this section is intended to help you increase your familiarity with the more uncommon vegetables, as well as to highlight the old standbys. The best way to learn about vegetables, however, is to spend some unhurried time around the well-stocked produce section of a natural foods store. Look, examine, and choose vegetables that are appealing. Take your purchases home, store them in the appropriate manner to maintain optimum freshness, consult a cookbook or two, and then prepare your selections with confidence. After that, congratulations—you have now joined the ranks of those connoisseurs who enjoy the greatest cuisines of the world, all of which treasure the priceless simplicity and goodness of fresh vegetables.

Botanically, vegetables can be divided into the following categories:

* Root (rutabaga)
* Tuber (potato)
* Bulb (onion, garlic)
* Leaf and Leafstalk (cabbage, celery)
* Flower (broccoli, cauliflower)
* Bud (Brussels sprout)
* Stem (asparagus, kohlrabi)
* Fruit (cucumber, bean, squash).

In this shopper's guide, we have grouped them into three categories, according to similar characteristics: root, tuber, and bulb; leaf and leafstalk, flower, bud, and stem; and fruit (vegetables that contain seeds). Mushrooms and bean sprouts appear at the end.

Although we recommend buying from local or regional growers whenever possible (in the summer, farmer's markets and roadside stands make it easy to do so), this is not always possible. Therefore we have included information on each vegetable's "origin"—where the greatest quantity is grown to be shipped to other areas of the United States. The place of origin is often California, Texas, or Florida.

The term "season" refers to the extended growing season of the place of origin. Local seasons will vary considerably depending on altitude and latitude, weather, climate, and so forth. Your state's land grant college, your county cooperative extension office, or your urban gardening group or market coordinator can give you guidelines for choosing vegetables that will be at their peak at any given time. Each state compiles this information, which can be had for the asking. Selection and storage hints are given for each vegetable, as well as nutritional information.

Root, Tuber, and Bulb Vegetables

In most instances it is better to buy roots that have their leaves attached, as this indicates freshness. Droopy leaves do not mean the root is spoiled. However, if root vegetables spend more than a couple of days between harvest and use, a loss of moisture and crispness will result if the leaves remain attached; they draw nutrients as well as water up from the roots.

Beets

Origin: Most commercial beets come from California, New Jersey, Ohio, and Texas.

Season: Beet roots are available year-round, the leaves from March to October. The peak of the season is from June to October.

Selection: The roots should be well shaped and firm, and possess a deep color. Smaller beets are likely to be more tender. Avoid spotted, scaly, or soft roots. When the leaves are sold separately from the root, buy those that are thin-ribbed; they are more tender.

Storage: If the leaves are intact, cut them off and use them as soon as possible. The roots will keep in the refrigerator wrapped in plastic for about three weeks, or in a root cellar for several months.

Nutrition: The roots contain vitamins A and C; the leaves, vitamins A and C, and calcium.

Burdock

Origin: Most commercial burdock is grown in California. Burdock grows wild in almost every state and can be dug up and eaten (consult a book about wild food foraging for details).

Season: Burdock is available year-round. The peak season for cultivated burdock is in the fall.

Selection: The root, which is generally long, thin, and dark, should be firm. It is best to avoid dried-up roots, although they can still be used. Burdock covered with soil keeps better than cleaned burdock. The smaller roots, up to one inch in diameter, are more tender. Large roots may be woody. The leaves are too bitter to be edible and are not sold in natural foods stores.

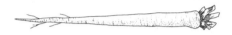

Storage: If placing burdock in the refrigerator, it is best to wrap it in a damp cloth. It will keep this way for several weeks provided the cloth is redampened occasionally. For longer storage wrap in newspaper, then plastic, and keep in a cool place.

Nutrition: Respected as a blood purifier and intestinal tonic, burdock supplies many minerals.

Carrots

Origin: Most commercial carrots are from California, Texas, Michigan, and Canada.

Season: Carrots are available all year.

Selection: Carrots should be relatively smooth and have a good orange color. Attached greens indicate freshness; they too may be eaten, although not everyone enjoys their bitter taste. Tiny carrots, of a mature dwarf or immature average-size variety, can be very sweet and tender, though in general size is not an indication of flavor. Rough, cracked, or pale carrots often lack sweetness. A green color at the top indicates sunburn and a bitter flavor. Avoid flabby, shriveled, and cracked roots. Also avoid carrots with over-the-hill greens, and trimmed carrots that are sprouting.

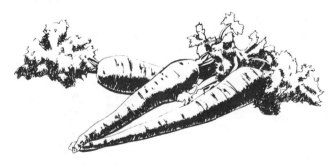

Storage: Cut greens off and use them, if desired, immediately. Store roots in the refrigerator in plastic at about 32° F and at high humidity (they will keep in a root cellar for months).

Nutrition: Carrots are very high in vitamin A.

Celeriac

Origin: Celeriac is a member of the celery family. Also called "turnip-rooted celery," it yields a large, roundish, turnip-like swelling, two to four inches wide, which has the odor typical of celery due to a volatile oil. Celeriac is very popular in continental Europe but not so much in England or the U.S. Commercial celeriac comes from California. In many areas, celeriac is also locally grown.

Season: Celeriac is available from September to April.

Selection: Celeriac roots should be firm. Press the top of the root as a check for internal rot, and avoid mushy roots. The smaller ones are usually more tender than the larger ones. Celeriac roots are usually boiled and eaten in salads or as a separate vegetable. The stems are not ordinarily eaten, being too bitter.

Storage: If wrapped in plastic and kept near freezing, celeriac should last up to seven days. In a root cellar, long-term storage is possible.

Nutrition: Celeriac contains phosphorus and potassium.

Daikon

Origin: Most commercial daikon is grown in California.

Season: Daikon is available year-round with peak availability from June to October.

Selection: Daikon, a white radish, is available in several varieties, the two most common being a tapered variety and a blunt-ended one. Both types should be firm. Ivory white color is desirable, as are smaller roots, for they are seldom woody. Daikon sometimes is sold with the leaves, which is a sign of freshness. The leaves are edible as well and should be a vibrant light green.

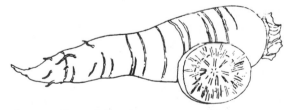

Storage: Store daikon in plastic and keep cold. If greens are attached, cut them off and use them as soon as possible.

Nutrition: The radishes contain vitamin C, calcium, potassium and phosphorus and have diuretic properties. The leaves have vitamin A and are high in many minerals. They aid in cleansing the blood of impurities.

Garlic

Origin: California fills most of the U.S. demand for garlic; the rest is imported from Mexico, Italy, Spain, and Peru.

Season: Garlic bulbs are available year-round.

Selection: Buy garlic loose, not prepacked. The bulbs should be firm, the skins unbroken. Avoid bulbs with green shoots emerging from the crown: they have been stored too long under poor conditions.

Storage: Keep garlic separate from other foods to prevent its odor from affecting them. Garlic can be stored at cool room temperature indefinitely, in a dry, well-ventilated place.

Nutrition: Garlic is a minor source of nutrients, but has strong bactericidal properties.

Ginger

Origin: Almost all ginger found in the United States comes from Hawaii.

Season: Fresh ginger is available year-round, although it is not sold everywhere.

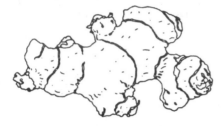

Selection: Buy ginger that is firm and plump for the best flavor. Small, greenish knobs growing from the main portion of the beige root are new growth and possess a milder flavor. There is no need to discard them. Avoid overly dried-out roots and those with moldy or discolored ends.

Storage: If kept in a cold and humid environment, ginger root will keep for several months.

Nutrition: Besides stimulating blood circulation, ginger is also a good source of minerals, most notably calcium, phosphorus, iron, and potassium. Made into tea, ginger is soothing to an unsettled stomach.

Jerusalem Artichokes

Origin: ''Jerusalem artichoke'' is the name given to the stem tubers of a plant which, despite its name, is closely related to the sunflower, a native of North America. ''Jerusalem'' is probably a corruption of *girasole,* the Italian word for sunflower. Also known as ''sunchoke,'' this plant was cultivated by Native Americans before the first Europeans arrived.

   The sweet taste of this vegetable is derived from inulin, a polysaccharide consisting of residues of fructose. Since inulin does not affect the blood sugar level, Jerusalem artichokes have been recommended for diabetics.

   Jerusalem artichokes are prepared in the same ways as the common potato—boiled, fried, or cooked in soups.

They can also be enjoyed raw in salads, having a crunchy sweetness reminiscent of carrots.

Season: Jerusalem artichokes are usually planted in the early spring and harvested in the fall or winter. They can also be left in the ground through the winter and harvested early the following spring. They store well and are available almost year-round.

Selection: Choose large, plump, crisp tubers, free of cuts and bruises.

Storage: Keep Jerusalem artichokes in the crisper of the refrigerator, where they should stay in prime condition for a week or longer.

Nutrition: Jerusalem artichokes contain vitamin A and B complex vitamins, plus iron, calcium, and magnesium.

Leeks

Origin: The leek is a subtle and sweet-tasting member of the lily family, to which onions also belong. Most commercial leeks come from California.

Season: Leeks can be found all year. The main season is from September to April.

Selection: Leeks are banked with soil for blanching and thus are white two to three inches up from the base. They are almost always sandy and must be well cleaned before use. The leaves should be tightly rolled and the tops fresh. Size is not an important factor. Avoid yellow or slimy leeks, and those that have been excessively trimmed.

Storage: Wrap leeks to avoid transfer of odor to other vegetables and store in the crisper of the refrigerator, where they will keep for three days or more.

Nutrition: Leeks contain calcium, phosphorus, and vitamins A, E, and C.

Lotus Root

Origin: Nearly all lotus comes from the Orient or Hawaii. Native Americans in the Northeast ate the seeds and roots of the American water lily, which is a close relative of lotus and can be found growing wild in many parts of the country.

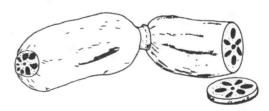

Season: Lotus root is available most of the year but is difficult to find. The peak season is late summer and fall.

Selection: Lotus root is strung together in approximately six-inch oblong segments of an ivory or brown color. When cut crosswise, hollow spaces are revealed, giving the section the appearance of a snowflake. Lotus root is rarely found with leaves or stems attached. The root should be two to nine inches long, and crisp enough so that it can be punctured easily by a thumbnail. Avoid bruised, rotten, or soft roots.

Storage: Store lotus in a cool and dry place.

Nutrition: Lotus root is not particularly high in any vitamins or minerals.

Onions, Shallots, Chives

Origin and Varieties: Onions, shallots, and chives, together with leeks (page 48), scallions (page 51), and garlic (page 48), are members of the lily family, often referred to as "kitchen lilies." There are nearly a dozen varieties of onion sold in the U.S. The main suppliers of commercial onions (including shallots and chives) are Texas, New York, and California. Following are the main available types and their best uses:

•*Pearl* onions are a tiny variety, usually white but sometimes yellow or red; good for boiling, pickling, braising, and creaming.

•*Yellow* onions are usually medium-sized and are the most versatile for cooking.

•*Spanish* onions are large, round, and yellow; they are mild and sweet, qualities that make them well-suited for slicing and eating raw.

•*White* onions come in a variety of shapes, sizes, and tastes. The small ones are often called boiling onions; the large, sweet, mild ones, sometimes called Bermuda, are good eaten raw.

•*Red* onions also vary in size, shape, and taste. The large mild ones are also often called Bermuda or, sometimes, Italian. Mild red onions are suitable raw.

•*Shallots,* the beautiful aristocrats of the onion family, grow in cloves, usually in twos, which are not connected by a thin skin as is garlic. Many traditional French recipes require shallots, and they can be used whenever onions are called for.

•*Chives* should be fresh and green; because their flavor and texture are so delicate, they are not usually cooked.

Season: Onions are available all year. The peak for Spanish onions is from September to April. The large red or white varieties, both often called Bermudas, peak from March to June. Shallots are less available during the summer months than at other times during the year. Domestic chives are rarely available commerically, but the heartier Chinese variety is often found in Oriental markets.

Selection: Purchase firm onions that are heavy for their size and that exhibit no sprouting. The outer skins should be like dry paper and have an even color. Shallots range in color from greyish- to reddish-brown, and should be plump, firm, and heavy. Avoid softness, mold, and sprouting. (If they start to sprout at home, snip the sprouts and

use them like chives.) Many people think that the smaller shallots are better-tasting. Avoid buying chives that are yellowed or wilting.

Storage: Keep onions and shallots in a cool, dry, and well-ventilated place. Do not refrigerate them. The smaller, firm, pungent types of onions will keep for months. The larger, milder types do not store as well. Shallots are somewhere between the two. Fresh chives can be wrapped in damp paper and stored in the refrigerator for a day. Better yet, grow your own in a pot on a sunny windowsill, and snip when needed.

Nutrition: The onion family is a good source of vitamin C.

Parsnips

Origin: Canada and Maine are the main parsnip suppliers.

Season: Parsnips are available year-round, with a peak from September to May.

Selection: It is best to buy parsnips in the late fall and winter after the frost has improved their flavor. Buy small-to medium-sized roots, unwilted, for best texture and flavor. The roots should also be heavy for their size and free from bruises. If possible, buy organically grown parsnips. Nonorganic parsnips are heavily treated with chemicals.

Storage: Parsnips will keep in the refrigerator up to three weeks; longer, if in a root cellar.

Nutrition: Parsnips are a source of vitamin A and minerals.

Potatoes

Origin and Varieties: California, Maine, and Idaho are the most productive potato-growing states. Though many varieties are available, five main types, classified by their shape and skin color, are sold in the United States: long whites, round whites, reds, long russets, and round russets. (Russets are characterized by a brownish, rough, scaly, or netted skin.) New round white, or early potatoes, are harvested when immature.

Season: Most potatoes are harvested in the fall and stored for year-round availability. New potatoes are harvested in the spring and are available in spring and summer.

Selection: Whatever the type, the tuber should be firm, heavy for its size, unwrinkled, and well-shaped. All potatoes should be free of large cuts, cracks, bruises, skinned areas, decay, and internal discoloration. New potatoes should have thin, glossy skin.

"Greening" is the result of chlorophyll formation, which occurs when potatoes are exposed to light. Since the green portions contain solanin, an alkaloid substance that

How to Select and Store Fresh Vegetables

When you shop for vegetables, one thing to be aware of is that *high density* is a desirable trait. It is usually a sign of maturity, freshness, and flavor. The lettuce, squash, or turnip you choose should feel heavy for its size. When you buy roots, choose firm ones. Rubbery, flexible carrots are past their peak of freshness. The same is true of fruit vegetables—they should be firm and their outer shells hard. As they age, soft spots develop in places where they have been bumped or bruised. Always look for a generally solid appearance and a vibrant color in leaf and leafstalk vegetables. Mustard greens, for instance, may be yellowish-green or green depending upon the variety, but the color in either case should be vibrant, the leaf crisp, and the appearance distinct. Feathery leafy greens should be especially crisp. Limpness in their case means loss of flavor and nutrition.

Storage at home is extremely important in preserving the vitality of vegetables. The first rule of home keeping is not to wash produce until you are ready to use it. Washing speeds up decay and is an invitation for mold to set in. The second rule is to plan your shopping so that you avoid long-term home storage—unless you know what you are doing and are equipped to do it. A home refrigerator does not provide the proper temperature or humidity for storage longer than a couple of days. Most refrigerators have a humidity of 40–50 percent. A crisper tray is somewhat helpful, because within its confines the humidity is raised above the level of the rest of the refrigerator, and the temperature is lowered by 3° F—to a point nearly adequate for most produce. But stuffing the crisper defeats its purpose. For the best results, buy vegetables for consumption within a day or two of purchase. In general, for refrigerator storage, roots should be wrapped in plastic and kept at temperatures close to freezing. All green leafy vegetables—from the most fragile lettuce to the hardiest cabbage—need to be kept near freezing and at high humidity.

Many vegetables, especially roots, can be kept unrefrigerated for months at a time during the colder seasons. This is useful if you buy large quantities of local produce at harvest time, or would like to. A root cellar, of course, is ideal for storage, but root-cellar conditions can be simulated by a cold room, as long as temperatures do not go below freezing. Materials such as sand or hay—dried or moistened to the right humidity—surround and separate the vegetables which are arranged in layers. Crates, plastic tubs, and even cardboard boxes can be used as containers.

An awareness of the best ways to select and store fresh vegetables will help you to derive the maximum nutrition and enjoyment from them. These simple guidelines may be summarized as follows: buy vegetables that are firm or crisp, vibrantly colored, and heavy for their size; avoid washing them until just before you use them; and avoid buying more than you will use in a few days unless you have a root cellar or a cool, humid storage area where you can arrange the vegetables without crowding them.

---

can be toxic, it is advisable not to buy any potatoes with green color. The green portion can be cut out, but the discoloration may be too extensive.

Potatoes with sprouts also contain solanin. Commercially grown potatoes are usually sprayed with sprouting inhibitors when they are packaged, and experimentation is underway using gamma rays for the same purpose. Nevertheless, if your potatoes have sprouts, cut them out, and use the rest of the potato (if it is firm).

Red potatoes are sometimes dyed and waxed to enhance their beauty, and legally this must be clearly marked. Some russet and white potatoes are clear-waxed as well. Although waxes are considered safe by the federal government, natural foods shoppers often choose to avoid buying waxed produce.

The specific gravity or relative density of the tuber indicates its best use. A potato with a higher specific gravity is more mealy and suitable for baking; one with a lower specific gravity is better for boiling. Since the specific gravity of potatoes is not labeled, most people go by the variety's reputation or consult their produce manager as to its best use. As a general rule, Idahoes, a russet type, are ideal for baking and mashing; new potatoes make the best salad.

Storage: Store potatoes in a dry, dark, well-ventilated, and cool (45–50° F) area. Do not store these tubers in the refrigerator as the low temperature will change the starch into sugar. To prevent greening, do not expose them to light. Potatoes will keep for several weeks at room temperature or from four to six months in a root cellar.

Nutrition: Potatoes contain vitamins as well as iron and phosphorus.

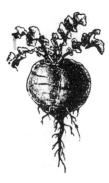

Radishes

Origin: California and Florida are the main radish

suppliers in the United States.

Season and Varieties: There are at least half a dozen varieties of radishes, and they can be loosely classified as either summer or winter radishes. Summer radishes, such as round white, round red, and icicle varieties, are smaller and more perishable than winter radishes. The common, cherry-sized round reds are the most popular radishes in the United States. Summer radishes are most available in late spring, though they can be found almost any time.

Winter radishes, such as Chinese, black, and daikon radishes, are bigger, although like summer radishes they may be either round or elongated. Chinese radishes are turnip-shaped and relatively mild in taste. Black radishes, an uncommon variety, are small but have a strong, pungent flavor. Daikon (see page 47) are a white, elongated Japanese variety that may grow over a foot in length.

Selection: The round red radish is usually sold topped and packaged, but it is generally fresher in bunches with the tops still attached. The leaves are edible, too. Buy all varieties of radishes firm, crisp, and small. Avoid those that are spongy or sprouting or that have black spots or cracks.

Storage: Radishes will keep in the refrigerator up to one week, sometimes longer.

Nutrition: Vitamin C, potassium, and magnesium are found abundantly in radishes.

Rutabagas

Origin: The rutabaga, a plant native to Eurasia, has a thick, bulbous root used as food. It is also called "Swedish turnip" and "swede." The vast majority of rutabagas on the market in North America come from Canada. Maine is the leading U.S. producer.

Season: Rutabagas are available starting in mid fall and throughout the winter.

Selection: These roots should be firm, solid, and heavy for their size. Avoid those that are waxed.

Storage: Rutabagas will keep in the refrigerator or in a cool room for up to one month, or in a root cellar for longer periods.

Nutrition: Rutabagas supply vitamins A and C, along with potassium, magnesium, and other minerals.

Scallions

Origin: Scallions, also called green or spring onions, are the immature plants of white onions pulled before bulb formation and sold in bunches. They can also (rarely) be young shallots. Florida and Texas supply most of the scallions on the U.S. market.

Season: Scallions are available year-round.

Selection: Scallions should possess a bright green color and appear fresh and tender. Avoid yellowed or slimy scallions.

Storage: Store scallions unwrapped in the refrigerator, or, like onions, in a cool, dry place. The tops will start to dry in a week or two; cut off the dry part and use the rest.

Nutrition: Minor.

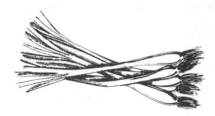

Taro

Origin: Also known as dasheen, taro is thought to have originated in China. Most U.S. taro comes from Hawaii. Taro should always be thoroughly cooked before eating.

Season: Taro is available year-round.

Selection: Choose taro that is plump and firm. Avoid softness, shriveling, and mold.

Storage: Store taro in a root cellar or in the refrigerator. Do not wrap it tightly.

Nutrition: Taro supplies calcium, phosphorus, iron, potassium, and vitamin A.

Turnips

Origin: Most commercially available turnips come from Canada and California. Both the leaves and roots are edible.

Season: Turnip roots are available all year with the peak harvest from September to March. Turnip greens are available from March to September.

Selection: As for all roots, look for turnips that are firm and heavy for their size. Reject coarse or very large roots. The leaves, if bought separately, should be unwilted, unspotted, and of a vibrant medium-green color.

Storage: Turnip greens will keep in the refrigerator for several days at 32° F, but it is best to use them as soon as you can. The roots should be stored separately from the greens. They will keep in a cool place for about one week, or in a root cellar for longer periods of time.

Nutrition: Turnips are a good source of vitamins and minerals. The leaves are an excellent source of vitamins A and C.

Leaf and Leafstalk, Flower, Bud, and Stem Vegetables

This group includes some of the most common and popular vegetables—broccoli, celery, lettuce, and spinach—as well as such overlooked but tasty ones as dandelions and watercress. Leafy vegetables in particular are among the most nutritious foods known.

Artichokes

Origin: California is the main U.S. supplier of artichokes.

Season: Artichokes are available year-round, with a peak in the spring.

Selection: Look for fresh green leaves and stems, and leaves that are closed tightly together, not spreading. Avoid blackening and softness or flabbiness. In winter, black tips may indicate frost damage, but this does not affect the rest of the artichoke.

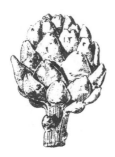

Storage: Refrigerate for a few days at high humidity.

Nutrition: Artichokes supply calcium, phosphorus, sodium, and potassium.

Asparagus

Origin: California, New Jersey, Washington, and Michigan are the chief asparagus suppliers.

Season: Asparagus season is from March to June, with a peak from April to June.

Selection: The color of this stem vegetable may be green or white. The tips should be closed and the stalk firm and compact. Asparagus that has open tips or is wilted is bound to be stringy. Angular or flat stalks denote woodiness; the smaller stalks are usually tastier. Avoid asparagus that has been sitting in water or has moldy or rotten tips.

Storage: When you store asparagus, the temperature should be below 40° F. Either the butt-end should be kept damp or the entire stalk placed in plastic. If the stalk goes limp, you can cut a piece from the bottom on the diagonal and stand the asparagus upright in water.

Nutrition: Asparagus contains vitamins A and C and iron (white asparagus has much less vitamin A).

Beet Greens

See Beets.

Broccoli

Origin: Botanically, broccoli is a member of the prolific *Brassica* genus, whose members include cabbage, cauliflower, kale, collards, turnips, rutabagas, Brussels sprouts, and Chinese cabbage. Most commercial broccoli comes from California.

Season: Broccoli is available year-round. The shortest supply is in July and August, the peak from October to April.

Selection: Broccoli's stalk and flower cluster are both eaten (the leaves are somewhat bitter). Clusters should be compact; the buds should be closed. The bud clusters can be dark green or purplish-green, depending on the variety. Avoid broccoli that has yellowed or wilted leaves or whose buds have opened and show tiny yellow flowers. The size of the head is not related to eating quality but wide stalks are often woody. Check the bottom of the stalks to make certain they are solid throughout.

Storage: Broccoli will remain fresh for up to a week in the refrigerator. Store it at around 32° F and at high humidity. To help retain moisture, wrap it in plastic.

Nutrition: Broccoli is a good source of vitamins A and C, and also contains riboflavin, iron, and calcium.

Brussels Sprouts

Origin: California, New York, and Oregon grow Brussels sprouts, but California produces more than all the other states combined.

Season: Brussels sprouts favor cool weather, and though they are available year-round, the best ones are harvested from October to February.

Selection: Look for small, compact sprouts that have a bright green color. Puffiness indicates a bland flavor. Wilted and yellow leaves mean ''over-the-hill'' produce.

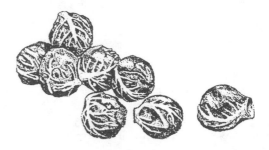

Storage: Do not wash sprouts until you are ready to use them. Remove any yellow leaves before storing. Brussels sprouts will keep for only a couple of days in most refrigerators at 32° F and 90 percent humidity.

Nutrition: Brussels sprouts are a good source of vitamins A and C, plus iron.

Cabbage

Origin: In the United States, Florida, Texas, California, New York, and New Jersey are the main suppliers of cabbage.

Season: The supply of cabbage is constant throughout the year.

Selection: "Food of the poor," cabbage yields more tonnage of crop per unit of land than any other vegetable. Try to find cabbages that have their coarse outer leaves in place, as this is a mark of freshness. Firm heads of cabbage, heavy for their size, are desirable. Avoid cabbages that have yellowing leaves or split heads, or are soft or flabby. Savoy cabbage is a winter variety with distinctive crimpled leaves. It forms a unique soft head whose inner leaves are particularly sweet and tender. Purple or red cabbages are similar to the more commonly available white and green varieties.

Storage: Cabbage does not fare well in dry storage as it will rapidly lose moisture, but it does well in root cellars. Keep at high humidity.

Nutrition: Cabbage is an excellent source of vitamins C and A and a good source of many minerals.

Cabbages, Chinese

Origin: The name Chinese cabbage is applied to three different vegetables—each of which also carries a slew of other names. For simplicity's sake we will call them nappa, green Chinese cabbage, and bok choy. California supplies most of the commercial crop.

Season: Not every store stocks these vegetables so they may be difficult to find regardless of season. Available year-round, they are most plentiful in summer and fall.

Selection: Nappa forms a tightly curled, oblong head. The outer leaves are usually white in the midrib and green along the edges. The inner leaves are white throughout. Green Chinese cabbage is more slender, similar to romaine lettuce, with a white midrib and green outer section. It is not as succulent as nappa nor is its flavor as mild. Bok choy, also known as Chinese celery, celery cabbage, and pak choy, has a thick white central stem that appears to be a stalk; the leaves on either side are dark green oval lobes. All three of these varieties should be as fresh as any other green. Ask the produce person to remove any outer leaves that are wilted or have brown speckles.

Storage: Chinese cabbages all keep well under refrigeration. Nappa and bok choy also do well in a root cellar.

Nutrition: All three types of Chinese cabbage are excellent sources of vitamins A and C and many minerals, including calcium.

Cauliflower

Origin: California and New York are the main suppliers of cauliflower.

Season: The cauliflower supply is fairly constant with a slight peak during the fall and a dip during summer.

Selection: The edible portion of the cauliflower is called the curd. It should be tightly clustered into a rounded mass as well as clean, firm, and of a white to creamy white color. If it is wearing a collar of outer leaves, these too should be green and firm. Size is irrelevant to quality; compactness and purity of color are better indicators. Avoid cauliflower that has open flower clusters, spotted curds (a sign of bruising), or a hollow core. Before buying cauliflower, turn it upside down and spot-check to make sure the stalk is solid.

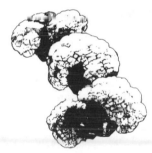

Storage: Store cauliflower in the refrigerator at around 32° F and at high humidity.

Nutrition: Cauliflower is a fair source of vitamins and minerals.

Celery

Origin: In the United States, California, Florida, Michigan, and New York are the main celery growers. Pascal celery, which is green in color, is the dominant variety on the market. Golden heart, a white variety, is seldom available.

Season: The supply of celery on the market is constant.

Selection: The leafstalk should be fresh and have a shiny luster. The stalks should be crisp and snap easily; avoid rubbery stalks. Thick stalks are often stringy.

Storage: Wrap celery in plastic and store it in the refrigerator, as you would a green leafy vegetable. Break off stalks only when you are ready to use them.

Nutrition: Celery contains vitamins A and B and minerals.

Chicory

Origin and Varieties: The chicories include green chicory, Belgian endive or witloof, and red chicory, or radicchio. All have a slightly bitter flavor and make fine salad ingredients. Chicory is closely related to endive.

Green chicory is more common in Europe than in the U.S. Some varieties are grown for their large roots, which are ground and added to coffee. Belgian endive or witloof is grown mainly in Belgium, although Canada produces some for the Western Hemisphere.

Season: Green chicory is rarely available, except for the variety called Catalonian, which is sometimes sold as dandelion greens, especially in the winter. Belgian endive can be found throughout the year, though it may be in short supply in the summer.

Selection: Green chicory, which resembles dandelion greens, should be fresh, crisp, and green. Avoid purchasing chicory with wilted leaves or rotting stems. Belgian endive, which looks like a tightly wrapped stalk rather than a leafy head, is grown in the dark to ensure its whiteness. As this whiteness accounts for its delicate flavor and high price, avoid green or brown Belgian endive. Loosely headed Belgian endive is also to be avoided. Radicchio, which is red and white, can be either round or long. Select crisp, fresh radicchio, with no browning or wilting.

Storage: Green chicory should be stored in the refrigerator at high humidity, like dandelion greens. Ideally, Belgian endive should be kept in its wrapping or wrapped in opaque paper to prevent greening. This vegetable will keep in the refrigerator for a day or two. Red chicory can also be wrapped and refrigerated for a few days.

Nutrition: The chicories contain vitamin A, vitamin B_1, and vitamin C.

Chinese Cabbage

See Cabbages, Chinese.

Collards

Origin: Georgia and Virginia are the chief suppliers, but other states grow collards as well.

Season: The supply of collards on the market remains fairly constant with a peak from January to April.

Selection: Collards should be fresh, crisp, and free of insect damage or discoloration.

Storage: Store collards at 32° F. Keep them wrapped in plastic to retain moisture.

Nutrition: One of the most nutritious vegetables known, collards are mineral-rich and very high in vitamins A and C. They are excellent for cleansing the blood.

Daikon Greens

See Daikon.

Dandelions

Origin: Commercial dandelions are grown throughout the South and Southeast. The winter crop comes from California and Florida.

Season: The supply of dandelions remains constant throughout the year.

Selection: At the market, there will usually be thick-leafed varieties of dandelion that are more tender and milder-tasting than what is growing in the backyard. The color of the cultivated dandelion is also lighter. Try to find leaves that have the roots at least in part still attached, as they will be more succulent. Avoid insect-damaged, wilted, or yellowing leaves.

Storage: Cultivated dandelion greens are extremely perishable. Store at 32° F with added ice.

Nutrition: Dandelions are perhaps even more nutritious than collards and act similarly to cleanse the blood.

Endive

The endives include escarole and curly endive. The endives and chicories are related, and share the same quality of bitterness.

Origin: California is a main supplier of endive, and local markets may also be good sources.

Season: The endives are available year-round, with a peak availability in March and April. Their quality may suffer in the summer.

Selection: Curly endive has a bunchy head with ragged leaves that curl at the ends, and a white center. Escarole has broader leaves that do not curl at the tips. For both, look for fresh, crisp greens, without wilt, rot, or discoloration. Smaller heads have better flavor.

Storage: Store in the refrigerator at high humidity for a couple of days.

Nutrition: The endives provide vitamins A, B_1, and C.

Kale

Origin: Most commercial kale comes from Virginia, Maryland, and New York.

Season: The supply of kale remains constant through the year with a slight peak from December to April.

Selection: Several varieties of kale are on the market. One day the kale you buy may be blue-green, finely curled, and small-stemmed; the next day it may be grey-green and nearly straight-edged, with a thick stem. No matter what the variety, kale should be fresh and its color uniform. Kale tastes best and is more tender after the first frost, so it's best to buy it in the late fall and winter.

Storage: Unlike most other greens, kale stores well. The temperature should be at least 40° F and humidity high.

Nutrition: Kale, like most leafy dark green vegetables, is nutritionally excellent, containing large amounts of vitamins and minerals.

Kohlrabi

Origin: Kohlrabi, a stem vegetable which is one of the varieties in the genus *Brassica,* comes from California.

Season: Although it is available from May through November, kohlrabi is most abundant in June and July.

Selection: Kohlrabi consists of an above-ground stem enlargement that resembles a green turnip. Its leaves, which are edible, shoot straight up. Buy small-bulbed kohlrabi, no bigger than three inches around, which have fresh-looking tops. The rind of the bulb should be easy to pierce with a thumbnail.

Storage: Wrap kohlrabi in plastic and store it as you would a root vegetable (either in the refrigerator or in the root cellar), except at a higher humidity. Kohlrabi will keep untrimmed in the refrigerator for about one week.

Nutrition: Kohlrabi contains vitamins A, C, and several B vitamins as well as calcium, phosphorus, and iron.

Lettuce

Origin: Iceberg lettuce is commercially grown in California and Arizona, which produce 85 percent of the annual crop. California also grows most of the romaine lettuce sold during the winter. New York and New Jersey are other major lettuce-producing states, but their crops are harvested during the summer. In the middle of winter, Mexican iceberg lettuce is usually imported to meet the large demand. Iceberg is by far the most widely cultivated variety of lettuce mainly because it withstands long transport and rough handling better than the other types.

Season: Romaine and iceberg lettuce are available all year. Other varieties are not grown for as large a market, and their availability tends to be regional or confined to the summer months.

Selection: Lettuces are divided into five categories: crisphead or iceberg; butterhead; leaf, looseleaf, or curly; romaine or cos; and stem.

The large tight heads of *iceberg* lettuce have pale green outer leaves, while the inner leaves are almost white. *Boston* and *Bibb,* which are butterhead types, were the most popular lettuces in the Eastern United States until iceberg was introduced in the 1920s. Boston lettuce forms a medium-size, medium-dense head; its green leaves are broad, smooth, and thick. If it is grown hydroponically, it is lighter and paler. Bibb lettuce forms a small soft head, with tender, dark green leaves. The butterheads are highly perishable.

•*Leaf, looseleaf,* or *curly* lettuces do not form into heads. The two most widely distributed varieties are "green leaf" (also called "salad bowl") and "red tipped," but it is almost impossible to find either in unwilted condition, as they are even more perishable than the butterheads.

•*Romaine* or *cos* lettuce has long, broad, upright leaves of a dark green color. Like the looseleaf varieties, romaine does not form into heads. New varieties which ship fairly well have been developed for the commercial market.

•*Stem* lettuce is very rare. Also called Chinese lettuce or celtuce, it is grown for its large stalk, which can be peeled and eaten raw, or cooked.

All lettuce should be crisp, blemish-free, and brightly colored. Avoid discolored or wilted lettuce.

Storage: All lettuce but iceberg can be washed in cold water, shaken dry, and stored in ventilated plastic bags in the refrigerator with excellent results. Iceberg will rot if it is stored even slightly wet, so make sure it is dry before putting it in the refrigerator.

Nutrition: Iceberg is nutritionally weakest. Darker green lettuces like romaine and Bibb contain vitamins A and C, and iron.

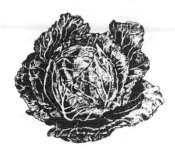

Mustards

Origin: In the United States, mustards are grown primarily in the South. Other commercial growers are California, Michigan, Indiana, New Jersey, and Arizona.

Season: You can find mustards all year. The season hits a peak in the months from December to April.

Selection: Mustards are pungent. Try to select young, fresh greens that have a bright color. Color and shape depend on variety, as mustards may be yellow-green or green, tightly crimpled or nearly straight.

Storage: Mustards are extremely perishable. Do not leave them unrefrigerated for very long. Store mustards in plastic at about 32° F, as you would collard greens.

Nutrition: Mustard greens, like kale, collards, and dandelions, are loaded with vitamins and minerals. They are an excellent source of vitamins A and C and of iron.

Parsley

Origin: Florida is a major supplier of parsley.

Season: Parsley is available year-round. The peak supplies are in October, November, and December.

Selection: Parsley is the most common herb in use today. In the U.S. it is generally eaten raw, but elsewhere it is also cooked as a potherb. Two distinct types are available, the curly-leaf variety, which is the most common, and the flat-leaf "Italian" parsley. Buy parsley that has a vibrant color, preferably dark green. Avoid yellowed parsley. The curly type should spring back from light pressure.

Storage: Store parsley wrapped in plastic in the refrigerator. It should keep for about three weeks.

Nutrition: Parsley is a highly nutritious food, containing exceptionally large amounts of vitamins A and C and minerals.

Spinach

Origin: Texas is the largest spinach producer but more than a dozen other states grow it commercially.

Season: Spinach is available all year. The peak season is in April and May.

Selection: Both crimpled and flat-leafed spinaches are available. Loose spinach is fresher than packaged. The leaves should be dark green and crisp, and the stalks should not be overgrown.

Storage: Store spinach in plastic at about 32° F, as you would collard greens.

Nutrition: Spinach contains reasonable quantities of vitamins A and C, plus minerals. However, it also contains large amounts of oxalic acid, which inhibits calcium absorption.

Swiss Chard

Origin: California is a main supplier, but local market gardens are also good sources of Swiss chard.

Season: Summer is the peak season for Swiss chard.

Selection: Swiss chard is a type of beet that doesn't form a bulbous root, but is grown for its broad, succulent leaves that can reach two feet in height; the fleshy stem is also edible. Usually dark green and yellowish green varieties are found, but there is also a rarer red variety. Purchase fresh leaves that have a uniform color. Avoid insect-damaged or discolored chard.

Storage: Store chard wrapped in plastic in the refrigerator at 32° F.

Nutrition: Swiss chard is an excellent source of vitamins A and C. It also contains other vitamins and minerals.

Turnip Greens

See Turnips.

Watercress

Origin: Florida is the major supplier of watercress.

Season: Watercress is available year-round, with a peak occurring in summer.

Selection: Watercress is sold in bunches. Look for bright green color and crispness of stalk. Wilted or yellowed leaves are a sign of age, bruises a sign of rough handling. Watercress that has flowered is peppery hot.

Storage: Watercress is best kept refrigerated, standing upright with its stems resting in a glass or bowl of water, but it can be stored like other greens. Avoid crushing watercress because it will bruise and decay. It will keep up to a week.

Nutrition: Watercress ranks with collards, dandelions, kale, and mustard greens in high nutritional value.

Fruit Vegetables

Two of the foods—corn and squash—that were mainstays in the diets of many Native American peoples are fruit vegetables. They're still favorites across the U.S., as are such other fruit vegetables as beans, cucumbers, and tomatoes.

Beans

Origin and Varieties: There are three main types of beans: those that are eaten in their entirety, seed and pod together, as with fresh green beans; those (known as shell beans) with tough pods which are discarded, such as cranberry, Lima, and fava beans; and those grown exclusively for drying (see pages 128–129).

•*Fresh green beans* are the immature pods of specially developed beans closely related to common dry beans such as pintos and kidneys; they are available in various shapes and sizes. Tiny French haricots; medium, snap, or string (now mostly stringless) beans; fat beans (pole beans); and yellow or wax beans are the main varieties. Florida is the major U.S. green bean supplier during the fall, winter, and early spring. In spring and summer the supply is local.

•*Lima* or *butter beans* come in small (baby) and large (Fordhook) sizes. They are usually shelled when they are sold and should always be well-cooked, as this reduces the amount of naturally occuring cyanide. Fresh cranberry beans are mainly grown in the Midwest and in New England.

•*Fava, broad,* or *Windsor beans,* recent newcomers to the United States, come in fat green pods and should be shelled and thoroughly cooked, as older pods and undercooked beans have been known to be toxic. One of the most popular foods of the Middle East, fava beans appear in spring in some Italian markets throughout the U.S.

Season: You can find fresh beans all year, but summer is the peak season. Occasionally, fresh chick peas, black-eyed peas, and pigeon peas (which, despite their names, are beans, not peas) are locally available. The cranberry season is brief, but cranberry beans, along with Limas and favas, are available year-round in their dried forms.

Selection: Fresh green beans should be plump and velvety, with the pointed ends fresh. The pods should snap readily. Smaller is usually better, no matter what the variety. Avoid shriveled, wilted, rusted, and bulging pods, as these signs indicate age. Lima beans should be in well-filled pods of a dark green color; the beans themselves should be plump, with tender skin of a green or greenish-white color. Fava and cranberry beans should also be in well-filled pods.

Storage: Fresh beans will keep for only a short time. Store them at about 45° F. As the humidity should be high, place the beans in a plastic bag to retain moisture. Shell Limas, cranberry beans, and favas just before cooking them.

Nutrition: Green beans contain some vitamin A (green beans have more more than wax beans). Shell beans contain protein and B vitamins.

Corn, Sweet

Origin: Florida and California are the main winter suppliers of sweet corn in the United States. Summer supply is local.

Season: Fresh corn is available year-round, with a peak from May to September.

Selection: Yellow and white corn, or a combination of the two colors, is available. Over 200 varieties are grown in the U.S. and new hybrids are developed constantly. Look for fresh green husks and fresh silk. Open the husk slightly and check to see that the kernels are plump and close together, in even rows. Generally, they should extend to the top of the cob. The kernels should be tender and milky, just firm enough to be punctured with slight pressure. If the kernels are very soft and very small, the corn is probably immature. Organic corn may be a little worm-eaten at the top, but most of the ear should be in good condition.

Storage: If possible, do not store sweet corn, but eat it right away, as the corn sugar quickly turns to starch. The ideal way is to pick it and eat it. If you must store corn, keep it very cold and at a very high humidity.

Nutrition: Sweet corn contributes some vitamins and minerals. Yellow corn has more vitamin A than white.

Cucumbers

Origin: Florida, North Carolina, South Carolina, and California supply cucumbers.

Season: Cucumbers are available year-round. The peak is from May to August.

Selection: Firmness and a good green color are the principal signs of fresh cucumbers. A dull green color or yellow tinge and a large size reveal old age. Reject those that are puffy, withered, or shriveled. Cucumbers are often waxed. If these are the only ones available, you may want to peel the skin. Pickling (Kirby) cucumbers should be small; the freshest ones have their spines still intact. Pickling cucumbers should not be waxed.

Storage: Store cucumbers at 45° F and average humidity.

Nutrition: Cucumbers contain vitamin A and iron.

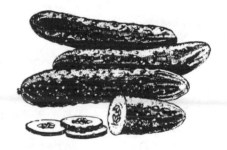

Eggplant

Origin: Eggplant, which is also called aubergine, originated in India and China. In the U.S., the commercial crop is grown mainly in Florida and New Jersey.

Season: The common large purple variety, the small purple (often called Italian), and the long, pale purple Chinese eggplant are available all year, with a peak in the fall. Other varieties are found mainly in the fall.

Selection: Eggplants can be purple, white, yellow-white, grey, or striped. Whatever the variety, they should be clear, plump, and glossy. Look for heavy, firm specimens with a fresh cap. Smaller is usually better; the common purple variety should be from 3 to 6 inches in diameter.

Storage: Eggplant may be wrapped and stored for a few days in the refrigerator at high humidity.

Nutrition: Eggplant does not have any outstanding nutrients.

Peas

Origin: The majority of the crop is frozen or canned, but fresh peas are shipped from California, Colorado, Washington, and Oregon.

Season: Fresh peas are available in the spring and summer.

Selection: Both shelling and edible pod types are on the market. Buy fresh, bright-green pods that snap easily. A yellowish-green pod shows overmaturity. Avoid swollen, speckled, mildewed, or limp pods. The edible pods of snow or sugar peas are picked before the peas are filled out.

Storage: Try to plan on not storing pods. They quickly lose the sweet flavor they're noted for. If you must store them, do so immediately at around 32° F. Do not shell peas until you are ready to use them.

Nutrition: Peas contain vitamins A and C, protein, and minerals.

Peppers, Sweet

Origin: The winter supply of sweet peppers comes from California, Florida, and Texas. In the summer, peppers reach markets from Southern, Midwestern, and Eastern growers.

Season: The season is fairly constant year-round, but it peaks slightly in summer.

Selection: Sweet peppers, often called bell peppers, may be green, green and red, or all red. Red peppers are actually ripe green peppers. Yellow ones are rare. In all cases the colors should be bright. The best peppers have a thick flesh and are firm to the touch. Avoid any with soft spots.

Storage: Stored like cucumbers, at 45° F and average humidity, peppers will keep up to a week.

Nutrition: Green peppers are a good source of vitamins A and C; red peppers contain even more of both vitamins than green peppers.

Pumpkins

Origin: Most of the pumpkin crop is sold fresh from local farms. Illinois, California, and New Jersey supply the off-season market.

Season: The pumpkin season runs primarily from September to December, with a peak in October.

Selection: Size is not much of a factor in picking pumpkins, but the smaller ones are often a bit more tender. The shape may be round or oblong. Look for a firm rind without soft spots and a deep orange color.

Storage: Store pumpkins whole. There is no need to refrigerate them.

Nutrition: Vitamin A is the chief nutrient in pumpkins.

Squashes

Origin: Squashes come in summer and winter varieties. The winter squashes are native to the Americas, but both summer and winter varieties are now grown throughout the United States. The supply will be local during the season. Florida is the leading off-season producer.

Season: Summer squashes are available all year. The winter squashes acorn, butternut, and buttercup are also available year-round. Peak for summer squash is late spring and summer. Winter squash peaks in the fall.

Selection: The summer varieties are fast-growing and picked while still immature so that their rinds are tender. Patty pan, zucchini, yellow crookneck, and straightneck are common summer types. Patty pan, which is bowl-shaped, should be no larger than four inches across. The others, which are more or less tubular, are best when about ten inches long. The rind should puncture easily with a thumbnail. Summer squashes should be firm and without soft spots or mildew.

Popular varieties of winter squash include acorn, buttercup, butternut, Hubbard, spaghetti, and Delicata. Kabocha, sometimes called Hokkaido pumpkin, is a winter squash similar to buttercup.

Winter squashes are slower than summer varieties to mature. They are harvested when the rind is hard, before the first frost. After the squash is harvested, it should be cured before it is stored, to further harden the skin and remove moisture. (Curing is not necessary for acorn squash, however.) If you buy a large quantity of squash to keep for the winter, ask if it has been cured (most squash is sold uncured). If not, set it in a warm place for a couple of days (if the warm place is outside in the sun, make sure that the squash is not resting on the ground, and cover it at night to protect against frost). If the skin of a squash is hard enough to resist being dented by your fingernail, then it is cured.

Buttercup squash should be a dull, dark green with orange markings; if it is shiny with yellow markings, it was harvested when immature. Check all winter squashes for soft spots or mold; a small soft spot on the outside can mean extensive deterioration inside.

Storage: Summer types should be refrigerated; they will keep up to a week. Winter squashes can be kept in any room that is not hot or humid. Check them periodically and remove any that show signs of mold, soft spots, etc.

Nutrition: Summer squashes are high in vitamins A and C, potassium, and magnesium; winter squashes have even more of these nutrients.

Sweet Peppers

See Peppers, Sweet.

Tomatoes

Origin: Florida and California are the top tomato producers and provide most of the winter crop, with California supplying most of the cherry tomatoes. Tomatoes are the leading imported vegetable from Mexico, usually in winter and early spring. In addition, they are the leading greenhouse vegetable and the principal crop grown hydroponically. In summer, local farms throughout the U.S. supply the majority of stores.

Season: Tomatoes are available all year. The peak season is summer.

Selection: Tomatoes should be firm, heavy for their size, and of good general appearance. Size is not a determinant of quality. Check to see if there are ridges at the stem end — these indicate mealiness. There is no such thing as a store-bought ''vine-ripened tomato.'' This marketing term means that the tomatoes are picked at the first hint of pink rather than before. They are then put into cold storage—which makes it impossible for them to ever truly ripen, even though they will turn red and become soft.

Storage: Tomatoes should not be refrigerated until they are fully ripened. To ripen, simply let them sit on a counter or windowsill for several days. When refrigerated they do best between 45° and 50° F.

Nutrition: A ripe tomato is rich in vitamins A and C, phosphorus, and potassium.

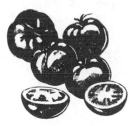

Additional Vegetables

While they don't easily fit into the three main categories covered in this article, two other vegetables deserve the produce shopper's attention. These are mushrooms and bean sprouts.

Bean Sprouts

Origin: The supply of bean sprouts is usually local.

Season: Bean sprouts are available year-round.

Selection: Select sprouts that look fresh and crisp, with tips that aren't dry and ends that aren't slimy. Mung bean sprouts are the most widely available, but many beans are sproutable. Seeds and grains can also be sprouted, although they are not commonly available in natural foods stores.

Storage: Store bean sprouts in plastic in the crisper of the refrigerator. To restore lost crispness, place in cold water with ice for half an hour.

Nutrition: Bean sprouts supply vitamin C.

Mushrooms

Origin: *Agaricus bisporus,* a close relative of the common edible field mushroom, *A. campestris,* is the type usually found in the market. It is grown in natural caves or specially designed windowless buildings, in sterilized composts. Pennsylvania and other Eastern states are the main suppliers.

Wild mushrooms now under limited cultivation in the U.S. include chanterelles, oyster mushrooms (sometimes called pleurottes), and the Japanese enoki and shiitake. Shiitake and chanterelles are also available dried.

Season: The common mushroom is found year-round, with peak availability in November and December.

Selection: The most important thing to consider when buying fresh mushrooms with a cap is the cap's condition. It should be tightly rounded, smooth, and unblemished. Opened caps mean age and a musty flavor. *A. bisporus* should be white or pale brown in color (dark brown signals oxidation or bruising). Tenderness does not depend on size, but short stems are preferable for economy's sake. The best-quality fresh shiitake is fleshy, with thick caps full of spores. The edges of the cap should curl under, not upward. There is some debate over whether the fall or spring crop yields the best-quality shiitake. Mushrooms of any variety should be firm and appear fresh, with no wilt or rot. Avoid mushrooms that have been treated with sulfiting agents such as potassium bisulfite, sodium bisulfite, and sulfur dioxide. These bacterial inhibitors affect flavor and may be toxic.

Storage: Fresh mushrooms keep for about four days in the refrigerator. Never wash or peel them before storing. Dried mushrooms can be stored in an airtight container, in a cool place away from light, for an indefinite period of time.

Nutrition: Mushrooms supply protein, along with phosphorus, iron, and other minerals. In addition, shiitake are rich in enzymes and vitamins.

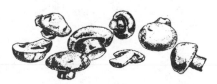

The Case for Regional Agriculture

Most of the fresh produce available in the United States today comes from three states synonymous with super-scale agribusiness—California, Florida, and Texas. Agribusiness runs the gamut of sins against nature from excessive use of chemicals to gross inefficiency (e.g., crops left in the fields to rot). The produce is fed a steady diet of fertilizers, fungicides, herbicides, and pesticides and there is very little hand-harvesting and packing—the emphasis is on mechanical harvesting, bulk handling, and assembly-line processing. Mechanical harvesting is rough and some vegetables are damaged during the harvest. Others remain behind in the fields, missed by the swift steel fingers. What isn't missed is dumped into a container and shipped to a packing plant, which is usually located miles away.

At the plant the first step is to cool the produce to remove "field heat." This is achieved by cold storage, vacuum cooling, or hydrocooling. Vacuum cooling is a relatively harmless mechanical process used primarily on lettuce. Cartons of produce are placed inside large metal tubes in which a strong flow of air is created. Evaporation-cooling swiftly reduces the temperature of the produce to about 32° F.

Hydrocooling seems on the surface to be a simple technique: a shower of icy water rains down on the produce as it moves along on a conveyor belt. This process, however, is also used as an opportunity to apply fungicides.

After cooling, the produce may be stored indoors for a while before it is again on the move—via assembly belt—to be sorted, washed, trimmed, graded, waxed, and showered with chemicals.

The final stop of the tour is packing, which accounts for the largest single cost incurred by the processors. Combined with repeated handling, it accounts for the largest chunk of cost to the consumer: more of your dollar goes for packaging and handling than for the cost of the goods. Packaging creates the additional problems of disposing of empty wire-bound crates, wax-treated fiberboard, and plastic sacks, none of which are as easily reusable as plain wooden crates.

More than half of all fresh produce is packaged into "consumer units" at some point during its journey to market. Refrigerated train cars carrying 160,000 pounds of radishes to the packing plant leave the plant with 320,000 half-pound packages. Most whole foods stores pass up prepackaged produce for crates, called "loose packs," which usually hold from 10 to 50 pounds per unit. Whether "loose pack" or "consumer unit," the produce is shipped from the packing plant to destinations across the nation. Large supermarkets buy directly from the processor. Smaller stores and wholesalers depend on brokers to buy produce and send it to them. A broker may handle the purchasing for twenty stores in one city or area of the country, and each store trusts that person to supply the quality of produce it desires. Large cities and dense population centers are served by produce markets where wholesalers, upon receiving consignments from their brokers, sell to smaller retailers, including most natural foods stores.

The long-distance transport of vegetables is handled by refrigerated train cars or trucks, and the effects on the produce of extended travel are usually minimal if all goes well. But all does *not* go well all the time; in severe winter weather, produce may freeze in transit, creating high prices and/or poor quality at the market. In every kind of weather, produce suffers once it is unloaded. It becomes subject to temperature variations, rough handling, and unsanitary conditions, all of which hasten deterioration. Even if the vegetables are kept refrigerated in the warehouse or produce market, the deterioration continues.

Loaded aboard a truck, once again the produce leaves the warehouse or produce market for delivery to the retailer, and more handling and storage. Produce from Florida is three days old by the time it reaches markets in the Northeast, and produce from California is nearly one week old. Even these estimates are conservative and apply only when optimum conditions prevail. When the market price is low, produce is often withheld and stored in the very train or truck it was shipped in until prices climb. Business tac-

tics like this tack an additional week or more onto the age of "fresh" produce.

Sometimes all this handling time allows the produce to ripen, but most often it leads to wilting and loss of nutrition. Measured for its nutritional value, produce past its prime has lost most of its vitamins A and C. Other victims of wilting are folic acid and carotene. Leafy vegetables are highly perishable and especially susceptible to vitamin loss.

In response to the problems arising from extended storage, a variety of techniques, beyond the usual measures of refrigeration and packing with ice, have been developed to suspend or retard decay. Some storage facilities keep vegetables in "controlled atmospheres," consisting of 97 percent nitrogen and only 3 percent oxygen, which greatly reduce the rotting that is caused by oxidation. The same technology applied to packaging replaces real air with nitrogen. The produce is called "nitrogen packed"; as nitrogen is an inert gas, this process appears to be harmless. A more old-fashioned method of preservation is waxing. Used on root vegetables, melons, apples, cucumbers, and winter squash, waxing retards spoilage and cosmetically enhances the produce. Cucumbers serve as an example of the effectiveness of this method. Pickling cukes (also known as Kirby cucumbers), which are not waxed because their purpose makes it impractical, begin to shrivel two or three days after they are first offered for sale. Waxed slicing cucumbers, on the other hand, hold up for nearly two weeks and are more apt to be done in by bruises than by shriveling. Most waxing materials are manufactured from vegetable oil, but the use of synthetic, petroleum-based waxes is growing.

Chemical sprays are also used for preservation. All are poisonous in large doses, although their use is supposedly monitored by the government. Be sure to wash all nonorganically grown vegetables (and fruits) before eating. Potatoes are sprayed when packed (unless marked "ecologically grown" or "organic"); in fact, it is wise to assume that the majority of commercially grown produce is in some way treated chemically after harvest in order to enhance its ability to withstand long-distance travel. The fact that the actual farm is in some cases three thousand miles from the consumer necessitates this practice. It also requires that huge volumes of gas and oil be expended to get the produce to market. For those who actively seek to reduce their reliance on fossil fuels and chemicals, a good place to begin is at the produce market.

This distribution system has had a marked imprint on the types and varieties of produce now grown. Vegetables and fruits that will stand up to the rigors of rough handling and long periods of transportation have been developed. Genetic changes induced by plant breeders include the thickening of skins and the standardizing of shapes: the thick-skinned, square tomato is a reality.

Of equal commercial importance is appearance. Fruits and vegetables are bred for good looks, and what can't yet be added genetically is applied after harvesting—coloring agents and wax being two examples. The drawback to picture-perfect produce is often a reduction of nutrients and hardiness. Flavor too is sacrificed in the pursuit of overall size and appearance.

Although not every farmer is bound by the dictates of fashion, all share in the same burdens of a tight economic squeeze and the necessity of finding a market for their goods, the appearance of which is an important selling point. The natural foods store is one market available to farmers who de-emphasize modern growing practices in favor of alternative methods aimed at soil improvement and plant health. But these methods may also produce an inferior-looking potato.

The produce at the natural foods store will often be tagged with descriptive subtitles that explain the farming practices used by the grower. The most common of these are "organic," "ecological," and "biodynamic." Most people have their own notion of what "organic" growing is and so do most farmers. Organic organizations are striving to set standards and have legislation passed that supports and defines organic agriculture. There is no standardized definition, though the California Or-

ganic Food Act (Section 26569.11 of the California Health and Safety Code) of 1979 set standards that have provided a starting point for organizations in other states. The California Certified Organic Farmers organization—CCOF—has even higher standards than the law requires.

In almost every part of the U.S. (California, Maine, Oregon, and a few Midwestern states are the exceptions), "organic" can mean just about anything and, except in the cases of highly reputable food companies that inspect the farms and test the soils and products they label as organic, many "organic" products undergo no inspection at all. Legislation is important to protect the conscientious organic farmers who suffer competitively from other growers who merely *label* their products "organic." (For more information on labeling and standards, see Chapter 6.)

Many organic farmers are conscientious and they, and the consumers who support them, are united by their desire to reestablish the natural order. They are willing to sacrifice cosmetic appearance and often pay higher prices for the sake of improving the health of soil, vegetables, and humans.

"Ecological" methods attempt to strike a balance between organic and conventional farming. Certain chemical fertilizers, pesticides, and fungicides are used in conjunction with compost and manure. The chemicals employed are non-persistent, which means they rapidly break down into organic compounds and disappear into the soil. Rather than putting the fields on a regular fertilizing and spraying schedule, regardless of need, the ecological farmer sprays and fertilizes only as the need arises. He or she may also farm by rotation of crops and by planting mixed fields—that is, not planting the same crop in the same field year after year, and not planting the entire field with one crop, but rather breaking it up into smaller patches of complementary vegetables. This last practice helps to confuse insects and foil disease.

"Biodynamic" agriculture is based on the principles of Rudolph Steiner and fits into the definition of organic farming spelled out earlier. Drawing from the three

worlds of animals, vegetables, and minerals, biodynamic composts are prepared and dug into the soil. This farming technique also relies on crop rotations, mixed planting, and natural sprays.

Compared with produce grown by the organic, ecological, and biodynamic methods, the bulk of the produce grown in the United States is polluted. But far and away the most contaminated produce is that which is imported from Mexico. In the United States, because of the work of environmentalists and concerned scientists, many dangerous chemicals such as DDT have been banned from farm use. However, these chemicals are still manufactured here and sold to other countries, Mexico included, which do not have stringent laws regarding them. Mexican farmers and laborers, sometimes ignorant of their toxicity or method of application, often harm themselves in the process of using them.

Almost everything that is grown in the United States is also grown in Mexico and exported to this country. U.S. farmers, citing unfair competition, are lobbying to make mandatory the inclusion of the country of origin on produce labels at the retail level. In the meantime, don't hesitate to ask the country of origin at your natural foods store.

With 60 percent or more of America's produce coming from three states, local farmers in the other states are faced with the difficulty of finding markets for their products. When you purchase locally grown produce, whether organic or not, you are not only helping the farmers of your area, you are helping to ultimately ensure the survival of your area's precious farmland. (Hundreds of square miles of excellent farmlands are lost yearly when farmers who own them are forced to sell out to housing or shopping mall developers.) In addition, local produce is fresher and, more likely than not, freer of chemicals than the best that agribusiness has to offer. Above all, the choice between organic farming and chemical commercial farming is one of philosophy and even politics. Your selection of produce is the equivalent of casting a vote for the type of world you wish to live in.

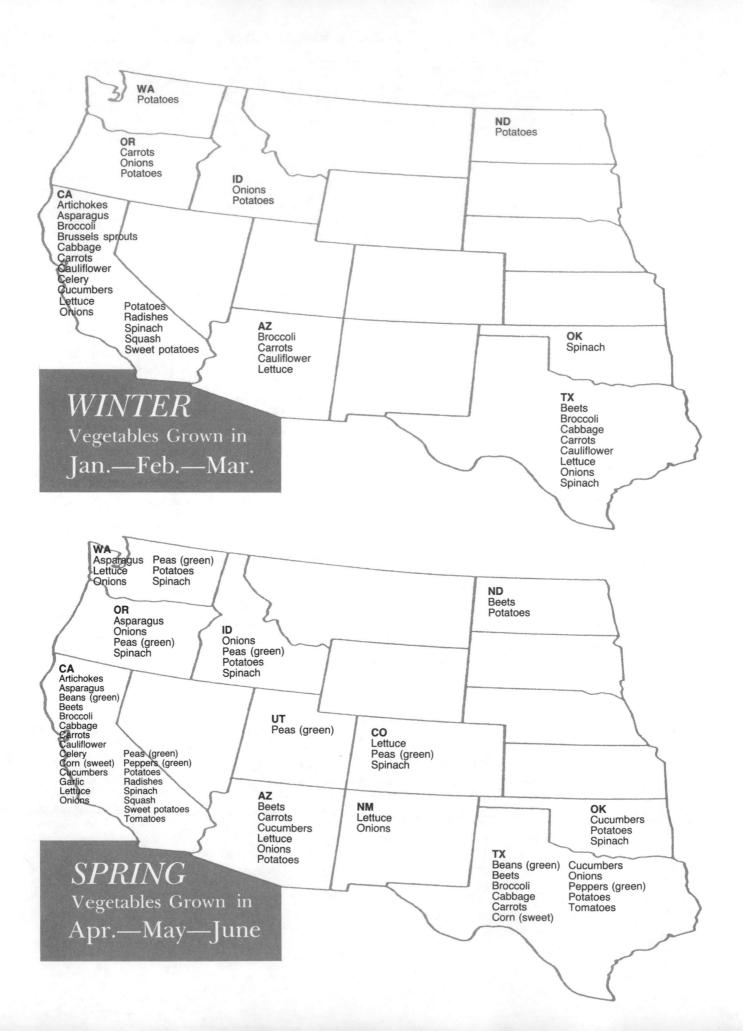

WA
Potatoes

ND
Potatoes

OR
Carrots
Onions
Potatoes

ID
Onions
Potatoes

CA
Artichokes
Asparagus
Broccoli
Brussels sprouts
Cabbage
Carrots
Cauliflower
Celery
Cucumbers
Lettuce
Onions

Potatoes
Radishes
Spinach
Squash
Sweet potatoes

AZ
Broccoli
Carrots
Cauliflower
Lettuce

OK
Spinach

TX
Beets
Broccoli
Cabbage
Carrots
Cauliflower
Lettuce
Onions
Spinach

WINTER
Vegetables Grown in
Jan.—Feb.—Mar.

WA
Asparagus   Peas (green)
Lettuce   Potatoes
Onions   Spinach

ND
Beets
Potatoes

OR
Asparagus
Onions
Peas (green)
Spinach

ID
Onions
Peas (green)
Potatoes
Spinach

CA
Artichokes
Asparagus
Beans (green)
Beets
Broccoli
Cabbage
Carrots
Cauliflower
Celery
Corn (sweet)
Cucumbers
Garlic
Lettuce
Onions

Peas (green)
Peppers (green)
Potatoes
Radishes
Spinach
Squash
Sweet potatoes
Tomatoes

UT
Peas (green)

CO
Lettuce
Peas (green)
Spinach

AZ
Beets
Carrots
Cucumbers
Lettuce
Onions
Potatoes

NM
Lettuce
Onions

OK
Cucumbers
Potatoes
Spinach

TX
Beans (green)   Cucumbers
Beets   Onions
Broccoli   Peppers (green)
Cabbage   Potatoes
Carrots   Tomatoes
Corn (sweet)

SPRING
Vegetables Grown in
Apr.—May—June

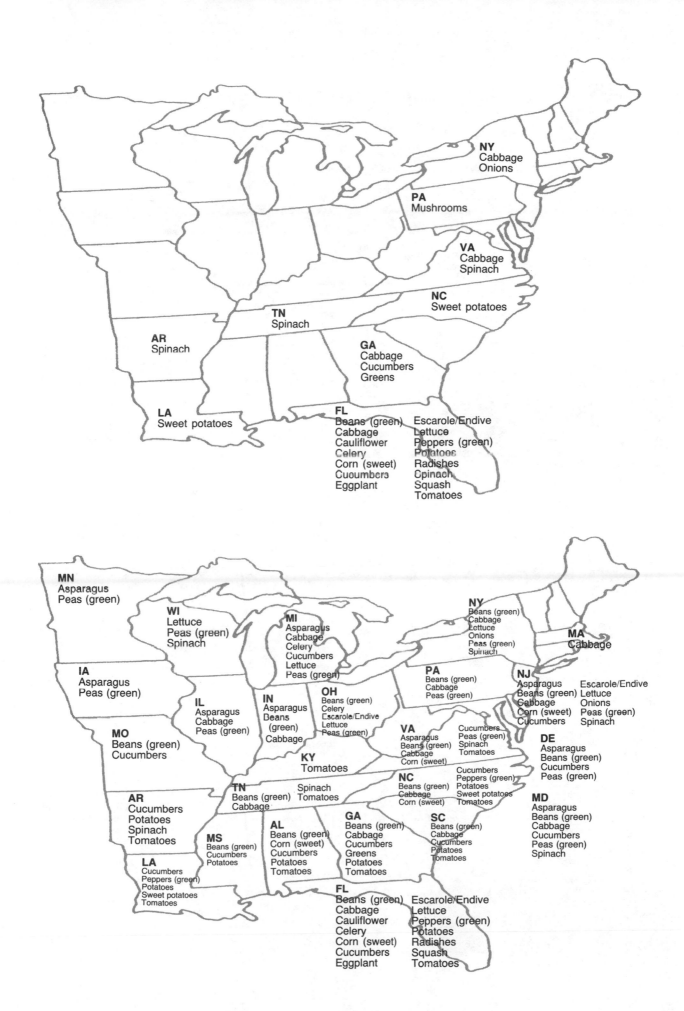

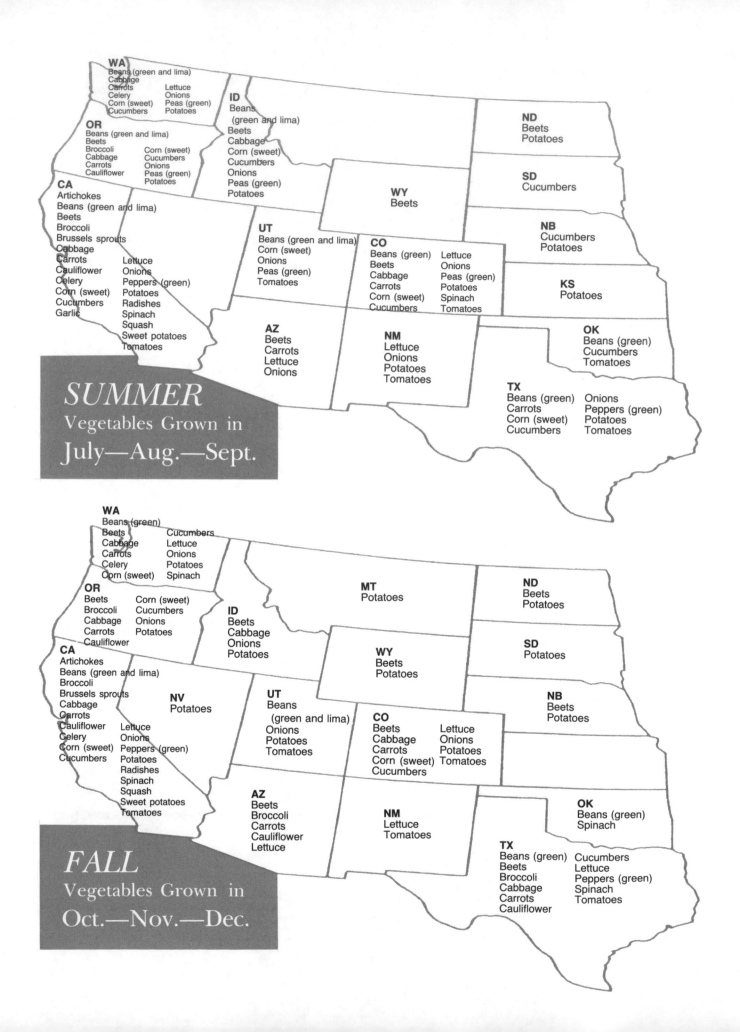

WA
Beans (green and lima)
Cabbage
Carrots   Lettuce
Celery   Onions
Corn (sweet)   Peas (green)
Cucumbers   Potatoes

OR
Beans (green and lima)
Beets
Broccoli   Corn (sweet)
Cabbage   Cucumbers
Carrots   Onions
Cauliflower   Peas (green)
    Potatoes

CA
Artichokes
Beans (green and lima)
Beets
Broccoli
Brussels sprouts
Cabbage
Carrots   Lettuce
Cauliflower   Onions
Celery   Peppers (green)
Corn (sweet)   Potatoes
Cucumbers   Radishes
Garlic   Spinach
    Squash
    Sweet potatoes
    Tomatoes

ID
Beans
(green and lima)
Beets
Cabbage
Corn (sweet)
Cucumbers
Onions
Peas (green)
Potatoes

UT
Beans (green and lima)
Corn (sweet)
Onions
Peas (green)
Tomatoes

AZ
Beets
Carrots
Lettuce
Onions

WY
Beets

CO
Beans (green)   Lettuce
Beets   Onions
Cabbage   Peas (green)
Carrots   Potatoes
Corn (sweet)   Spinach
Cucumbers   Tomatoes

NM
Lettuce
Onions
Potatoes
Tomatoes

ND
Beets
Potatoes

SD
Cucumbers

NB
Cucumbers
Potatoes

KS
Potatoes

OK
Beans (green)
Cucumbers
Tomatoes

TX
Beans (green)   Onions
Carrots   Peppers (green)
Corn (sweet)   Potatoes
Cucumbers   Tomatoes

SUMMER
Vegetables Grown in
July—Aug.—Sept.

WA
Beans (green)
Beets   Cucumbers
Cabbage   Lettuce
Carrots   Onions
Celery   Potatoes
Corn (sweet)   Spinach

OR
Beets   Corn (sweet)
Broccoli   Cucumbers
Cabbage   Onions
Carrots   Potatoes
Cauliflower

CA
Artichokes
Beans (green and lima)
Broccoli
Brussels sprouts
Cabbage
Carrots
Cauliflower
Celery   Lettuce
Corn (sweet)   Onions
Cucumbers   Peppers (green)
    Potatoes
    Radishes
    Spinach
    Squash
    Sweet potatoes
    Tomatoes

ID
Beets
Cabbage
Onions
Potatoes

NV
Potatoes

UT
Beans
(green and lima)
Onions
Potatoes
Tomatoes

AZ
Beets
Broccoli
Carrots
Cauliflower
Lettuce

MT
Potatoes

WY
Beets
Potatoes

CO
Beets   Lettuce
Cabbage   Onions
Carrots   Potatoes
Corn (sweet)   Tomatoes
Cucumbers

NM
Lettuce
Tomatoes

ND
Beets
Potatoes

SD
Potatoes

NB
Beets
Potatoes

OK
Beans (green)
Spinach

TX
Beans (green)   Cucumbers
Beets   Lettuce
Broccoli   Peppers (green)
Cabbage   Spinach
Carrots   Tomatoes
Cauliflower

FALL
Vegetables Grown in
Oct.—Nov.—Dec.

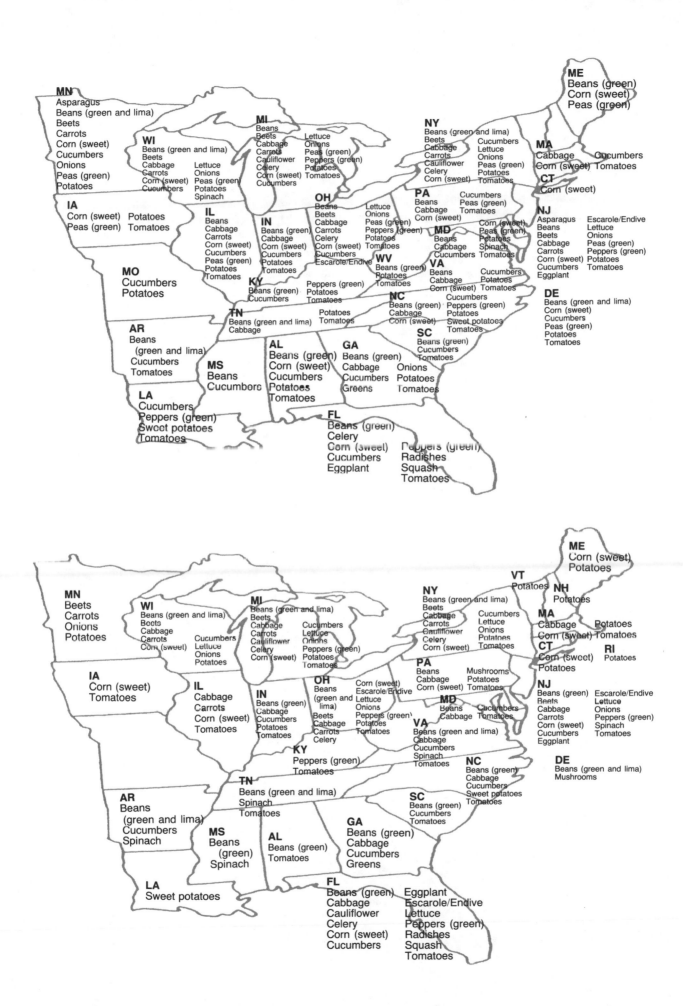

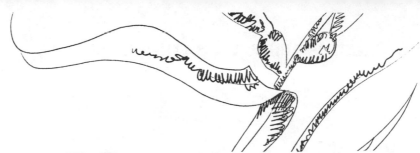

5. SEA VEGETABLES

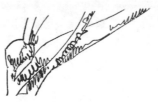

Sea vegetables have an image problem. Their most common name, seaweeds, makes them sound unappetizing. People think they taste bad, and even their appearance and texture can be unsettling to those new to eating them. Recently, another limitation to their acceptance by the general public has arisen. That is the question of whether sea vegetables, which are often raised off the shores of industrialized countries, contain potentially harmful levels of pollutants.

Fortunately for those who have long been taking advantage of the sea vegetable section of the natural foods store, this image problem is largely undeserved. As David Wollner points out in the following story, sea vegetables have traditionally been appreciated by coastal peoples both because they can be very appetizing and because they are high in some important nutrients. Also, as Thom Leonard points out, a recent independent laboratory test sponsored by *East West* had encouraging findings about the levels of heavy metals in both Japanese and Atlantic Coast sea vegetables. This section of the *Shopper's Guide* also includes tips from Ken Burns on using sea vegetables in the kitchen. We hope this chapter will inspire people to add these valuable foods to their daily diet, and perhaps lend a hand in the promotion of a new, more positive image for sea vegetables.

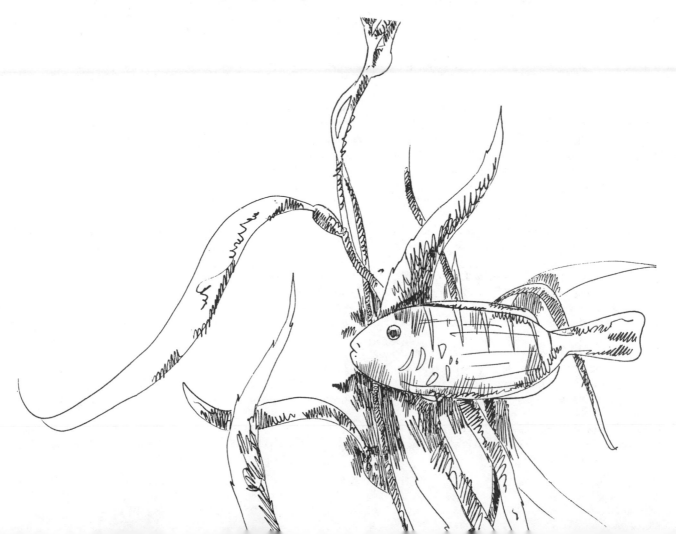

A Guide to Sea Vegetables

Captain Nemo was watching me. I asked him no questions, but he read my thoughts. "Most of these dishes are absolutely new to you," he said, "but eat them without anxiety. They are wholesome and nutritious. Since I have renounced the foods of earth, I am never ill. My crew eat the same food, and they are all healthy."

"You mean that all these dishes come from the sea?" It was still hard to accept.

"Yes, professor. I cast my nets in tow and pull them in ready to snap. Sometimes I hunt on the ocean floor, which appears to be inaccessible to man, and stalk the game that dwells in my submarine forests. My flocks, like those of Neptune's shepherds, graze without fear on the immense prairies of the ocean. I have vast properties, sown by the hand of the Creator, and cultivated by me."

—Jules Verne
Twenty Thousand Leagues Under the Sea

The bounty of the sea offered to Monsieur Aronnax by the indomitable Nemo comes as no surprise to us today. The nations of the world are turning their sights to the fertile pastures of the ocean in a search for new sources of food. One they may find is really an old one: the seaweeds. Virtually all seaweeds are edible but only a few are harvested for human consumption for their superior taste and nutrition. These are often referred to as sea vegetables. Though these plants have gone largely unrecognized by the modern world, they have been eaten for centuries. Humans have taken advantage of sea vegetables wherever they have lived near the sea. To regard them as a recent Oriental import is a misconception, as natives in Ireland, Scotland, Wales, Iceland, coastal sections of Europe, Scandinavia, Russia, the Americas, and the South Pacific eat seaweeds to this day. Nevertheless, across North America, only a daring few have struck out on their own to include sea vegetables in the modern diet. It is too bad that the thought of eating sea vegetables seems strange to many people, for these plants really are culinary delicacies of the first order, and in addition are extremely nutritious.

In one form or another we have all been using sea vegetables, even eating them, all of our lives. Sea vegetables, disguised by laboratory nomenclature, are and have been important ingredients in baked goods, ice cream, cheese, and processed meats, as well as in medicines and cosmetics.

Origin of Sea Vegetables

The term "seaweed" defines the marine algae. (Algae are photosynthetic plants, and include land and fresh-water types as well.) The marine algae are among the most ancient life forms on earth and probably were the first cellular life to exist. They have remained primitive due to the relatively small amount of change in their ocean environment. Everyone who lives near the sea knows of the moderating influence of the ocean on air temperature. This is because the ocean temperature changes more slowly and varies much less than the land temperature does. Ocean temperature depends on the temperature of the core of the earth, not on that of the air. Skin divers tell how a gale of tumultuous waves on the water's surface is only a pleasant breezy current a few yards below. And a marine scientist can supply data showing that below a certain depth the ocean temperature remains practically constant, changing only in broad zones as one descends to the bottom. Compared to the land and land plants, the ocean and oceanic plants do not experience so severe or so direct a degree of change. The ongoing evolution of the ocean is a tortoise's plod compared to the jack-rabbit leaps made on land.

Unlike land plants, most sea vegetables are largely *undifferentiated*, that is, they have a minimum of tissue types within each plant. Although the leaf or frond (blade), stem (stipe), and root (holdfast) are markedly different in shape, the tissue which composes each is the same. The holdfast does not extract nourishment like a root but acts only as an anchor for the plant. Nourishment is taken through the entire plant surface directly from seawater and is converted by the plant into organic compounds. The first signs of differentiation are present in the later-developing sea vegetables. In these plants, reproductive activity is specialized to certain areas, though it is still accomplished through primitive means of fragmentation, sporing, and gamete production.

One of the richest sources of minerals is the sea vegetable. And just as land plants relay the energy of the earth, taking their nourishment directly from the soil and passing it along to animals and humans, sea vegetables contain and transmit the energies of the sea.

Health Benefits from Sea Vegetables

As the direct transformation of sea brine and a natural reserve of the sea's mineral wealth, sea vegetables compare favorably with land vegetation. Sea vegetables are well endowed with calcium and phosphorus, and rank extremely high in magnesium, iron, iodine, and sodium. They also contain vitamins A, B_1, B_{12}, C, and E, as well as proteins and carbohydrates. In some instances their vitamin content is comparable to the richest land vegetable sources. Sea vegetables purify the blood as they contain alkalizing minerals that negate the acidic effects of a modern diet. They have proven effective in ameliorating cancer, rheumatism, arthritis, high blood pressure, constipation, diarrhea, worms, ulcers, bronchitis, emphysema, asthma, gall, kidney, and bladder stones, genito-urinary ailments, nervous disorders, and thyroid and other endocrine system malfunctioning. Sea vegetables also help dissolve the fat deposits that can accumulate from the overconsumption of fatty and oily foods. The alginic acid found in the brown sea vegetables (kombu, wakame, kelp, and hijiki) turns toxic metallic elements in the intestines into harmless salts that can be discharged from the body. This quality is also an advantage for anyone just beginning to adapt to whole foods, as it allows for better absorption of nutrients by the intestines. If all this weren't enough, tests conducted at McGill University and later duplicated elsewhere have shown that sea vegetables actually remove radioactive strontium-90 from the body.

Of all the vitamins found in sea vegetables, the one that stands out most is vitamin B_{12}. B_{12} is a rare but essential vitamin necessary for proper functioning of the neuro-muscular system; a deficiency results in pernicious anemia. Sea vegetables (along with fermented soy products and spirulina—a fresh-water algaean cousin) are an important vegetable source of B_{12}.

Testing Sea Vegetables

As we change our diets to include more healthful and natural sources of food, we wonder about contamination from harmful environmental pollutants. It has been discovered that exposure to heavy metals—lead, arsenic, cadmium, and mercury, among others—leads to a variety of health problems. In small quantities lead is a powerful neurotoxin, and mercury even more so; cadmium is known to be a carcinogen. As sea vegetables have the capacity to collect and concentrate available heavy metals, it is important to know in what quantity, if any, they are present in the sea vegetables that we eat.

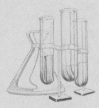

Over the years I have heard more doubts expressed about the cleanliness of Japanese sea vegetables than about any other food, and understandably so. The Japanese islands are small, densely populated, and industrialized. The Minamata Bay incident in the late 1960s, in which consumption of contaminated fish resulted in methyl mercury poisoning, did little to assuage these doubts. A less widely publicized occurrence of heavy-metal-induced disease took place in Toyama Bay, when water polluted with cadmium from an upstream mine was used to irrigate rice paddies. Itai-itai (ouch-ouch) disease resulted in significant skeletal deformities, predominantly among postmenopausal women. The same river that irrigated the Toyama Bay rice paddies also flows into Toyama Bay itself. And that bay's waters are circulated along the coast of Japan into major sea vegetable harvesting areas.

These incidents suggest that there might be health dangers associated with regular consumption of Japanese sea vegetables. In order to take a closer look at the sea vegetables in question, we first contacted Muso Syokuhin Co., Ltd., the trading company that supplies Eden Foods with their Japanese imports, sea vegetables included. They sent us a copy of "Contents of Heavy Metals in Foods: Extents and Average Contents of Heavy Metals in Vegetable Foods," the report of a study conducted by the Osaka Prefectural Institute of Public Health published in 1977 (see Table 1). However, the sea vegetables tested were not Muso products and had been collected prior to February 1977, so the levels reported are not indica-tive of the levels of heavy metals found in the sea vegetables sold today in natural foods stores in the United States. Westbrae Natural Foods sent us lab reports of tests done in 1977 on samples of their arame, hijiki, kombu, and wakame. The samples were of products available to U.S. customers, but tests conducted almost ten years ago don't tell us much about what's in the food we eat today. Heavy metals in water and atmospheric pollution will vary over a period of time, as will absorption rates in the various sea vegetables.

Table 1: Osaka Study

Parts per million (micrograms per gram)				
	As	Cd	Pb	Hg
Kombu	56.7	0.59	0.92	0.02
Nori	NR	0.17	0.33	0.02
Wakame	NR	0.57	0.92	0.26

Average metal contents in sea vegetables tested by the Osaka Prefectural Institute for Public Health, 1977. (Only kombu was tested for arsenic content.)

NR = analysis not requested.
As = Arsenic; Cd = Cadmium;
Pb = Lead; Hg = Mercury.

Table 2

Report to East West Journal
From Skinner and Sherman Laboratories Inc.   29 April 1983

Project Description

Analysis of nine (9) samples of edible seaweed for arsenic, cadmium, lead and mercury content.

Sample Identification

1. Eden Kombu, one 2.75 oz. package.
2. Erewhon Kombu, one 2.75 oz. package.
3. Eden Nori, three 0.8 oz. packages.
4. Erewhon Japanese Nori, three 0.9 oz. packages.
5. Eden Wakame, one 2.75 oz. package.
6. Erewhon Wakame, one 2.75 oz. package.
7. Atlantic Kombu, one 4 oz. package.
8. Wild Atlantic Nori, two 1 oz. packages.
9. Alaria, one 4 oz. package.

The above samples were received on 19 April 1983 and 20 April 1983.

Method of Test

Official Methods of Analysis of the Association of Official Analytical Chemists (AOAC), Thirteenth Edition, 1980, Chapter 25.

Metals were determined by atomic absorption spectroscopy.

RESULTS

| | Parts per million (micrograms per gram) | | | |
Sample	Arsenic	Cadmium	Lead	Mercury
1. Eden Kombu	23.0	0.1	0.8	0.022
2. Erewhon Kombu	41.0	0.3	0.8	0.005
3. Eden Nori	NR	0.2	0.5	0.005
4. Erewhon Nori	NR	0.4	1.1	< 0.005
5. Eden Wakame	NR	0.2	0.8	0.017
6. Erewhon Wakame	NR	0.2	0.8	< 0.005
7. Atlantic Kombu	64.0	1.3	0.5	< 0.005
8. Atlantic Nori	NR	1.6	3.1	< 0.005
9. Alaria	NR	2.6	0.9	< 0.005

NR = analysis not requested.
< = less than.
Source: Skinner and Sherman Laboratories, Inc., Waltham, MA. Reprinted by permission.

It appeared that there was no current data available on possible heavy metal contamination of sea vegetables, so we decided to select samples from the shelves of natural foods stores and have them tested by a qualified laboratory. We purchased samples of Japanese kombu, nori, and wakame from two American distributors, Eden and Erewhon. We also bought Atlantic kombu, wild nori, and alaria (a wakame-like seaweed) distributed by Maine Coast Sea Vegetables. Due to our limited budget and the cost of accurate analysis we were unable to select more samples from other distributors or to have other varieties such as arame and hijiki tested. However, Eden and Erewhon represent the products of the two major Japanese suppliers of natural foods to the United States, Muso and Mitoku. Most of the Japanese sea vegetables sold by U.S. natural foods distributors are supplied by one of these companies.

We asked the laboratory to test for levels of cadmium, lead, and mercury in all the samples, because these metals were included in the two analyses we had already seen and seemed to be the ones that people were most concerned about. We tested for arsenic only on the three samples of kombu. The presence of the metals was determined by a method known as "atomic absorption spectroscopy." The results are given in Table 2.

The first surprise was the relatively high levels of cadmium in all of the Maine sea vegetables and the high level of lead in the Maine wild nori. Maine, with its empty, windswept beaches and wild surf crashing on rugged rocks, seems pristine in comparison to industrial Japan. And the Maine Coast Sea Vegetables are harvested not near Portland where most of the state's industry is, but "down east," in the vicinity of Acadia National Park. Why the high levels of cadmium in the Maine samples? Are these levels potentially dangerous? Are the levels found in the Japanese seaweeds safe? Suddenly I realized that none of these numbers meant anything to me.

A dozen phone calls later I discovered that I was not alone in my ignorance. Officials with the Massachusetts Department of Public Health, the Francis Stearn Health and Nutrition Center in Cambridge, and the Food and Drug Administration (FDA) could tell me little about acceptable levels of arsenic, cadmium, lead, or mercury in foods. The FDA representative with whom I spoke said that seafood was allowed to have up to one part per million (ppm) of mercury, but made it very clear that this was for fish, not edible seaweed, and that the FDA has established no safe levels for any of the four potential toxins in any other food. I later read in a toxicology text that the legal limit for mercury in fish was 0.5 ppm. So maybe even the FDA doesn't know what it knows.

I called Shepard Erhart at Maine Coast Sea Vegetables and told him of our findings and everyone's ignorance. He immediately contacted the Maine Department of Natural Resources and the University of Maine at Orono. No one was surprised at any of the levels. It seems that the cadmium in the Maine sea vegetables is not from industrial pollution but from minerals in the granite rocks along the coastline. There was no explanation for what I thought was a high level of lead in the nori, nor did anyone express any concern.

George Seaver of Atlantic Laboratories in Waldoboro, Maine, finally came up with some solid information. The Food and Nutrition Board of the National Research Council publishes the *Food Chemicals Codex (FCC)* which lists requirements for food ingredients. Included in the list is kelp, "brown algae of the genera *Macrocystis* and *Laminaria*." Kombu, wakame, and alaria are all brown algae. Both the Maine and Japanese kombu are of the genus *Laminaria*. So it appeared that finally we'd be able to interpret our data.

When I told Seaver the results of our analysis, he said that everything seemed

pretty normal, although the tests we had requested really didn't fit into the *FCC* guidelines, as the *FCC* requires that *total* heavy metals in kelp not exceed 40 ppm (there are individual tolerance levels for lead and inorganic arsenic, however). We didn't test for total heavy metals, but after reviewing our lab report, Seaver thought that our samples would probably fall below that figure. All our samples, even the Maine nori, are well within the 10 ppm *FCC* limit set for lead. (There is no *FCC* requirement for either cadmium or mercury, but since all our samples had mercury levels far below even the lower reported limits for fish there appears no need for concern in that quarter.)

The *FCC* requires that kelp not exceed 3 ppm of *inorganic* arsenic. Our test was for total arsenic, not just the inorganic portion. But most of the arsenic found in sea vegetables occurs as *organic* compounds that are indigestible and therefore not potentially toxic. Since it is only the inorganic forms that pose any problems, our reported arsenic levels are meaningless except in comparison to other tests.

Robert P. Beliles, in *Toxicology: The Basic Science of Poisons*, reports that in the absence of specific regulations an interim action guideline for food and beverages of 0.5 ppm cadmium has been established. In their dehydrated state all of the Atlantic sea vegetables we tested exceed this level. However, when reconstituted, as they are usually eaten, dried sea vegetables absorb five to seven times their weight in water. Thus, soaking would reduce the *concentration* of cadmium in the Maine sea vegetables so that all would fall below this suggested guideline. The Japanese sea vegetables we tested came in at less than 0.5 ppm.

There may be another factor to consider when determining an acceptable level for cadmium. Because sea vegetables live in a saline environment, they must have a means of controlling the entry and exit of inorganic ions in order to maintain proper mineral balance. The substance primarily responsible for this function in brown algae (alaria, arame, hijiki, kelp, kombu, wakame) is called alginic acid. Seibin and Teruko Arasaki, in *Vegetables from the Sea* (Japan Publications, 1983), point out that alginic acid binds certain metallic ions to itself and that no known intestinal enzyme digests it. They conclude, "Heavy metals taken into the hu-

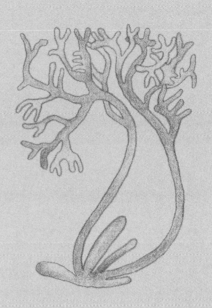

man body are rendered insoluble by alginic acid in the intestines and cannot, therefore, be absorbed into body tissues."

In addition, studies by a research team at McGill University in Montreal have shown that alginic acid will help to remove radioactive strontium from the body. A subsequent report by the same group extended this effect "to other metal pollutants such as barium, cadmium, and zinc." The same mechanism that enables the brown algae to absorb heavy metals in the human body governs their behavior while they live in the ocean, hence the concentration of cadmium in the Maine sea vegetables. In light of the binding quality of alginic acid and the indigestibility of the compounds it forms with metals, including cadmium, it may be useful to differentiate between organic (indigestible) and inorganic (potentially toxic) forms of all heavy metals, as in the case of arsenic.

In conclusion, neither lead nor mercury approach tolerance levels in any of our samples. Although there are unanswered questions about actual levels of inorganic arsenic and whether we should consider total or inorganic cadmium when determining safe levels, there seems no immediate need for concern about the moderate consumption of either imported or domestic sea vegetables. When we take into account the research at McGill, it appears that sea vegetables, rather than being a source of heavy metals in the diet, may actually serve to cleanse the body of these toxic elements.

However, the real value of our doing this study has been learning what isn't known or understood. We initiated it because of concern over modern industrial heavy metal pollution in Japanese waters. We discovered that metal contents (except mercury) are actually higher in the Maine sea vegetables, and that the source, at least in the case of cadmium, is not industry but ancient veins in the coastal granite. That there is a distinction made between organic and inorganic arsenic levels leads us to ask if the same distinction should not be extended to other metals. Why are there no established levels for cadmium? Because it isn't a problem? Or because no one understands sea vegetables well enough to make a decision?

You'll have to make your own decisions, but I had a cup of wakame and split pea soup with my lunch today and a strip of Maine kombu cooked in a stew of fresh garden vegetables for supper. Both were delicious.

A Guide to Sea Vegetables

Sea vegetables present a variety of flavors for the palate, each one unique and with its own variety of uses. Sea vegetables do not taste salty, being in fact only 2 to 4 percent salt. Neither do they taste fishy. They have been described as "nutty" or "beanlike," or even as tasting like celery or grapes. Although many imported sea vegetables may seem exotic at first, dulse has always been a staple in Eastern seaport markets. And the speed with which sushi bars have become popular in the United States indicates that at least one sea vegetable—the exquisitely beautiful nori—has easily found a niche in some North American diets.

The Japanese have collected sea vegetables for centuries and have made the farming, processing, and grading of them into a refined art. Most sea vegetables are rated according to the time of the year they are harvested, the factor that determines succulence and price. When the sea vegetables are dried, however, the appearance of ones collected in May and of ones collected in December may be identical. It is therefore necessary for you to choose a brand you can trust. Japanese sea vegetables packaged under natural foods company labels are top quality. They are also the most expensive. Non-natural foods importers usually bring in lesser quality seaweeds—some of which may have undesirable additives—that sell for less. You get what you pay for. Locally harvested sea vegetables are our hope for the future. Companies in Eastern Canada and Maine, and on the west and northwest coasts of the U.S., have sea vegetables on the market that are excellent products.

Sea vegetables can be added to soups and salads, cooked alone or with land vegetables, and even brewed into teas. Their versatility in the kitchen is as wide as the ocean. When added to beans, they have the unique ability to shorten the cooking time. They add flavor to and promote the digestibility of most foods and accentuate the natural tastes of the vegetables, beans, and grains with which they are cooked.

Brown algae account for the majority of edible sea vegetables worldwide. Most of the others are red, although a few other colors are represented as well.

Brown Algae

Arame

Arame is a Japanese sea vegetable. When dried, it has a taste and texture similar to that of hijiki, but with a milder flavor. It also lacks that sea vegetable's deep lustrous color. After harvesting, arame (*Eisenia arborea*) may be cooked for

Composition of Sea Vegetables
per 100 grams (3½ ounces)

Sea Vegetable	Protein (gm)	Fat (gm)	Carbohydrate (gm)	Calcium (mg)	Phosphorus (mg)
Agar-agar	2.3	0.1	74.6	400	8
Arame	7.5	0.1	60.6	1170	150
Carragheen	—	1.8	—	885	157
Dulse	—	3.0	—	567	22
Hijiki	5.6	0.8	42.8	1400	56
Kelp	—	1.1	—	1093	240
Kombu	7.3	1.1	54.9	800	150
Nori	35.6	0.7	44.3	260	510
Wakame	12.7	1.5	51.4	1300	260

gm = grams; IU = International Units;
mg = milligrams

Dash indicates that data is not available.

several hours to soften it, and then dried in the sun. Naturally a wide blade, arame is sliced into thin strands for packaging.

Arame can be added to soups or served as a vegetable side dish to complement rice or other grains. It is a source of protein, fat, vitamins A, B₁, and B₂, and many minerals and trace elements.

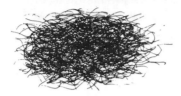

Arame

Hijiki

Hijiki, *Hizikia fusiforme,* found primarily in the Far East, contains the most calcium of any of the widely eaten sea vegetables, 1,400 mg per 100 gr dry weight. This is considerably more than milk, which checks in at 100 mg/100 gr, and slightly more than wakame (1,300 mg/100 gr).

Hijiki is a popular food in the Orient. Folk legend holds it to be excellent for maintaining healthy hair, and its shining black strands remind one of the beautiful tresses of the Far East.

Hijiki is very tough in its natural state. After harvesting, it is dried, steamed for four hours, and dried again. It is then soaked in the juice of arame to darken its color, sundried, and packaged. As with all dried sea vegetables, cooking rehydrates hijiki; as it expands to about five times its dry volume, be careful not to start out with too much.

In addition to ample amounts of calcium, hijiki contains large quantities of protein, vitamins A, B₁, and B₂, iron, and smaller quantities of other minerals.

Kelp

The kelps make up a large family of brown algae. They grow mainly in the northern latitudes near the shoreline, although some types grow in the southern waters of Africa, South America, and the South Pacific. Kelps show more differentiation than any other sea vegetables. The most widely distributed, *Pleuraphycus gardneri,* grows at the low-water mark on rocky shores from temperate to frigid zones in the Atlantic and Pacific. The name kelp is European in origin and originally referred to the ash derived from burning brown algae, which was used to make soap and glass.

Kelp has many industrial uses. Algins—water-absorbent compounds—are derived from the cell walls of kelps and are used as stabilizers, thickeners, emulsifiers, and suspending agents.

Like many sea vegetables, kelp can be eaten fresh but is usually dried. It is sold whole, granulated, or powdered. Granulated and powdered kelps are used as condiments or flavorings. Whole kelp can be eaten in salads, used as a wrapping for a variety of fillings, pickled, steamed, or boiled. The various kelps are rich sources of vitamins, minerals, and many trace elements.

What is sold in the natural foods stores as kelp (Atlantic kombu) is mostly *Laminaria longicruris* (oarweed). "Horsetail" on the east coast and "Pacific kombu" on the west is *Laminaria digitata.* These laminarias are similar to Japanese kombu. They cook more quickly and tenderly than the imports that are available.

Kombu

Kombu is the Japanese name for several species of brown algae, most often of the genus *Laminaria.* Dashi-kombu, tororo-kombu, Rishiri-kombu, ma-kombu, and so forth, all indicate the specific type and/or how it is processed before packaging. Dashi is a broad flat strip used primarily for soup stock; tororo is kombu that has been shaved with a knife to obtain thin slivers that are sometimes marinated in rice vinegar; Rishiri-kombu is a dashi-kombu from the

Iron (mg)	Sodium (mg)	Potassium (mg)	Vit. A (IU)	Vit. B₁ (mg)	Vit. B₂ (mg)	Niacin (mg)	Vit. C (mg)
5.0	—	—	0	00	0.00	0.0	0
12.0	—	—	50	02	0.20	2.6	0
8.9	2892	2844	—	—	—	—	—
6.3	—	—	—	—	—	—	—
29.0	—	—	150	01	0.20	4.0	0
—	3007	5273	—	—	—	—	—
—	2500	—	430	08	0.32	1.8	11
12.0	600	—	11000	25	1.24	10.0	20
13.0	2500	—	140	11	0.14	10.0	15

island of Rishiri, and ma-kombu is another variety of dashi-kombu. Ne-kombu is the dried root (holdfast) of kombu.

A strip of dashi-kombu at the bottom of a pot of rice or vegetables will help to keep them from sticking to the bottom, while at the same time enhancing the flavors of all the ingredients. Added to a pot of beans, kombu helps them to cook faster and renders them more digestible—testimony to its mineral properties. Kombu is especially delicious with root vegetables; it should be soaked first for fifteen minutes, then cooked beneath the vegetables until tender.

The proportion of nutrients varies with the type of kombu and the time at which it is harvested, but all kombus are highly endowed with vitamins, minerals, and protein.

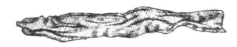

Kombu

Wakame and Alaria

Japanese wakame, *Undaria pinnatifida*, is collected in the cold northern waters off the island of Hokkaido. In the Orient, wakame is sold fresh during the early spring when it is tenderest, but during the rest of the year (and in the United States) it is available only in dried form. During the drying process, it is treated with ash or blanched and processed in other ways to preserve it. It may also be shaved or roasted. Mekabu, the spore-producing portions near the wakame holdfast, are prized as delicacies in Japan.

Alaria esculenta, harvested in North America on the east and west coasts, has qualities similar to wakame but is not as tender. Both alaria and wakame are best when harvested from plants with small midribs or stipes (stems). After drying this is difficult to detect, so you have a choice between putting your faith in brand names or ending up with a chewy salad or vegetable dish. Wakame and alaria are sold in natural foods stores, and the health food brands are good-quality products.

Dried wakame and alaria can be added to soups or cooked as vegetables with other vegetables or tofu. Baked, they can be crumbled and used as a garnish. Wakame can be soaked for five minutes then added, uncooked, to salads. This highly nutritious sea vegetable is a good source of protein, iron, calcium, sodium, magnesium, and other minerals. It also contains vitamins A, B_1, B_2, and C. Alaria is high in vitamin K and all the B vitamins, including B_{12}. It is also high in the minerals iodine and bromine.

Wakame

Red Algae

Agar-Agar

Agar is a versatile, tasty gel that will set at room temperature. It is traditionally made in the Orient by rinsing, cleaning, sun-bleaching, and rerinsing *Gelidium amansii*, a red algae. Then it is boiled and poured through filters and into frames. Once in the frames the mixture is freeze-dried, thawed, recleaned, and redried, producing feather-light translucent bars. The agar flakes available from some importers are trimmed from bars, and thus are virtually identical in quality and gelling strength. (Agar powder is made from a similar seaweed but has undergone more processing.)

Agar gel has been used in the home for centuries. It is effective as a mild laxative. It is the basic ingredient in a dessert which the Japanese call *kanten*. This light, healthful, and delicious gelatin is made by dissolving agar in juice, simmering, and adding slices, chunks, or balls of fruit. Vegetables, water, and seasonings may be substituted for the fruit and juice to make a refreshing aspic.

Agar-agar is rich in iodine and trace elements.

Carragheen or Irish Moss

Carragheen—so named after a coastal town in western Ireland—is a red sea vegetable that grows in the temperate waters of the North Atlantic. Also called *Irish moss*, and known scientifically as *Chondrus crispus*, carragheen is known primarily for its gelling properties, yielding a softer gel than that of agar-agar. It can be boiled down for its clear gel to make puddings, jellies, and gelatins, or cooked fresh as a stew vegetable. Served as a thick drink with lemon and a natural sweetener, carragheen is recommended as a tonic for the respiratory system. It is also noted as a healer of diarrhea, urinary disorders, and chronic chest infections. Carragheen is a good source of vitamin A, iodine, and many other minerals.

Dulse

Dulse, *Palmaria palmata*, is probably the sea vegetable that appeals the most to North Americans. Eaten by coastal people in northern latitudes of the Western World, it is known by many names—*dillisk* in Ireland, *sol* in Iceland, *water leaf* in Scotland. A red algae which grows from the mid-tide mark to below the low-tide mark, it is harvested from late spring to early fall. Most dulse on the market comes from Canada's east coast. Even some American collectors buy and distribute Canadian dulse and consider it a superior product. Canadian dulse is a thinner, lighter-colored plant that cooks up more tenderly than its American counterpart.

Dulse is not a stranger or newcomer to this continent, where it was harvested by people of Irish, Scottish, and Welsh descent. Sailors often rolled raw dulse into a tight wad and chewed it like tobacco.

Dulse can be eaten fresh—and when it is used that way, it really spices up a salad. Because of its unique and delicious flavor, dried dulse has long been a favorite ingredient in relishes, breads, soups, fritters, oatmeal, and fermented beverages. Many dulse-lovers snack on the dried sea vegetable, just as it comes from the bag.

Dulse is an excellent source of iodine and phosphorus and is high in protein, fat, and vitamin A. It also contains vitamins B_6, B_{12}, C, and E, and numerous minerals.

Nori or Laver

Nori, various species of the genus *Porphyra*, is a red sea vegetable usually sold dried and pressed into sheets. Unlike other sea vegetables, which are generally collected wild from the sea, Japanese nori is cultivated. The traditional cultivation process begins in early autumn. Bamboo poles are sunk into the muddy bottoms of shallow inlets at low tide. Rope nets are strung on these poles, the rope being wound of a special braid that encourages spore attachment and facilitates harvesting. Then spores are scattered over the water. From late November to March the ripe nori is taken from the nets by hand: bundled-up farmers release the nori and it falls into wicker baskets. This fresh nori is washed and chopped into small fragments, which are stirred in a vat. A dipper ladles measured amounts onto porous bamboo mats. Any excess liquid drains away, leaving only nori fragments. These are spread out evenly on the mat and then the whole lot is hung on racks to dry. The thin sheets of nori which result are removed from the mats, folded, and packaged for market.

Although the basic process has remained the same,

modern technological innovations have been introduced. The nets are supported by floats rather than poles; giant ''vacuum cleaners'' harvest the fronds, and other machinery has made the process less labor-intensive.

In Ireland, porphyra species are known as *sloke* and in Scotland and Wales as *laver*. Gaelic people of the British Isles have long made flat breads from flour and porphyra. The resulting cakes are known as laver bread. Wild nori, harvested off the coast of Maine and on the Pacific coast, is sold dried for use as a vegetable side dish or condiment. In the Far East nori is also boiled to produce a gel in cooking, but most often it is wrapped around rice balls, used for sushi, or lightly toasted and cut into strips for garnishes. High-quality nori possesses a deep color and brilliant luster, while lesser-quality nori is dull and flat. Nori is exceptionally high in vitamin A and protein. It also contains other vitamins, minerals, and trace elements.

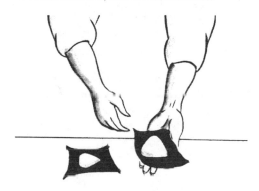

Nori sheets are used to wrap rice balls.

Sea Vegetables in the Kitchen

Here are a few basic but tasty recipes that will get people started using sea vegetables in the kitchen. One good experience with a delicious sea vegetable dish will lead to a desire for another. The sea vegetables themselves will teach you how they should be cooked.

The sea vegetables in order of easiest to hardest to cook are dulse, Irish moss, wakame or alaria, and kombu. Gentle boiling will be enough for the first two; stronger, more prolonged boiling for wakame or alaria; and either strong, longtime cooking, or pressure-cooking for kombu. Sauteing kombu first also helps. In general, the standard natural foods cooking methods of steaming, boiling, pressure cooking, sauteing, and tempura will allow us to cook any sea vegetable—the entire spectrum will open up.

For a full-fledged treatment of the cooking of sea vegetables, I recommend *The Seavegetable Book* by Judith Madlener (Crown, 1977) or any of the macrobiotic cookbooks by Cornelia Aihara, who uses a lot of sea vegetables in her cooking. (Maybe that's because she goes out to the ocean and gathers them herself.)

Red Kidney Beans with Kombu

1 cup red kidney beans
2 medium-sized fronds of dried kombu
2 medium-sized carrots
1 large onion

Soak the kombu and beans separately for one hour before cooking. Pour off the water from soaking beans, add six cups of fresh water, and put into a pressure cooker without the top on or into an enameled

cooking pot over high heat. Cut reconstituted kombu into rather large pieces and add to the cooking beans. Chop up carrots and onion and add. If you are using a pressure cooker, after the beans have boiled for ten minutes, put the top on and pressure cook for 45 minutes. If using enameled pot, cook over a lower flame for 1½ hours. In either case, at the end add sea salt or shoyu to taste and cook ten minutes longer. Serves six.

If you have trouble eating beans because of gas or because your beans often come out starchy, then this recipe, which eliminates both those problems, is for you. The glutamic acid of the kombu efficiently breaks down the starch in the beans while its alkaline minerals neutralize the sulfur in them that is the chief culprit in the formation of gas.

Dulse/Shoyu Broth

1¹/₂ quarts water
²/₃ cup of dried dulse
4 medium-sized scallions
shoyu
1 lemon

Begin heating the water in a soup pot. Then chop dulse or tear it up with your fingers and add to the water. Chop scallions, keeping the white part separate from the green, and add the white part to the water. Add shoyu to taste or until a clear, light-brown color is obtained. Add one-half of the green part of the scallions and allow broth to gently boil for five minutes longer. Squeeze the lemon and add the juice to the soup. Chop the remaining green scallion tops finely and when the soup is served, add as a garnish. Serves six.

Besides being simple and easy to make, this broth is beautiful in appearance and very tasty. It is especially satisfying in the spring and summer.

Lettuce/Wakame/Orange Salad

3 medium-sized fronds of dried
wakame
1 medium-sized head of lettuce
1 large bunch of red radishes
3 oranges

Soak the wakame until reconstituted, cut into salad-sized pieces and boil in water for ten minutes. Drain and allow to cool. Either cut or shred lettuce into salad-sized pieces and put into a salad bowl. Chop radishes. Combine wakame, lettuce, and radishes in salad bowl. Peel two of the oranges, cut them into small chunks, and add to the salad. Squeeze the other orange. Add a few pinches of sea salt to the juice and pour it over the salad as a dressing, then mix. Serves four to six.

This small riot of color is accompanied by a similar riot of taste. For some reason, oranges combine well with sea vegetables, particularly wakame. Dulse or sweet kombu may be substituted for the wakame.

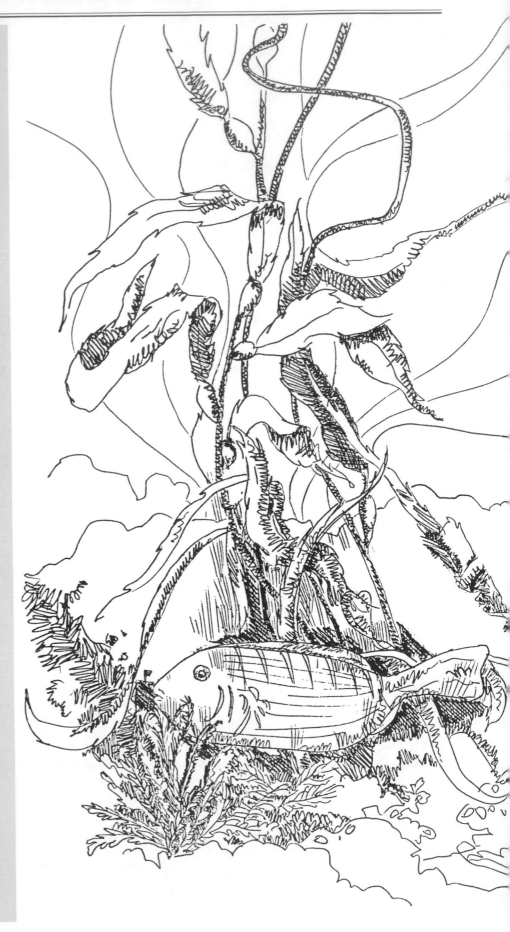

6. LABELING & STANDARDS

Recently, more than twenty national consumer organizations formed a coalition for an odd purpose: to urge the Council of Better Business Bureaus to *ignore* the Federal Trade Commission! At issue was a voluntary program aimed at halting deceptive advertisements. The Council, which annually reviews more than 100 national advertising campaigns in response to complaints by consumers and local Better Business Bureaus, often obtains voluntary agreements from advertisers to modify or discontinue deceptive ads. In an annual meeting of the Better Business Bureaus, the chairman of the FTC felt it was necessary to tell the Council, "You have become a powerful regulator" and warned the group "to resist the temptation to overregulate." Consumer groups then had to urge the Better Business Bureaus not to go along with the FTC's new laissez-faire approach to regulating deceptive ads.

Obviously, when the very agency that is supposed to be most concerned with the job of protecting consumers from fraudulent product claims becomes a spokesperson for benign neglect of that job, shoppers must take on more responsibility for determining the truth and falsity of advertising and packaging claims. This is especially true for consumers of natural foods, since some of the companies may be transient or so small as to easily slip through regulatory attention. Buzzwords are tossed about casually, chief among them "natural" and "organic," and food labels may include unfamiliar ingredients and terms. Determining what level of standards has been applied to any particular food can be a confusing task.

The stories that will follow in this chapter hopefully will begin to make this task easier for you. First we take a look at a very commendable movement underway in the natural foods industry: the efforts to develop procedures for certifying when fresh produce or other products are really organic. Definitions and standards for organic foods are still being worked out, but the many certifying agencies in operation and being planned are encouraging signs for concerned consumers. Also in this chapter, we offer some pointers for reading a food label and deciphering the small print, and define some of the more common additives that might be found even in natural foods. We've also included information to help you evaluate the many natural sweets on the market today—especially the increasingly popular frozen dairy-free desserts. Hopefully, a little self-education won't cause the FTC to become worried about *your* powers!

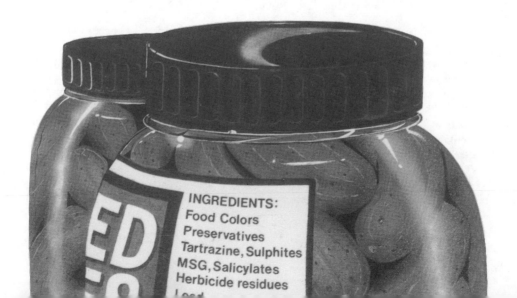

INGREDIENTS:
Food Colors
Preservatives
Tartrazine, Sulphites
MSG, Salicylates
Herbicide residues

"Yes, But Is It *Really Organic?*"

A veteran produce buyer for a major San Francisco natural foods outlet says he's heard some pretty diverse definitions of organic food. "One farmer," says Rainbow Grocery's Stuart Fishman, "told me his onions were organic because they grew in dirt. Another said he felt he could use any chemical he wanted as long as his soil fertility increased. That meant, I guess, that if he got a soil test and it showed his nitrogen and phosphorus content were up, he could call his crop organic.

"I had a supplier tell me organic meant 'no DDT.' And an orange grower believed that since he sprayed simazine between his trees instead of directly on them, his oranges were organic."

In the infancy of the modern-day organic food movement, it was not uncommon, Fishman says, for a crop to be called organic based on "rumors and the farmer's 'good vibes.'" And it probably didn't hurt if a grower tied his hair back into a ponytail.

Today the organic food industry works hard to police its trade and it takes more than rumors to merit an organic label in most natural foods stores. Yet many of the problems of certifying organic foods persist. Eager to sell their produce at premium prices, some farmers and retailers invent their own definition of organic. Few laws restrict organic labeling and where they do, enforcement is almost unheard of.

Organic growers throughout this and other countries worry about their product's reputations. To shore up the credibility of organic foods, members of the trade have formed certification agencies that define organic standards and certify those farms that meet them. At least three dozen such agencies operate in the U.S. and Canada under names and acronymns that for the most part are familiar only to a small percentage of natural foods shoppers—CCOF in California; Eden in Michigan; Tilth in Washington and Oregon; FVO in Connecticut; OCIA in Pennsylvania; Bear Creek in Wisconsin, to name a few.

Certification, though, is no snap answer to all of organic farming's problems. For one thing, it's costly. Different groups still disagree on what an organic farm should be. Neither can they concur on the best way to certify—by inspecting the farm or by testing the foods. Some even think certification is the wrong short-term goal, that the emphasis should be on helping chemical-dependent farmers move *toward* an organic system, which may take years to reach. Some worry that certification might squeeze out transition farmers who find their high-priced uncertified crop outsold by cheaper chemical food and by fully certified organic items. Transition farmers are the future of the organic movement, after all.

Eyeing all this carefully are corporate market researchers who could at any time decide to unveil their version of organic food for a purity-hungry public. Unfortunately, when organic growers themselves cannot agree upon a definition of organic, it's doubtful that the "organic" labels of food processing giants would be that meaningful. If Stuart Fishman cringes at the various definitions he's heard, he might find that organic labels turned loose in the supermarkets of America, like the word "natural" has been, would set new standards for labeling doubletalk.

Organic Nerve Gas?

When few laws govern the use of "organic" on labels, who's to say what's organic? Beginning chemistry students learn that organic compounds simply contain carbon derived from a living organism. Organic matter, says the *Encyclopedia Britannica*, includes many naturally occurring substances in varying stages of alteration, from decaying vegetation to crude oil. Organic phosphorus compounds, which contain molecules with at least one atom each of carbon and phosphorus, include certain insecticides (for instance, Malathion™) and chemical warfare agents (nerve gases).

Few agronomists would have the nerve to do so, but it's

possible to stand behind the specious reasoning that everything in nature is natural, or organic, if it even exists, and that whatever we extract from the earth or can manufacture from its raw materials traces its origins to living, organic matter. Anti-ecologists have been known to hide behind one form or another of that logic.

Before the organic movement, the term "organic" in farming referred to the presence in soil of large amounts of decomposed, soil-enriching plant material, or humus. Dr. Rudolph Ballentine wrote in *Diet and Nutrition* (Himalayan Publishers, 1978) that in nonorganic soils, fertility is supplied by manufactured chemical compounds, like potash, nitrates, and phosphates—inorganic compounds that dissolve in water and are absorbed directly into plant roots independent of the soil's life systems, including its diverse microbial population.

Ballentine pointed out that these inorganic compounds, which farmers several decades ago began using extensively as fertilizers, are thought to diminish a plant's innate absorption powers, thereby forcing it to become dependent on synthetic chemical nutrients. Since these artificially nourished plants show less-than-normal resistance to insects and diseases (which is also the result of other factors such as monocropping), it's become necessary to spray insecticides and herbicides.

Crops that are merely unsprayed are sometimes incorrectly called organic, regardless of the soil condition in which they grow. Many unsprayed crops, however, are grown on weakened, artificially fed soil. People who assume that organic foods must look pale and bug-eaten don't realize that plants raised in healthy soil are decidedly more appetizing than those which are not.

Certification—
A Comparison

Farmers laying some claim to organic methods remain nearly a non-factor in American farming—totaling roughly 40,000 farms out of a total 2.4 million. Organic farms produce $100 million worth or crops annually out of a total $150 billion. Many of these 40,000 farms have adopted just one or a few ecologically sound practices. It's estimated that less than 5,000 meet the standards of one of the three dozen certifying agencies in this country and Canada.

These agencies are mostly regional trade associations that offer farmers a crop certification program as well as help in shifting from chemical-intensive to organic methods. Standards for their certifications vary, but a critical requirement often is the implementation of a soil-building program, including composting, rotation, and green manuring. Other standards evolve to suit local regulations, regional attitudes, or immediate business needs. For instance, the length of time that the land must be free of fertilizers and pesticides may range from one to several years. Or the method for verifying whether a farm meets organic standards can be a perfunctory agreement signed by the farmer or it might include a rigorous on-site inspection by an independent panel of farmers and consumers.

In 1984, members of the organic community met in Toronto and decided that the variety of certifying standards, combined with today's huge interregional shipments of crops, necessitated their agreement on a minimal standard and a seal of approval that retailers, distributors, and consumers everywhere could recognize as a trusted organic label. Out of that meeting emerged the Organic Food Producers Association of North America, or OFPANA.

OFPANA seeks to become the certifier of certifiers. In February 1986, its members met in southern California to discuss the guidelines to which a certification group must adhere to gain OFPANA endorsement. These guidelines cover both organic standards and verification procedures.

OFPANA may seem presumptuous in setting trade standards for a whole continent, but its support is broad—among its 3,000 members are numerous industry leaders. One is Michael Marcolla, whose family in 1947 founded Mercantile Development, Inc., of Westport, Connecticut, a diversified international company which began distributing organic products through its natural foods division in 1979. MDI formed Farm Verified Organic (FVO) to monitor and certify the quality of organic products that it exports to Western Europe. Today FVO operates a certifying program for many MDI organic foods grown on over 100 farms.

Marcolla probably wouldn't complain if FVO became the country's foremost certification agent, but he endorses OFPANA (he's its treasurer) and recognizes the need for it. When distributors throughout the U.S. buy from California farmers, they might find the boxes marked, "Organically grown in accordance with Section 26569.11 of the California Health and Safety Code," a statement required by California law in order to make an organic claim. But California's law probably doesn't meet all the regional standards (legal and otherwise) throughout the country. And people certainly don't have the time to become familiar with California's and other states' laws.

OFPANA's objective is to unify the many certifying agencies with an agreement on minimal organic requirements. By introducing a universal seal to the public, OFPANA hopes to gain public confidence in organic labeling. It will not be easy, however, trying to get a consensus from the various regional groups, each having its own philosophical and sometimes legal standards. So far, four states have passed legislation and about six more are developing some, so the complexity of trying to standardize organic principles is only going to increase.

A comparison of FVO's standards with those of California Certified Organic Farmers (CCOF) illustrates the difference among certifiers. FVO maintains a ten-point check list of requirements, summarized as follows:

- Soils must be treated according to standards for at least three years.
- No chemically fortified soil-enrichment ingredients.
- Rotation required for annual crops.
- Insect control limited to predatory insects, insect disease cultures, and attractants.
- Weed control by crop rotation or by hand cultivation.
- Rodent control only with rodents' natural enemies, repellents and traps.
- Fungal and bacterial disease controlled without chemically fortified ingredients.
- Drying done naturally or at temperatures no greater than 160° Farenheit.
- During storage, only diatomaceous earth (composed of algae cell walls) allowed for fumigation.
- All production must meet USDA and FDA standards and all applicable state organic codes.

CCOF's 200 certified farms must meet the minimum requirements of California's organic farming law, which covers both vegetable and animal products. While most organic farmers think the 1982 California statute has provided badly needed order to the state's organic farming industry, some see it as a compromise bill. Among its requirements are the following:

- No synthetically compounded fertilizers, pesticides, or growth regulators.
- A twelve-month abstention from synthetics from time of planting.
- Only materials extracted solely from plant, animal, or mineral-bearing rock substances may be applied.

Certain exceptions are allowed, such as Bordeaux mixes, soaps, and detergents. (The use of Bordeaux mixes—copper sulfate and lime fungicides—is one of the controversial California compromises.) Other provisions also reflect a more lenient policy. Pesticide residues are permitted in amounts up to ten percent of EPA tolerance levels, mainly to accommodate farmers whose crops pick up neighbors' drifting sprays. Also, production of the seeds from which organic foods are grown is unrestricted, thus allowing seed fumigation.

CCOF's standards are not identical to the California code (CCOF requires a soil-building program, which California law does not), but their certification requirements approximate this somewhat permissive law.

The backbone of most certification programs is an inspection and enforcement procedure. FVO and CCOF both ask farmers for data about their land and farming methods, including fertilizer programs, rotations, irrigation, soil building, pest control, and land history. If the farm qualifies and if a soil test is acceptable, a farm visit is then scheduled.

Responsibility for CCOF's farm inspection rests with its

separate chapters, which are autonomous units made up of at least three farmers bound by the CCOF state constitution. All chapters devise their own certification procedures, but they must meet the minimum CCOF state requirements: an annual on-site inspection performed by a member of the chapter's certification committee; an annual soil test to verify the maintenance of humus; and, when a questionable or hazardous condition exists, a chemical analysis of soil, water, or plant products.

CCOF's chairman of state certification standards, Eric Gliessman, says one of CCOF's shortcomings is the inconsistency of its inspection procedures. Even though all chapters (there are now ten) must follow state rules, Gliessman feels that "the farm visit should be standardized. Now we have variation with the chapters."

Gliessman also admits that no attempt is made now to routinely test whether a farm is within the ten percent residue allowance level. "The expense of doing that," says Gliessman, "is prohibitive."

FVO's verification includes on-site inspection by regional farm groups who work under FVO's appointed consultants. Where farm groups aren't established, FVO may enlist the help of another regional certifier like CCOF. The on-site inspection report is then studied by FVO's five-member "Independent Evaluation Panel," comprised of farmers, consumer representatives, and an outside consultant. FVO, like CCOF, performs residue testing whenever a problem is suspected.

Packing Organic Food in Chemical Cardboard

Some people think certifying programs should rely more on residue testing. By testing foods for specific chemical residues, an examiner theoretically can get reliable evidence of a farmer's compliance. Also, one might learn if farmland is picking up drifting sprays, or blowover.

If an on-site examiner is somewhat inexperienced at spotting signs of chemical use, or is biased, then the residue test may indeed be more reliable. But when inspectors know what to look for, they might learn more. FVO's Marcolla, who selectively employs residue testing when on-site data is inconclusive, says, "If, in a twenty-acre field, one strip is clean as a whistle, is it because of blowover or is it a section that the insects just didn't reach? Insects usually begin infestation at the edge of a field, so a clean strip there suggests blowover, whereas one in the center of the field might mean the insects simply hadn't made it to that point." Residue tests cannot make judgments like that.

Ken McMullen, vice president of OFPANA, agrees that if you know what to look for, a farm visit is an invaluable verification tool. "I can tell a lot from the equipment the farmer uses," McMullen says, "and the way the land is laid out. I've done enough farming myself to be able to spot things and ask the right questions."

McMullen also is aware of the limits of on-site inspections. Toxic substances can find their way into food at many points along the journey from soil to dinner table. "Often the farmer is not the guilty one," he says. "It could be the shipper or packager or the processor. At every stage of handling, each party with control over a product must protect it from spoiling. If, for instance, the hopper cars used by shippers carry fumigated foods in addition to organic ones, traces of the fumigants may be picked up by the organic stock. Also, in storage areas, cockroaches and mice are often controlled with toxic substances. Or packagers introduce preservatives to the cardboard to increase shelf life. The farmer has no control over these things, and may not even know they are done."

Even if food is protected from contaminants until it reaches the store, store employees can mix up organic and nonorganic foods. "We need to examine the whole food chain," says McMullen, "from the soil to the plate."

Another loophole in on-site inspection is the possibility that a farmer will deliver crops not grown on the farmer's land, the land that has been certified. If a farmer has a bad crop, he or she could ask a neighbor for help in filling a contract. Of course, certification agencies disallow such a practice, but on-site verification can do nothing to prevent this abuse. Residue testing might.

An Oakland, California company has recently begun the most comprehensive residue testing program ever. Ohlone (pronounced "oh low knee") is a small food distributor named after a tribe of Northern California Native Americans. Stan Rhodes, the founder of Ohlone, holds a Ph.D. in chemistry and has twelve years' experience in the organic foods business. He explains that Ohlone will rate foods based on the results of two categories of testing—one for residues of pest control substances and the other for nutritional content. Ohlone will screen for all classes of pesticides, as well as for toxic metals, fumigants, and other chemicals.

A sample from every crop will be tested. Ohlone spokesperson Linda Brown contends that the federal government today tests just 3 percent of products for sale, and 3 percent of those are found contaminated or rejectable, meaning that a significant amount of the food reaching supermarkets fails to meet the EPA's already lax standards.

Ohlone products will carry a silver or gold label. To qualify for the silver label, a food must have toxic residues no greater than one-tenth of the current EPA tolerance levels. Ohlone will test for major vitamins and minerals one expects to find in the food. If a food's weighted nutritional index is superior—greater than 100 percent (of exposed amounts)—and its pesticide levels are one-one-hundredth or less of EPA tolerance, it will get a gold label. Consumers, says Rhodes, will receive detailed point-of-purchase information on key nutrients and pesticides for each crop of food.

Such a program could have great public appeal—people love to shop comparatively—but skeptics have questions.

They say residue testing does not directly address soil-building, which organic farmers consider the cornerstone of sustainable agriculture. According to Eric Gliessman, "some sprays break down on the plant [and tests won't show them], but the soil still picks them up. A good chemical farmer knows when to stop using the sprays so they aren't picked up by the fruits and vegetables. But they still enter the soil. The entire ecology is affected, to say nothing of the farmers who use the chemicals."

Rhodes answers that if a product scores well in both the residue and nutrition tests, it's very likely the soil is healthy. "We've found that farmers using these substances drastically downgrade the nutrition of the foods. So it's true, the soil is degraded. But in the process the nutrition of the food is compromised." Rhodes says that a farmer raising a gold label Ohlone food will, by necessity, have maintained high-quality soil.

Another question is how conclusive residue tests can be. Marcolla says, "In Germany we were required to test for DDT. We spent a great deal of time and money testing for various hydrocarbons, and it became confusing. The differences between the organic and the nonorganic weren't so clear-cut. DDT, it was found, was everywhere." Presumably Ohlone's test instruments can distinguish between moderate and very slight toxicity (which is the basis of its service). Nevertheless, it's unknown whether scientific tests can capably judge all aspects of a food's value.

Finally, residue testing's biggest drawback may be the cost. Most everyone in the certification business says that the tests are too expensive to be widely practical. Brown and Rhodes both reply, however, that the program will be "consumer driven" and will add an average of just pennies to retail costs. Brown says studies show that consumers are willing to pay more for substantiated organic foods. In May, Rhodes announced that the program was ready to begin with the initial participation of twenty-five growers and ten stores.

The Public's Role

The costs for any certification, either residue testing or on-site inspection, will be felt by shoppers. CCOF presently operates on a meager $15,000 annual budget, which it collects from farmers who pay one-half of one percent of revenues. But CCOF now runs almost solely on volunteer labor. (Gliessman contributes up to twenty hours a week to CCOF, after the sixty or more he toils in his own fields.)

If certification is ever to become widespread, workers must earn salaries to administer the programs. Put another way, the store prices must support them. So far, organic foods haven't appealed to more than a small fraction of Americans. Perhaps peoples' reluctance to buy organic products stems from the uncertainty of uncertified foods, combined undoubtedly with their higher costs. (Some organic farmers are showing that it can be less expensive to farm organically, but so far the distribution of most organic products is too limited to compete with chemical-intensive farming.) It remains to be seen which factor might be depressing public interest in organic foods more—disbelief that they're truly organic, or the high cost.

This brings to mind the possibility that big corporations might soon test the organic waters. Leaders in the organic movement say that large grocery store chains are now making inquiries. With its economies of scale and efficient distribution networks, a chain of stores could certainly sell cheaper than distributors of organic products have so far. Such stores would need, however, a greater supply of organic crops than is now produced. They would need to contract with farmers whom they might ask to grow crops that are somewhere between organic and all-out chemical. This possibility concerns those in the organic industry. They feel these foods will simply be called organic even though the farmland from which they'll be taken will be anything but sustainable.

It's reminiscent, they say, of the way "natural" foods swamped the supermarkets. Once people learned that whole grains and fiber and other foods in their natural form were healthy to eat, food companies pushed "natural" up and down the aisle of every grocery store in the land, even when ingredients in these products often were about as natural as plastic.

Despite fears of organic principles becoming adulterated, many conscientious farmers today subscribe to something less than a gold label organic philosophy. On Integrated Pest Management farms, for example, growers try to use natural insect controls by timing their planting to miss the insects' life cycles or by introducing the pests' natural enemies. As a last resort, however, they will use synthetic chemicals. They also use some chemical fertilizers—what they must to produce a crop and stay in business.

The goal of sustainable agriculturists is to regenerate healthy soil on farms where no synthetic fertilizers are needed and where plant resistance to pests and diseases is high. Dr. Garth Youngberg, executive director of the Institute for Alternative Agriculture in Beltsville, Maryland,

shares this goal. Youngberg is well known in organic farming circles as the man who struggled in the Department of Agriculture during the Carter administration for passage of organic farming legislation, only to see his efforts fail and his position topple when the Reagan administration came in. (The 1985 farm bill has provisions for organic farming research, which Youngberg says is an exciting and encouraging development.) Youngberg's enthusiasm for lofty organic goals is tempered somewhat by the need, he says, "to build bridges."

"How do we establish organic farming in the minds of [mainstream] farmers?" Youngberg asks. "This is what we're trying to do [at the Institute]. Some farmers are not looking to become certified organic farmers, but instead to simply cut back on chemical-intensive practices because they're so expensive. For some, just to put a hay crop or a legume into rotation is a big chance and can make a difference. It's a beginning."

Youngberg and certification groups are not at odds, by any means. They're pushing in the same direction, and most certifiers in fact give lots of help to farmers who want to switch but who aren't sure how to start.

In the final analysis, it's likely that the meaning of "organic" will remain fuzzy for quite some time. Stan Rhodes says, "We cannot look at this as a black and white thing. We need to see it as a continuum." There are, and will continue to be, foods that are more organic than others. And the public, therefore, will continue to face decisions—whether to pay more for food that claims to be organic—and whether to believe the claims. But instead of shunning organic products altogether, out of frustration over misrepresentation, what shoppers can do to promote sane agriculture is to buy organic products and insist that stores furnish documentation to back up the organic claims. Buying from stores that have taken the trouble to verify the representations made by organic growers will be a vote for a sustainable future. An active, insistent public will do more to crystallize the meaning of organic farming and promote its goal than anything else.

How to Read a Food Label

Deciphering the Small Print Can Be a Healthful Habit

Mitch Mainstream pulls up to his local supermarket with visions of constructing the perfect strawberry shortcake. Scanning the shelves for a topping, he spies Creme-O brand "whipped dessert product." "Contains real cream!" the label manages to promise with a straight face. Perfect. Into the shopping basket it goes. Not till Mitch is well into his second helping of dessert does he happen to glance at the list of ingredients in Creme-O. Oh, it has real cream, all right. But that's the only natural ingredient to be found. The remaining emulsifiers, artificial colors, thickeners, and synthetic flavors are enough to stock a small chemistry set. Mitch does a slow burn. He's been had.

Halfway across town, Polly Progressive has just bicycled over to her local natural foods store. Polly generally avoids supermarkets, placing her trust in the deep down honesty of whole foods. Today she's in a mood to experiment. So when she spots a package of Tofu Tasties, "the delicious meatball substitute," she can't wait to pedal home to give them a try. Poor Polly. Had she read the fine print, she would have realized that her ersatz meatballs contained whole wheat bread crumbs, brown rice, vegetables, spices—and not a speck of real tofu. Soy isolate, the protein portion of soybeans, was as close as it got to the food Polly presumed she was buying.

You wouldn't expect it, but whole foods devotees sometimes face the same difficult buying decisions as shoppers with more conventional tastes. There's but one way for those of us at the point of sale to know what's inside a box, bag, or can of food: the label. Regardless of how natural the food is, some labels serve as accurate representations of what lies within, disclosing every ingredient and even offering nutrition data to help health-minded consumers plan a sound diet. Others fall considerably short of telling the whole story, omitting ingredients, using euphemisms for chemical additives that might alienate shoppers, and tossing around words like "natural' and "organic" with all the dignity and restraint of a used-car salesman.

Thus, labels can mystify and even mislead as often as they inform. And for the typical shopper, a stroll through a natural foods store can give rise to all sorts of questions.

How much salt can be in soy sauce for it to be called "low sodium"? If a whole wheat bread maker adds the barest trace of a preservative to increase shelf life, is it all right not to list it on the label? When a box of sesame crackers claims "all natural ingredients," does it mean they are unprocessed? Grown without pesticides? Not synthesized in a lab? Some of the above? None of the above?

The key to knowing precisely what a label is and isn't telling you is understanding the art, the business, and a little bit of the law behind modern food labeling.

Naturally Unclear

Where would food marketers be these days without the word "natural"? A lot less rich, for one thing. Marketing professionals have studied the surveys that show anywhere from 60–75 percent of Americans perceive natural foods as nutritionally superior to and safer than processed foods. Food manufacturers know that America's romantic fixation with simpler, less complicated lifestyles is being manifested in changing diets: more whole grains, fresh fruit and vegetables, poultry and fish; less salt, sugar, fat, red meat, and chemical additives. But most of all, they realize that good nutrition—even the semblance of good nutrition—pays. Half the respondents in one poll said they would be willing to pay 10 percent extra for a natural food. That can add up to quite a sum.

And so we find modern-day food packages festooned with "natural" claims: "natural ingredients," "natural flavors," "natural colors." Occasionally things get a little out of hand. One brand of chicken frankfurters claims to be "made only with ground natural spices," and sugar is now being promoted as a "natural sweetener."

If you haven't guessed it already, the little known truth about the word "natural" is that it is virtually meaningless. The Vermont cheddar in your natural foods store probably has a strong case for a "natural" label, but Kraft is using the same word successfully and without federal challenge to promote Cheez Whiz and Velveeta, two foods

Monosodium Glutamate

Monosodium glutamate is a naturally occurring form of glutamic acid, an amino acid, that is extracted from certain vegetables and grains. It is long famous for gracing Asian dishes with a special brand of crystalline magic. Virtually every expert you talk with agrees that MSG adds a certain "zing" to many foods. But hardly anyone agrees on how the spice actually works.

The MSG industry claims that MSG replaces the glutamates in food that are lost during storage, processing, and cooking. This theory, though, does not explain why MSG enhances the taste of chicken, which unlike other foods loses no natural glutamates.

Other food chemists think MSG joins with other chemicals and magnifies them. With MSG, one expert told *The New York Times*, "More messages go to the brain." But that doesn't fully explain why MSG works with some foods (meat, poultry, fish, and vegetables) but not with others (sweet, acidic, or dairy foods).

A third contingent says MSG brings an entirely new fifth taste to the human palate, adding to the well-known quartet of sweet, sour, salty, and bitter. This explanation is favored by the Japanese, who early in this century isolated MSG from sea vegetables. The Japanese call this fifth taste "unami."

In China, where MSG is known as *wei ching* or *wei chen* ("essence of taste"), many chefs recommend that the spice be used sparingly if at all. Overdoing it makes all the flavors in a dish taste the same. Besides, the high sodium content and the unpleasant allergy-like reactions of MSG-sensitive diners make it prudent for cooks to rely on the colorful flavors of the food itself.

that are so highly processed they don't even meet the federal government's definition of cheese.

Back in the late 1970s, attorneys at the Federal Trade Commission (FTC), the agency that polices advertising claims, tried to nail down a reasonable definition of what constituted a natural food, finally deciding on the twin criteria of minimal processing and lack of artificial additives. But after three years of staff work, FTC's commissioners abandoned the regulation before it was adopted, claiming the issue was too complex. While even food industry experts did indeed disagree on such crucial questions as how much processing qualifies as "minimal," many people who were closely involved with the effort believe the rule was dropped for political reasons. Dr. Kate Clancy, a former FTC nutritionist, said, "The people who came to the FTC in 1980 made it clear that they didn't want to regulate food claims of any kind. To them, any amount of regulation was overregulation."

Thanks to the FTC cave-in, "natural" and terms such as "organic" and "health food" have no legal meaning, leaving food companies to use them however they wish. FTC chairman James Miller says even Coca-Cola could probably be labeled natural and organic.

The Food and Drug Administration, the arm of the government that oversees the composition and labeling of foods, also uses little of its formidable clout when it comes to regulating healthful-sounding label claims. FDA's policy is so generous ("something clearly synthesized in a lab can't be labeled natural," one spokesman explained) that in recent years, the agency has taken action against only two products for making an unfounded "natural" claim.

The sad truth is that, at least for the time being, the words "natural" and "organic" are no guarantee that a product has been minimally processed, contains no artificial ingredients, or has indeed been grown organically.

There are efforts underway within segments of the food industry to create more effective self-regulating policies with regard to these terms, but it is always a good idea to check the ingredient list to make sure a food's lofty image has a firm footing in reality.

A Tale of Two Labels

The federal government has devised a fairly elaborate labeling system that's designed to enable consumers to make intelligent, informed food purchases. It works like this.

Let's say you're at the breakfast table one morning facing the same old bowl of cereal when you suddenly get a flash of inspiration to market a new breakfast product: a fruit and whole grain cereal for joggers called Crunchy Runnola. You scurry about the kitchen in a creative frenzy, selecting just the right ingredients for your new taste treat, and when it comes out of the oven all fragrant and toasty brown, a sure winner, you turn your attention to a label.

First, you'll need to have an *ingredient label*, listing the ingredients in descending order by weight: oats, wheat germ, honey, rice bran, sunflower seeds, corn oil, dates, dried apricots, sea salt. You can be as descriptive as you want with the ingredients as long as you stay within the truth. Instead of just plain oats, for example, you can use "organic, steel-cut oats," which sounds more impressive. Since the words "organic" and "natural" have no established definition, you might want to set aside space on the label to explain how you are using them. One chain of natural foods stores defines its products as "100% natural with no additives, preservatives, refined sugars, hydrogenated oils, artificial colorings, or artificial flavorings." Your definition may coincide with this one or differ; it's up to you as the manufacturer.

Aside from listing the ingredients, you may have to

declare certain information about Runnola's nutritive value. Under current laws, if you make a nutrition claim or if you add any vitamin, mineral, or protein to a product, you have to include a *nutrition label*. This gives a breakdown of seven vitamins and minerals (vitamins A and C, thiamine, riboflavin, niacin, calcium, and iron, in that order), calories, protein, carbohydrate, and total fat per serving. These are mandatory. Other information—on sodium content, cholesterol, and saturated/unsaturated/polyunsaturated fat breakdown—is optional. So if you decide that your Runnola could use an added measure of vitamin C, or you want to mention on the label or in ads that the vitamin B₁ in Runnola's rice bran helps athletes convert carbohydrates to energy, you'll have to spring for a full (and relatively expensive) laboratory analysis.

Every ingredient that is deliberately added must be declared on the label, no matter how miniscule the amount. What's more, any substance that might have been added to a raw ingredient must also be mentioned. If the bright orange color of your dried apricots was preserved with sulfur dioxide, you've got to let customers know about it even if you didn't do the actual preserving.

There are various other requirements to abide by as well. Your label can claim that Crunchy Runnola is a "significant source" of a nutrient (say, protein or iron), but only if a single serving contains at least 10 percent of the Recommended Daily Allowance of the nutrient. This rather generous rule stops a manufacturer from deciding that 2 percent sounds significant. Individual manufacturers, do, however, establish the serving size, so you have a bit of leeway here.

And if you want to list the sodium content, FDA has special rules on how to go about it. In the unlikely event that a bowl of Runnola contains less than 5 mg of sodium, you can call it "sodium-free." If a serving has 35 mg or less, you can use the term "very low sodium." With 140 mg or less, "low sodium." If your product has at least 75 percent less sodium than comparable breakfast cereals, you can use "reduced sodium." These rules, which went into effect on July 1, 1985, do not force a manufacturer to list sodium levels, as some consumer advocates have urged. They do provide a set of working definitions for the roughly half of the food manufacturers who use nutrition labels, many when it's not required.

Now that you appreciate how complex a food label can be, you're probably longing for simplicity. "All I want to do is market my little Crunchy Runnola," you sniff. "Isn't there any way to avoid jumping through all these hoops?"

As a matter of fact, there is, but there's a catch. Because of a loophole, the FDA lets some foods slip through the federal dragnet without ingredient labels. (As we'll explore in detail below, anyone who makes a staple food from a standard recipe—mayonnaise, ketchup, canned vegetables, milk, ice cream, margarine, and some breads—doesn't have to list the ingredients. As a result, even whole wheat bread, that granddaddy of natural foods, can come onto the market bearing fourteen or more optional ingredi-

ents and additives, none of which have to be disclosed.*) Nor do you have to carry a nutrition label as long as you refrain from making health claims. Breakfast cereals aren't on the FDA's freebie list, but the agency says it will consider special requests for exemptions on a case-by-case basis.

Uncle Sam Writes a Recipe Book

By some accounts, the Chicago meat-packing houses immortalized so memorably in Upton Sinclair's 1906 novel *The Jungle* merely typified conditions throughout other sectors of the food industry. Everywhere, farmers were watering down milk; cheese makers were collecting moldy, unsold cheeses, grinding them up, heating them, and repackaging them as "processed"; coffee manufacturers were fashioning fake whole coffee beans out of sawdust.

To end some of the deception, the government stepped in with recipes called "standards of identity." Standards of identity are rules that define what can and cannot be in a product before it can be called a certain food. The standards set forth minimum levels of desirable ingredients and maximum levels of not-so-desirable ones. Raisin bread must by law contain at least 50 percent raisins by weight, while ice cream can have no more than .5 percent thickening agents.

Identity standards not only dictate quantity, but quality. The standard for canned pears describes an elaborate ripeness test that demands piercing the fruit with a rod attached to a 100-gram weight.

Standards of identity are also designed to prevent a manufacturer from passing off as a whole food one that has been highly processed. For instance, only plain orange juice with seeds and excess pulp removed can be called "orange juice." If the juice has been heated to kill microorganisms and boosted with concentrated orange juice, it must be called "pasteurized orange juice." "Orange juice from concentrate" means a once-frozen, reconstituted, and possibly pasteurized product to which frozen orange juice, orange oil, orange pulp, and sweeteners all may be added. With fruit juice as in other foods, the simpler the label designation, the more unprocessed the product.

---

*To whole wheat flour, bread makers can legally add the following types of ingredients without identifying them on the label: moistening ingredients (water, milk, and/or dairy products); yeast; salt; shortening, with or without lecithin and mono and diglycerides; egg products; sugar, corn syrup, or other sweeteners; "enzyme active preparations" that change starch into sugars; lactic-acid-producing bacteria; non-wheat flours (up to 3 percent); yeast nutrients and calcium salts (up to .25 percent); ground, dehulled soybeans (up to .5 percent); azodicarbonamide, a "flour-maturing" agent (up to .0045 percent); dough strengtheners and conditioners (up to .5 percent); spices, and "other ingredients that do not change the basic identity of the food."

Standards of identity obviously can't be written for each of the untold thousands of foods in commerce—the task would be overwhelming. So the FDA has stuck to 263 of the most popular items, a decision that has important implications for natural foods shoppers. A number of whole foods lie considerably outside the American mainstream. Thus there are no identity standards for soy products such as miso, tofu, tempeh, and tahini; sea vegetables like kelp, kombu, and dulse; meat alternatives; ice cream substitutes; unfiltered juices; unprocessed oils; and a host of others. And because there are no standards, consumers have very little protection against an unscrupulous manufacturer who may be selling a questionable food in a natural wrapper merely to cash in on the back-to-nature phenomenon. As things now stand, Bogus Foods, Inc. could market a soyburger that contains five soybeans and a lot of filler, with only an outside chance of being nabbed by the FDA.

The government has toyed with the idea of extending identity standards to natural foods, but the issue creates a minor furor in Washington every time it is brought up. The 17,000-member National Health Federation is one of several organizations that thinks such natural foods standards would be a mistake. A "health civil liberties" group, the N.H.F. argues that because foods with identity standards don't have to declare their ingredients, most manufacturers of those foods tend to use just enough of a given ingredient to satisfy the standard. If the law says wheat and soy macaroni has to contain at least 12.5 percent soy flour, rare is the manufacturer who will use more. That's the Federation's first objection—that the standards encourage lowest-common-denominator mediocrity.

Their second point has to do with consumer information. Without a clarifying label, shoppers would have no way of selecting the most nutritious macaroni even if a manufacturer did happen to use more than 12.5 percent soy flour.

Third, the Federation says standards of identity discourage innovation. Clinton Miller, president of the member-funded consumer group, puts it this way. "What if a soyburger had to contain 80 percent soybeans by law, and someone discovered that a patty made with 50 percent soybeans and 50 percent lima beans gave people a better overall mix of amino acids? Under the present law, they'd have to label it an artificial soyburger even though it was nutritionally superior." Miller says identity standards have prevented natural foods from gaining a foothold on the national market, citing a case where peaches sweetened with honey had to be labeled "imitation" because the standard for canned peaches allowed only sugar or corn syrup. "With that kind of label, those peaches just couldn't sell."

There are obvious solutions to the identity standards problem. The FDA could force all manufacturers to disclose all ingredients, along with both the amount used and the amount required by law, so consumers could judge for themselves a manufacturer's integrity. The agency could also certainly show greater flexibility in expanding the wording in its standards, such as allowing "sweeteners" in canned peaches instead of dictating only sugar or corn syrup.

The paucity of identity standards does mean shoppers must place a great deal of reliance on manufacturers, rather than Uncle Sam, to ensure that whole foods are indeed "whole." While many natural foods firms pursue their trade with integrity, some clearly do not. Labels can help you distinguish between the two.

Scrutinizing ingredient and nutrition labels can be a healthy habit. This helps take a great deal of the guesswork out of grocery shopping. Nutrition labels can help you translate product ingredients into the nutrients your body needs. They can also help you avoid those products high in fat, sodium, sugar, and other bad actors your body could do without. Natural foods generally contain far fewer chemical additives than processed foods, and many of the substances you will find on ingredient labels are quite safe. Use the accompanying glossary of terms to help decipher any ingredients that may be foreign to you.

INGREDIENTS

A Glossary of Common Food Additives

Unless otherwise noted, the following food additives are generally recognized as safe by the federal government and food researchers, at the levels of consumption common in the average American diet. Marked with asterisks (*) are those additives which some scientific research indicates it is best to avoid excessive consumption of during pregnancy. Also, in many cases full testing for chromosomal damage, birth defects, allergic reactions, interactions with other additives or food ingredients, and so forth, has yet to be completed.

Beet Powder. Dehydrated or powdered beets. Used as a food coloring.

Beta-Carotene. A naturally occurring source of vitamin A in fruits and vegetables; used as an orange or yellow food coloring.

Calcium Sulfate. A firming agent added to tomato products, canned vegetables, and other foods; also a dough conditioner for baked products and flours. Since it absorbs moisture and hardens quickly, it has been tied to intestinal obstruction in some people.

Carrageenan. A vegetable gum extracted from Irish moss, or carragheen, a sea vegetable found along the coasts of Canada, Maine, Britain, Scandinavia, and France. It emulsifies (prevents from separating) and thickens food products.

Citric Acid. A tart, strong acid present naturally in high concentration in fruits and berries. Commercial citric acid is made by using a fungus to ferment beet molasses; a small amount is also isolated from pineapple byproducts and from low-quality lemons. Citric acid is added to jellies and preserves, canned fruits and vegetables, carbonated beverages, fruit juice drinks, and other products as a fruit flavoring and adjuster of acid/base balance. Excess consumption may interfere with calcium absorption.

Fructose. A sugar naturally occurring in many fruits; as an additive, often derived from corn syrup and highly processed.

Locust Bean Gum (Carob Bean Gum). A substance extracted from the seed of the carob tree, an evergreen cultivated in Mediterranean countries. It is used to blend ingredients and to prevent ice cream, sauces, and salad dressings from separating; it also improves texture.*

Guar Gum. A complex sugar extracted from the seed of the guar plant, a legume similar to the soybean plant. It thickens frozen fruit and drinks. Found in baked goods, salad dressings, and dairy products.*

Gum Arabic. A tasteless, odorless, colorless dried gummy extract taken from the acacia tree, which is grown in Africa, the Near East, India, and southern United States. It thickens candy, helps dissolve citrus oils in drinks, thickens the texture of ice cream, and helps other food ingredients blend together smoothly. People prone to allergies may have reactions from gum arabic.*

Gum Tragacanth. The dried discharge from a wild shrub found in the Middle East. Used as a thickener and emulsifier in sherbets, salad dressings, and candy. The FDA classifies it as "generally recognized as safe" but it has been held responsible for occasional allergic reactions.*

Hydrolyzed Plant Protein (HPP), Hydrolyzed Vegetable Protein (HVP). Protein obtained by the chemical splitting of soybean or peanut meal or recovered when wheat and corn are milled. Most HPP and HVP come from soybeans. They are used as flavor enhancers and are sources of meat-like flavor in soup mixes, gravies, and chili. They are fairly high in sodium content.

Lactic Acid. As an additive, usually produced by chemical synthesis or through the bacterial fermentation of a carbohydrate such as corn sugar. Lactic acid is used to give tartness and flavor to some desserts and carbonated juices. It also conditions dough and stabilizes some wines.

Lecithin. A compound derived from the processing of soybeans, egg yolk, or corn; it breaks up fats and protects them from spoilage. Naturally present in many foods.

Pectin. Present in most plants, it is a type of fiber that gives strength to cell walls. Most commercial pectin is derived from citrus peels and the residue from apple pressings. Pectin is added to foods, ranging from jellies to ice cream, to thicken or blend them.

Sodium Bicarbonate (Baking Soda). Used as a leavening agent in baking powder and to lighten or raise dough in bakery products such as crackers, cookies, and prepared cake and muffin mixes. It is produced by reacting carbon dioxide with soda ash, a white powder sometimes extracted from sea water but more often produced commercially. Sodium bicarbonate is high in sodium (821 mgs per teaspoon).

Whey. The watery part of milk after its principal protein, casein, is removed. Whey can be processed to obtain lactose (milk sugar) or lactalbumin, an amino-acid-rich protein. Dried whey solids, found in ice cream, baked goods, and milk products, are 75 percent lactose and 13 percent lactalbumin.

RESOURCES

For more information on these and other food additives, the following reference books may be useful.

- Robert L. Berko, *Food Additives Explained*, Consumer Education Task Force Research Center (PO Box 336, South Orange, NJ 07079), 1983, 79 pp.
- Nicholas Freydberg and Willis Gortner, *The Food Additives Book*, Bantam Books, 1982, 717 pp.
- Michael F. Jacobson, *The Complete Eater's Digest and Nutrition Scoreboard*, Anchor Press/Doubleday, 1985, 392 pp.

Rating the Natural Sweets

Despite Their Image of Wholesomeness, Not All Natural Desserts and Snacks Are Healthful Foods

Sweets are virtually irresistible to most of us, no matter how many tugs of war they set off between appetite and conscience. Taking candy from a baby may be easy, but asking a grownup to give up carrot cake is a different matter altogether.

Enlightened eaters realize, of course, that sweets are studded with perils. Their two most villainous components—sugar and fat—are blamed for hundreds of thousands of cases of debilitating, sometimes fatal disease. Whether for health reasons or political ones many of us, seeking refuge from the hypersweet world of gruelingly overprocessed commercial desserts and snacks, have seized on natural sweets as a way to satisfy our cravings without sacrificing our principles. With their emphasis on whole grains and unrefined sweeteners, natural sweets enjoy a reputation of not only being less damaging to our health than those overprocessed commercial products, but of even making a positive contribution. Our perception of wholesomeness is more than just intuitive; advertisements straddling the theme "good food that's good for you" are *de rigueur* in the natural foods industry. But how well do whole grain cookies, ice cream substitutes, natural candy bars, and related delectables live up to their billing? What follows is an overview of some of the most popular natural sweets distributed nationally in the United States.

The Best Sweets Money Can Buy

No proper survey of commercial sweets can begin without mentioning one food that stands head and shoulders above the rest. If you're looking for a sweet that satisfies the most finicky nutritionists, stroll past the aisles of whole grain cookies and granola bars and on into the produce section.

The sugar in fruit is principally fructose, which, unlike sucrose (table sugar), in its natural form is absorbed by the body gradually enough to stave off the sharp rise in blood

sugar that often follows the consumption of refined sweets.

Refined sugar, whether from cane or from beets, is hard on the teeth, and it doesn't do much for the waistline. Some studies have shown a link between high sugar intake and an increase in blood fat and subsequent thickening of the arteries (arteriosclerosis). Refined sugars also lack the minerals and trace elements found in genuine raw sugar (that is, sugarcane juice with just the water evaporated out). Cane cutters in the South African province of Natal habitually chew sugarcane, but their teeth don't seem to suffer much, and diabetes is virtually unknown. Physicians have theorized that something in unrefined sugar juice (perhaps the mineral molybdenum) serves a protective function that's lost when sugar is refined.

It's the desire to cash in on precious nutrients that has natural foods shoppers reaching for snacks sweetened with honey or maple syrup. The fact is, though, most natural sweeteners offer little nutritional advantage. With the exception of molasses—the dark syrup left over when white sugar is extracted from sugarcane—none of the more popular sweeteners (honey, fructose, maple syrup, brown and turbinado sugar) provide more than the tiniest traces of vitamins and minerals. What they do provide is empty calories.

Rice syrup and barley malt, two grain sweeteners, do feature the advantage of being closer to whole foods than other sweeteners. They are produced when naturally occurring enzymes convert the starch in the grains to sugar. Rice syrup contains more vitamins than barley malt; it's also about 3 percent protein. But on the whole, neither product offers enough nutrients to be called truly nutritious. Grain syrups are only 70–80 percent sugar. They are also high in complex carbohydrates, which the body metabolizes more slowly than the simple sugars found in honey, maple syrup, and other products. According to Cheryl Mitchell, Ph.D., a sugar chemist with California Natural Products, these two factors explain why grain syrups cause less of a sugar high than other sweeteners.

As important as nutrition is, it's not the only thing at

stake when we mull over how snacks are sweetened. Geopolitical considerations take us far beyond the nutritional composition of sweeteners to the consideration of their origin. In many developing nations, cash crops such as sugarcane and cocoa have supplanted nutritious foods. The small farms that once supported the dietary need of much of the local population have become profitable plantations where multinational concerns employ local labor to produce luxury foods often priced beyond the reach of indigenous peoples. Honey, rice syrup, barley malt, and the like are generally produced here in the United States or are imported from Japan and other lands where the cash crop mentality hasn't led to such severe local trauma. Thus, while snacks featuring alternative sweeteners may be of no great nutritional boon, buying them can contribute in a small way to a more just global economy. (For more information, see "A Guide to Natural Sweeteners," page 177.)

When Is a Natural Sweet Unnatural?

In addition to considering the choice of sweetener used, there are other factors that should determine whether a product deserves to be called a "natural sweet." The term "natural" is loosely defined and recklessly used in the marketplace today. Market surveys repeatedly show that consumers prefer so-called natural foods to ones laden with chemicals and preservatives. Food companies of all stripes and sizes are jumping on the bandwagon, with mixed results for the consumer. Is a dessert product "natural," for instance, merely because it forgoes artificial flavors and colors? To what extent is the degree of processing or the ultimate healthfulness of its main ingredients important?

Take Haagen-Dazs ice cream, for example. Its ingredients say cleanness and simplicity: fresh cream, skim milk, pure honey, egg yolk, natural vanilla. But in your dish a half-cup serving translates into a tablespoon-sized dollop of honey and a whopping 17 grams of butterfat. That's one-quarter of the amount of fat an average adult should consume in an entire day, according to federal guidelines.

And then there are the obvious transgressions against the concept of natural sweets. For instance, nothing says "natural" like granola bars. Unless they're made by a large company like Quaker, that is. We counted thirty-four ingredients in Quaker's Chocolate, Graham, and Marshmallow Chewy Granola Bars, including artificial flavors, synthetic color (blue), and no less than seven sweeteners.

The Natural Sweets Hall of Fame

GLENNY'S BROWN RICE TREAT

The ads sound a bit too good to be true. Here's a snack that contains no added salt, honey, oils, or dairy products. It's "lower in fat than any other candy or nutrition bar in the world." Its ingredients are hypo-allergenic, and it uses a sweetener that breaks down during digestion more slowly than sugar, honey, or maple syrup.

Glenny's pulls off this minor miracle by sticking to just two ingredients: crisp brown rice and whole grain barley malt. That's how, when other snacks are singing the fat and sugar blues, Glenny's can market its products as "the macrobiotic snacks Japan wants from America."

BARBARA'S COOKIES

Barbara's claim to fame is a line of ten cookies sweetened only with concentrated fruit juices. Some seem positively packed with imaginative ingredients. For example, Barbara's Three-Fiber Bran Cookies feature whole wheat flour and wheat bran; soy oil, oats and raisins; pineapple, pear, and peach juices; apple and pea fiber; cinnamon, salt, and soda.

Barbara's products carry an occasional surprise. At 11 grams of fat per ounce, the peanut butter cookies are among the oiliest around. But when they're good, Barbara's cookies are great. We found several—Tropical Coconut, Oatmeal Raisin, and Fruit and Nut—that averaged just 2.5 grams of fat per ounce, a nice bonus to add to the assorted benefits of whole grains and natural fruit juices.

ARROWHEAD MILLS WHOLE GRAIN BRAN MUFFIN MIX

We were curious to see how this bran muffin mix stacks up against fresh-baked bran muffins from scratch, so we brought out the cookbooks. Where recipes in such fine cookbooks as *The Tassajara Bread Book*, *Laurel's Kitchen*, and *The Enchanted Broccoli Forest* call for one type of grain (wheat flour and wheat bran), Arrowhead Mills' mix goes two better with the addition of whole corn flour and whole soy flour. With the exception of sweet whey, a milk constituent that, according to the company, gives the muffins smoothness and body, the remaining ingredients (baking powder and sea salt) could be found in any kitchen. The suggested additions of oil, honey or molasses, an egg, and water gave the mix muffins nutrition comparable to all three home-baked versions, and the taste is fine as well.

JUST JUICE FROZEN BARS

Once in a while you run across a product that's so honest you want to hug it. Here's one. It's a frozen treat called Just Juice. What's in it? Just juice. Well, almost. Natural foods purists may object to the presence of a small amount of guar gum, a harmless vegetable-based thickener. But considering the kinds of ingredients one finds in mainstream sweets—not to mention some natural ones—things could be far worse.

Small natural food companies, no doubt aghast by the excesses of more commercial firms, often offer sweets that seem premised on a great respect for wholesomeness and integrity. One glance at the ingredient label is usually enough to unravel how these manufacturers go about creating their more healthful alternatives.

Take graham crackers. Nabisco makes a mainstream version; Health Foods, Inc. of Des Plains, Illinois markets a whole foods version under the label Mi-del. Nabisco uses a mix of enriched bleached flour and whole wheat (graham) flour. Mi-del uses 100 percent whole wheat. Nabisco's crackers get their sweetness mostly from white sugar, with ''corn sweetener'' (probably corn syrup) and some honey thrown in to justify the name ''Honey Maid.'' Mi-del uses honey and unsulfured molasses. Where Nabisco uses inexpensive artificial flavors, Mi-del uses oil of lemon—the real thing.

And so on down the line. Refined, synthetic ingredients are exchanged for unrefined, less processed ones. What results in many cases is a much improved product.

But what happens when item-for-item substitution simply gives us whole foods versions of the same troublesome ingredients? Some sweets are so handicapped nutritionally that even the translation from commercial to more natural ingredients is little improvement.

Candy bars are a classic example. The makers of natural candy bars promise high nutrition without guilt, or as one company, Absolutely Nuttin' Ltd., puts it, ''Good food in the guise of a candy bar.'' ''It's the perfect marketing ploy,'' says Bonnie F. Liebman, nutritionist at the Washington, D.C.-based Center for Science in the Public Interest. ''Disarm the consumer who feels pangs of conscience about eating sweets, and let temptation take over. The sale is closed.''

The typical natural candy bar features carob instead of chocolate, and honey or another natural sweetener instead of white sugar. Is the difference really great enough to make candy bars good food? Not likely.

Carob powder beats out chocolate's cocoa powder in terms of caffeine content (0 milligrams vs. chocolate's 6 milligrams per ounce) and fat content (less than .5 grams vs. 3.5 to 5.5 grams in cocoa powder). But by the time manufacturers add enough oil to turn carob powder into carob coating, and mix in all the remaining ingredients, they can end up with candy bars that contain the same degree of fat as their commercial analogs. Carob-based Carafection bars have as much fat (7 grams per ounce) as the popular chocolate-coated Baby Ruths. Mellow Mocha, a Golden Temple product that features the fatty trio of almond butter, cream, and butter, contains 9 grams of fat, the same as a milk chocolate candy, Mr. Goodbar. And Celebration, a carob-coated ''peanut-butter fudge'' creation from Robinson's Foods, has over 10 grams of fat per ounce. That's more fat than you find in a Reese's Peanut Butter Cup.

It gets worse. The fat that's added to carob powder is usually palm kernel oil, which is more than 80 percent saturated and thus one of the worst fats you can eat.

Similarly, some carob bars contain as much sugar (in the form of honey, turbinado sugar, and so forth) as chocolate bars. Carafection and Natural Nectar's 100% Bar are two carob-based products that join chocolatey successes like Butterfinger and Milky Way in the dubious distinction of offering the equivalent of 4 or more teaspoons of sugar per ounce. (The typical carob bar weighs anywhere from 1 to 1¹/₂ ounces.)

There are a few bright spots here and there. For instance, a Sunfield Foods product, Lanzi's Carob Cashew Nut and Rice Crunch, not only contains no added sugar—a fairly common claim among natural candy makers—but boasts of having no added sweeteners of any kind. Cashew nuts and crisped rice are the predominant ingredients, followed by carob powder, nonfat milk solids, fractionated palm kernel oil, lecithin, and vanilla.

Some carob bar makers have embarked on a mission of high ideals, shunning chocolate, dairy products, and refined white sugar and seeking out a variety of fruits and nuts, alternative sweeteners, and nontraditional flavorings such as cinchona bark and sea salt. They make products with clear merit, no matter how you slice them. Socially, they're more responsive to consumers who may like to indulge in an occasional candy bar but who either cannot eat (because of food allergies) or prefer not to eat (because of a dietary preference) certain ingredients. Politically, their presence on the market challenges the giant candy makers by empowering disenfranchised consumers who seek more wholesome products. The problem is that many of the alternative candy bars have the same nutritional drawbacks as conventional ones: lots of sugar and fat.

Re-Thinking Sweets in a Natural Context

Natural sweets need to be thought of not as me-too imitations of existing sweets, but as opportunities to depart from tradition. What Sunfield Foods—originators of the unsweetened candy bar—did for carob, other manufacturers could do for their own products.

That's what happened in 1976 when members of an intentional community (a 1980's commune) called The Farm opened a natural foods store and soyfoods restaurant in San Raphael, California. The group had been experimenting with ways to turn honey-sweetened soymilk into a frozen confection that was just as tasty and smooth and satisfying as ice cream, but without the dairy products. They named their brainchild Ice Bean, and it marked the beginning of a small revolution in the frozen dessert world. Ice Bean's success spawned a whole new family of soy-based products. According to Bill Shurtleff, who with Akiko Aoyagi has written the definitive text on the industry (*Tofutti and Other Soy Ice Creams*, Soyfoods Center, 1985, 2 vol.), yearly production of soy ice creams in 1985 stood at around 2.3 million gallons—over $39 million worth—and had climbed by 600 percent in the previous two years.

Shurtleff says such meteoric growth has attracted a fair share of forked-tongued entrepreneurs. "The soy ice cream market is riddled with deception," claims the soy-foods advocate. Indeed there are numerous examples of products that stray from the whole foods ethic.

Despite the excesses (see "Frozen Dairy-Free Desserts: A Comparison," on page 92), soy ice creams can be good food. For instance, Ice Bean's honey-vanilla flavor offers the taste of vanilla ice cream with 25 percent fewer calories, less than half the sugar, and a scant one-third of the sodium. The fat in Ice Bean is comparable in quantity to ice cream, but it is less harmful to the cardiovascular system because it is only 15 percent saturated, as compared to milk fat's 63 percent.

Frozen soy desserts contain an average of 23 percent fewer calories than ice cream by one reckoning, and they contain no cholesterol, no lactose, and no animal products. Some brands have their faults, but the best of these new confections stand as nice examples of how re-thinking the assumptions that underlie conventional treats can produce more healthful alternatives.

The thick, creamy base of Rice Dream from Imagine Foods, Inc., is made by a process that, like grain syrup production, takes advantage of sugar producing enzymes. Nutritionally, Rice Dream is similar to ice cream, but its fat is safflower oil (8 percent saturated) rather than milk fat. Standard ice cream makers rely on butterfat for a richly textured product, whereas the rice fiber in Rice Dream helps it achieve the same pleasing consistency.

Nutrition labels are important for helping keep your diet within a range considered healthful. If you're crazy about granola bars but you're watching your weight, the caloric and fat data let you select intelligently from among several brand names.

When it comes to some natural sweets, however, nutrition data alone is not enough. The reason is that some whole food natural sweets offer nutritional profiles strikingly similar to commercial ones. Take a look at the accompanying profile from two boxes of apricot fruit leather.

One of these products contains apricots, pears, and a dab (2 percent) of honey. The other contains apricots from concentrate, pear puree concentrate, malto-dextrin, sugar, natural flavor, partially hydrogenated soy oil, citric acid, mono and diglycerides, and artificial color. Can you tell which is which? (Stretch Island Fruit Leather, a whole foods product, is Product A; Fruit Corners Fruit Roll-Ups, a Betty Crocker label, is Product B.)

Scanning the ingredients can give you a good picture of how well a product delivers beneficial nutrients that aren't required to be listed on the nutrition label. If one cookie contains whole wheat flour and the other uses unbleached white, you can probably count on the former to provide more fiber even though that kind of information isn't explicitly given on the package.

Nutritional Profile

| | Product | |
	A	B
Serving Size	1/2 oz	1/2 oz
Calories	45	50
Protein	1 g	0
Carbohydrate	10 g	12 g
Fat	1 g	1 g
Sodium	10 mg	5 mg
Vitamin A	4% *	2% *
Calcium	2% *	—
Iron	2% *	—
Vitamin C	—	—
Thiamine	—	—
Riboflavin	—	—
Niacin	—	—

* percent of Recommended Daily Allowance

Item: New Morning Honey Graham Crackers boasts of containing a blend of whole amaranth and oat bran, two grain products celebrated for their wholesomeness. Amaranth, "the staff of the ancient Aztecs, contains more protein than all other grains," reads the package. "The quality of that protein, and its ability to meet human protein needs, exceeds that contained in soybeans or even milk." Oat bran, on the other hand, is renowned for its dietary fiber and a probable connection with reduced cholesterol levels in the blood.

It's hard to tell how much of these two grain wonders are actually in the cookies, but if the ingredient list is accurate, it can't be more than a pinch. Ingredient lists start with the most prominent ingredient by weight and work their way down to the least prominent. In this case, the principal ingredients are whole wheat flour, honey, unsulfured molasses, and soy oil. Then come sodium bicarbonate and aluminum bicarbonate, two leavening agents. Next on the list is lecithin, a natural emulsifier used in very small amounts to help mix together the ingredients. And finally, just before we get to the last ingredient, oil of lemon, we come to "whole amaranth and oat bran," our protein- and fiber-rich friends. The distributor for this company wasn't able to divulge the exact figures but we estimate that New Morning's graham crackers contain about the same amount of protein and fiber as Nabisco's.

Mix with Care

Anyone who has ever kneaded a loaf of whole grain bread knows how deeply satisfying it can be to prepare whole foods from scratch. For those of us who would prefer not to root around for measuring spoons while the phone is jangling and the cat is eating another fern, prepackaged mixes offer the next best thing: the convenience of conventional mixes married to the wholesomeness of real food.

Mixes give consumers more power to determine the composition of food than any other natural sweet. Many provide the basics—flour, leavening, and spices for a muffin mix, for example—and then let the customer add oil, pureed fruit or tofu, and other wet ingredients to round out the product. The system is a boon for people who would rather tailor a product to their own exact needs than have to accept the judgment of a corporate taste-tester (or accountant) as to how much honey should go into the spice cake.

For all their advantage there's a small hitch to some natural mixes. We didn't realize it until we had bought four banana bread mixes—two natural and two conventional—to see how they measured up. As expected, the quality of the ingredients in the whole foods version was vastly superior to the best that Pillsbury and General Mills had to offer. Enriched bleached flour will never hold a candle to whole wheat pastry, unbleached white, whole barley, and whole oat flours—the four-star combination used by Arrowhead Mills.

Nutrition labels for the products looked similar at first glance. All four seemed to offer about the same amount of calories, protein, and other nutrients. Then we noticed the fine print. The breakdown for the two conventional mixes included egg and milk, the ingredients that consumers were instructed to mix in at home. The numbers for the two natural mixes (by Fearn and Arrowhead Mills) were for dry mix only, a fact that Arrowhead Mills neglected to mention on the label. When we recalculated the figures based on the manufacturer's suggested additions (oil, honey, eggs, vanilla, bananas), the natural mixes faded a bit. On the average, they had slightly more protein and a bit less sodium than the conventionals. But serving for serving, they contained twice the calories (286) and nearly three times the fat (11 grams).

But it wouldn't make sense to imply that the new figures significantly undermine the superiority of the natural mixes. Their ingredients are too beneficial, and no one needs the additives and assorted boosters that they leave out. But there's ample room for improvement. One obvious recommendation to mix manufacturers: make sure that buyers can clearly tell how much nutrition they're getting, in both dry and prepared forms. Suggestion number two: give customers greater options. There's more than one way to prepare a bran muffin, but you wouldn't know it by looking at some package instructions. Can customers reduce the oil they add by half and still get good results? Can they safely use fruit juice or barley malt in place of honey?

Making Sense of It All

Reach into a bag of natural sweets and you'll find a tangle of contradictions. On one hand, there are so very many products that stand a cut above commercial sweets on the basis of more wholesome ingredients—whole grains, fruits, nuts—and the distinct absence of unsavory additives. On the other, we find little recognition that the fats and sugars in natural confections can promote heart disease and obesity and dental decay just as readily as conventional ingredients.

Lots of natural sweets are substantial improvements over the standard stuff. The choice of ingredients for many of these products shows thought and care. By the same token, our tour of Snack Land has taken us past candy bars that promise nutrition without guilt—and can't deliver—to frozen soy confections that pack just as much sugar, fat, and calories as the most sumptuous ice cream, and to whole grain cake mixes whose labels don't include half the ingredients.

The message to consumers seems fairly clear. Natural sweets are, on the whole, an improvement over commercial ones, but not with every type of product and perhaps not to the extent that many of us assume. Whole grain cakes, soy desserts, carob bars, and the rest of the natural sweets family line up along a continuum. Some are so barren that not even natural ingredients can save them from the nutritional trash heap. These products remain afloat on the strength of persuasive promotion and an undeserved reputation for wholesomeness.

The natural sweets industry needs to gravitate toward the more responsible end of the product continuum. Many companies are headed in the right direction, but they all need to arrive. Until they do, we may be able to walk into natural foods stores and breathe a little easier, but we can't for an instant afford to shut our eyes.

Frozen Dairy-Free Desserts: A Comparison

Only a few years ago tofu and soymilk frozen desserts were a novelty, made by a few small companies for regional distribution. Today, according to *The New York Times*, "The frozen tofu wars will be won or lost in suburban supermarket freezers, right next to the ice cream." Obviously, much has changed rapidly. As of mid-1986, there are at least six nationally distributed tofu or soymilk-based brands, several more regional products, a couple of frozen natural fruit confections, and one frozen rice dessert as well. Industry analyst William Shurtleff says that the non-dairy frozen dessert market is worth almost $40 million yearly, and is growing by 600 percent each year.

One consistency among the many

brands is that they usually refrain from using artificial flavors, colors, stabilizers, and preservatives. They also generally favor such sweeteners as honey and fructose (usually in the form of high fructose corn syrup, or HFCS) over cane sugar or corn syrup made from chemically purified cornstarch. Without once more jumping into the sweetener debate (see "A Guide to Natural Sweeteners," page 177), suffice it to say that in our opinion honey is at least marginally better on a number of counts than cane sugar or corn syrup, and that HFCS has little to recommend it over either of the latter. Also, keep in mind during the following review of products that leading natural foods chains such as Bread & Circus and Mrs. Gooch's will not carry fructose-sweetened products.

Non-dairy frozen desserts often have nutritional benefits compared to most ice creams, which are generally higher in fat, calories, and sugar content. In addition, dairy products contain cholesterol, while fruit- and grain-based frozen desserts are cholesterol-free.

To help the consumer sort out the healthier, more whole products from among the dozen non-dairy frozen desserts considered here, we've created three categories in the competition for the crown: the Pretenders, the Contenders, and the Champs. Among the factors we take into consideration are ingredients, degree of processing, taste and texture, appearance, and nutritional qualities.

THE PRETENDERS

The Pretenders to the crown are mostly slickly promoted products that pay mere lip-service to such concepts as "natural." They tend to use such highly refined products as HFCS and, instead of tofu or soymilk, "soy protein isolate."

The most visible Pretender is, of course, **Tofutti** by Tofu Time of Rahway, New Jersey. The name is ingenious, the marketing aggressive, and the distribution (it's available in 22,000 stores in forty-eight states) thorough. Created in 1981 by New Yorker David Mintz, Tofut-

ti's success has been nothing short of astounding. However, there's little to recommend Tofutti over the average ice cream. The exact amount of tofu in it is not publicly available, but industry insiders estimate it at a mere 2 to 9 percent. Most of Tofutti's soy comes from soy protein isolate, and it is sweetened with HFCS.

Tofulite from Barricini Foods of Oyster Bay, New York, is the commercial form, blended for the supermarkets, of the original Ice Bean. There are a lot of options to choose from—six flavors, pints, soft serve (four flavors), three-gallon tubs—but ingredient quality is lacking. Cane sugar is second only to water and is ahead of tofu on the ingredient list. Corn syrup is also used. Not surprisingly, the sweetness is cloying and overpowering.

Tofruzen, a product of Tofu Today in Englewood, Colorado, appeals to similarly immature taste buds and it too rates a Pretender. It's available in pints, soft serve, and bulk, in about a half dozen flavors, including some innovative ones like

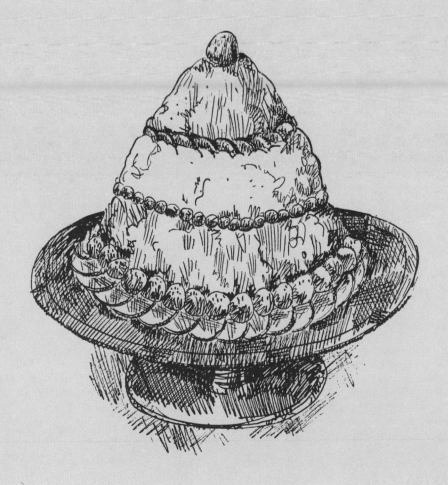

Chocolate Peanut Crunch. The first ingredient in all Tofruzen flavors is "tofu dessert base." This brilliant and misleading marketing ploy allows Tofu Today to get the word tofu in the first ingredient on the label, whereas if tofu were ranked by actual volume it would appear much further down the list. In fact, tofu is even the last ingredient in the "dessert base," which contains water, corn syrup solids, HFCS, soy oil, soy solids, and tofu. The addition of natural fruits, fruit concentrates, lecithin, and guar gum typically rounds out the label.

THE CONTENDERS

The next group of frozen desserts are a cut above the Pretenders, offering better ingredients and usually a better nutritional profile. Industry pioneer **Ice Bean** by Farm Foods (now a division of Barricini), for instance, is sweetened with honey, although its main soy source is usually not tofu but whole soybeans, either as a spray-dried powder or as a bulk liquid. (Farm Foods recently began offering three tofu flavors of Ice Bean, which they say are made with tofu instead of soymilk.) Ice Bean comes in a wide variety of forms, flavors, and sizes: nine honey flavors, three tofu flavors, soft serve, three-ounce cups, and sandwiches. At about two dollars per pint, it is one of the best buys among the alternative frozen desserts.

Le Tofu is made by Brightsong Foods of Petaluma, California, a well-established tofu products company. It uses 15 percent organic tofu instead of soy powders, and all-natural flavorings, such as Dutch cocoa, pure vanilla, and real strawberries, but this is another case of an otherwise quality product being dragged down by its choice of sweeteners: fructose and corn syrup solids, in addition to honey.

Acorn Natural Foods Italian Ice from Chicago, Illinois, is one of the new natural sorbets on the market. It comes in five flavors, from the old standby Lemon to an appetizing Blueberry Lemon-Lime. Ingredients are simple, usually fruit puree, puree from concentrate, or juice from concentrate, along with honey and guar gum and carob bean gum as stabilizers. The result is a tangy, refreshing taste, and a nutritionally very attractive product. In comparison to Nouvelle Sorbet (see below), however, Acorn's falls short.

The makers of **Penguinos** first introduced this tofu and soymilk dessert in their Rochester, New York, soyfoods restaurant, where it was received with pleasure as a soft-serve confection. Today Penguinos comes in four flavors and is distributed nationally. It is sweetened with honey, and with flavors such as pure Dutch unsweetened cocoa contributing to the mix, the result is smooth and pleasing overall.

THE CHAMPS

Only the highest-quality ingredients, and the brightest, freshest taste combinations qualify a dessert for ranking among the Champs.

Tofreezi, for instance, is some 75 percent tofu and soymilk by volume, uses honey and fruit for sweetness, and contains natural flavorings. Its extensive use of rich soy ingredients, instead of isolates or powders, makes Tofreezi, from Metta Tofu Products, Denman Island, B.C., Canada, one of the highest in fat and calories (and thus a close call for inclusion among the Champs), but this richness comes through in a superior, fully satisfying dessert.

An imaginative alternative to both soy- and fruit-based frozen desserts is **Rice Dream**, from Imagine Foods of Palo Alto, California. This is a rice-based confection that is distributed nationally and is quite popular among natural foods aficionados. It is sweetened with maple syrup and a form of amasake, a fermented rice product that is especially easy to digest. Other ingredients, from toasted almonds to sea salt, are also high-quality. (For more on this innovative dessert, see page 181.)

Two frozen fruit desserts round out the Champs. The first, **Yodolo** from Olympus Industries in Spokane, Washington, we've tasted only in soft-serve and thus can give only tentative listing here among products available in consumer servings. The soft-serve Yodolo is made from just fruit, flavors, and gums, with no added sweetener, and the taste is heavenly. If the hardpack version is similar (it's due out soon), Olympus will have another winner.

The top-of-the-line sorbet that we know about is **Nouvelle Sorbet** from the Nouvelle Ice Cream Corp. of San Raphael, California. Nouvelle Sorbet is a creamy, chilled fruit puree now available in five flavors. Its ingredients are simple: fruit and fruit juices, spring water, and fruit pectin. There's no fat and only 80 calories in a four-ounce serving. Light and clean on the palate, this is a frozen dessert both gourmands and health-conscious people can easily love.

The Nutrition Face–Off

Product (per 4 oz)	Fat (g)	Calories	Sodium (mg)	Sweetener	Basic Ingredient
Tofutti	8-12	210	60-130	HFCS	tofu, I.S.P
Tofulite	7-10	150-180	50-90	cane sugar, corn syrup	tofu
Tofruzen	8	162	10	corn syrup, HFCS	soymilk powder
Ice Bean	4-8	110-150	44	honey	soybeans, tofu
Le Tofu	6	128	28	fructose, honey, corn syrup	tofu
Acorn Sorbet	0	na	na	honey	fruit juice
Penguinos	10	131	2	honey	soybeans, tofu
Tofreezi	14	247	85	honey	soymilk, tofu
Rice Dream	5-6	130-150	80	amasake, maple syrup	cultured rice
Nouvelle Sorbet	0	80	na	apple juice	fruit

na: *not available*.

* percent of Recommended Daily Allowance

7. FRUITS

Sweet and succulent, fresh fruit surely deserves a place of honor in the natural foods diet. What better snack is there than a crisp, tart apple or a juicy, ripe peach? Fruits can also make excellent alternative sweeteners, from raisins in cereal to blueberries in pancakes.

Fruits are so appealing and versatile, in fact, that they are becoming an increasingly significant proportion of the American diet. Total fruit consumption in the United States is up to over 200 pounds per person per year, compared to around 140 pounds at the turn of the century. However, most of this growth in fruit consumption in the U.S. has been in the form of processed fruit, especially orange juice. Sometime in the late 1950s, Americans began consuming more processed fruit than fresh. Today, most of the fruit eaten in America continues to be either sliced, diced, canned, juiced, jarred, jellied, frozen, sweetened, or concentrated.

The real attractions of eating fruit, though, are most evident when it is fresh and locally grown. It is then that cherries are sweetest, melons juiciest, strawberries their most flavorful. Also, nutrient levels have not begun to fade, handling has been kept to a minimum, and storage has not had a chance to play havoc with flavor and texture.

For many years, shopping for fresh fruit was perhaps threatening to become a lost art as processed fruit took over and fresh fruit in the supermarket began to be dyed, waxed, and wrapped in ways that camouflaged the fruit's true state. Nevertheless, today it is possible to get good-quality fruit. The information and techniques that follow can help anyone to become an astute fresh fruit shopper. In the main section, we have divided fruits into three categories—temperate, subtropical, and tropical. For each fruit, we look at its most common place of origin, the season in which it is most available, how to select for freshness and ripeness, how best to store, and special nutritional considerations. There are also shorter stories on dried fruit, fruit spreads, and the new breeding technologies being used by the fruit industry. In addition, we will also take a critical look at Americans' increasing fondness for tropical and subtropical fruits such as oranges and bananas, and discuss the range of chemical treatments that might accompany a fruit's trip from the orchard to your table.

Especially if you've been part of the trend away from fresh, locally grown fruits, we'd like you to come rediscover what apples, berries, apricots, melons, plums, and other fruits can add to a natural foods diet.

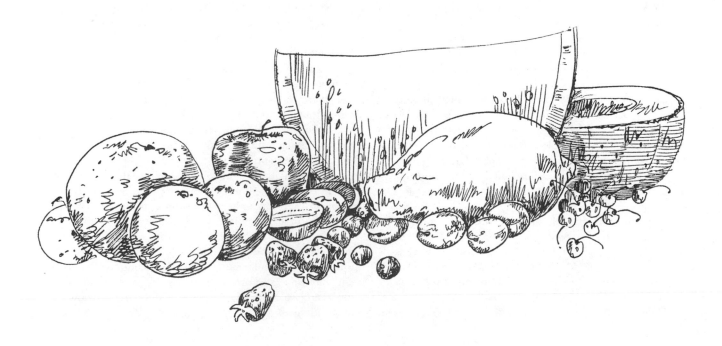

A Guide to Fruits

From ancient times, people have appreciated the beauty and deliciousness of fruits. The word ''fruit'' can be traced to the Latin *fructus*, meaning ''enjoyment, means of enjoyment, fruit.'' The English word ''fructify'' means to impregnate, fertilize, or cause to bear fruit.

Botanically speaking, it's proper for sex to occupy a discussion of fruits because fruits are an integral part of the reproductive system of angiosperms, the flowering plants. It is estimated that angiosperms evolved about 100 million years ago, 96 million years ahead of the human race. Angiosperms today are the most developed of all plants. Their species comprise about 250,000 of the 350,000 plant species on earth, and include the cereal grasses. While many plants reproduce only asexually, propagation of angiosperms is achieved in nature through fertilization of the flower's female organ—the pistil—with pollen from the male organ—the stamen. Riding the winds or the feet of insects, pollen grains are carried from stamens to pistils. The subsequent union produces seeds—the packages of new life—which are safely suspended within a fleshy, ripened organ of the pistil known botanically as the ovary. We know these swollen ovaries of angiosperms by such names as apples and peaches, grapes and berries, oranges and plums.

To a botanist, a fruit is the ripened ovary, fleshy or dry, surrounding the seed. The wheat ''berry,'' which is ground into flour to make bread, botanically is not a berry (by definition, a berry is a fleshy fruit) but it *is* a fruit—the edible, starchy fruit of a grass. In a grain, the fruit and the seed coat are united, making it difficult to separate the two except by milling. Most of us have been reminded that a tomato is not a vegetable but rather a fruit—a ripened ovary containing seeds. So is a pepper. The definition we will use here, however, is a functional and dynamic one: a fruit is any edible part of a plant that people eat for the sweet taste.

Though humans had gathered wild fruits for over 99 percent of their history, the advent of cultivation 10 thousand years ago reduced the need to forage. Planting seeds became a widespread practice; as exploration increased, seeds accompanied travelers, which meant new homes for many plants.

Colonists took pear seeds from the Caucasus mountain ranges, between the Black and Caspian Seas, to Europe and then to North America. Peach seeds traveled from China to Persia to Europe, and in the 16th century Spanish colonists introduced the peach plant to the village of St. Augustine in what is now Florida. The sweet cherry, taken from its native habitats in Asia Minor and Persia, took up residence in Greece. Apricots, originally from China, were introduced to Europe during the time of the Roman empire. They were brought to California by the early mission fathers of Spain in the 18th century.

Few fruits eaten by Americans today are indigenous to North America. In fact, the European colonists are believed to have found only three major wild fruits here—blueberries, cranberries, and grapes. Three-and-a-half centuries ago the French explorer Samuel de Champlain observed American Indians near Lake Huron gathering blueberries for winter storage. After the blueberries dried in the sun, they were beaten into a powder and then added to parched meal, resulting in a dish called *sautauthig*. Other Indians used persimmons in the making of bread. In her book *Wild Fruits* (Contemporary Books, 1983) Mildred Fielder writes that persimmon flour was made by grinding the seeds and then adding the sweet pulp. The seeds were also ground and roasted to make a beverage, and the pulp sometimes ended up in a kind of cookie or as beer. Fielder's fascinating accounts of the many native fruits growing wild throughout North America is a journey into a dreamworld teeming with wild sweet crabapples, blite goosefoot berries, black chokecherries, lemonade sumac, and countless others that are generally overlooked today.

Carbohydrates, mainly the simple sugars fructose and sucrose (along with some fiber), are the principal nutritional components of all fruits. Fruits contain small amounts of many other nutrients as well; of these, vitamins C and A and the mineral potassium tend to be the most noteworthy. Fruits either lack entirely or are sorely deficient in protein, complex carbohydrates, fats, and B vitamins. Some contain moderate amounts of vitamin E, niacin, folic acid, and magnesium. All in all, fruits are an unreliable source of balanced nutrition. For nutrients presently known to sustain the human body, whole grains, legumes, and vegetables are better providers. In the following descriptions of the nutrients of fruits, only those that ap-

High Tech in the Garden

Today, produce sections in supermarkets across the United States are daily filled with a streaming supply of fruits that are a long reach from the crabapples and chokecherries of the Indians and early colonists. Most of the fruit we buy now has been either transplanted or imported from foreign lands. Some of the transplants have struggled in their new environments. However, farmers and scientists for several centuries have labored to perfect the hybridization and asexual reproduction of plants to the point that new varieties can survive many conditions previously intolerable to their species. Since wild varieties often show more disease resistance, farmers will graft branches of new hybrids, selected for other qualities, onto wild stocks, chosen for their hardiness, and end up with what Dr. Miklos Faust of the U.S. Department of Agriculture calls "the beauty of Miss America and the toughness of a pro football player in one package."

Strong and pretty, maybe, but not as tasty, as Jack Watson, Area Extension Horticulturist at Washington State University, explains: "The Red Delicious apples sold today are obtained through selection. When a good fruit is found, the limb is grafted. The Red Delicious in the stores aren't like the original ones found in nature, which were a muddy brown apple. Those would never make the grade in Washington, they wouldn't sell. What we sell are selected for color and for early color, to the exclusion of taste. The newer variations get red before the fruit is ripe and they're picked earlier."

Sometime after the practice of agriculture began with the deliberate saving of seeds, humans began to select seeds of plants with favorable characteristics. In Europe, this practice did not become refined until the 18th century, after which crop yields became much greater than in the Middle Ages. As Barbara Evelyn Nicholson informs us in *The Oxford Book of Food Plants* (Oxford University Press, 1969), "From the late nineteenth century onwards, this process was greatly speeded up by the development of the modern science of genetics. Now man began not only to select parent plants, but to make hybrids between species and varieties, to search the world for plants with promising characteristics, and even to create new genetic variations by treating plants with chemical substances or bombarding them with x-rays." Modern techniques of bioengineering enabled plant scientists to isolate single genes and implant them elsewhere, creating new varieties with increased efficiency.

Current hybridization practices tend to cater to commercial growers who supply supermarkets with produce. Plants are bred for uniform shape and ripening time, ease of harvesting by machines and of storing and shipping, responsiveness to synthetic fertilizers, and color. Taste, nutritional value, and other qualities valued by home gardeners and by consumers are often not taken into account.

pear in exceptional amounts will be mentioned. If nutrients are not mentioned, it may be assumed that the fruit is nutritionally about the same as most others—composed primarily of simple sugars, with some fiber, vitamin C, vitamin A, potassium, and a few other vitamins and minerals in small amounts.

Eaten at the right time, in the right climate, and in moderation, fruits are the best natural sweeteners. They contain a minimal but wide range of nutrients that clearly help in our metabolism of them—no other sweetener is as well endowed. And if it's true that the enjoyment of food plays an important role in maintaining good health, then the succulent and irresistible deliciousness of fruits surely affords them a place of honor in the natural foods diet.

Temperate Fruits

Apples

Origin and Varieties: The apple's original home may have been around the Caspian Sea, or in Switzerland, where carbonized apples have been found in prehistoric lake dwellings. The wild crabapple, *Malus pumila*, is the parent species of our cultivated apples. As apples grown from seed are not like their parents, most cultivation is done by grafting a scion to a rootstock.

In the first half of the 19th century, John Chapman, a preacher and nurseryman, traveled from Pennsylvania through Indiana and Ohio, selling, giving away, and planting apple tree stock. The barefoot Chapman wore an inverted mush pan hat, an old burlap bag shirt, and ragged trousers. This gentle and beloved eccentric, however, was a knowledgeable nurseryman; the apple-tree stock that he supplied to the Middle West helped pave the way for the pioneers of the 19th century. He also gave birth to the legend of Johnny Appleseed.

Very few varieties of apples are widely marketed. Eight principal ones—Red Delicious, McIntosh, Golden Delicious, Rome Beauty, Jonathan, Winesap, York, and Stayman—account for 75 percent of commercial production. Nevertheless, many other varieties are sold on a limited basis. The Granny Smith is an Australian dessert apple imported during our winter; it is also raised in the United States on a limited scale. Gravensteins are an exceptionally delicious apple grown in northern California's Sonoma County. They were originally found in the Duke of Augustinberg's garden at Gravenstein in Holstein, Germany. In northern California they're one of the first to hit the market (late July) and some apple lovers in that area claim it's all downhill after that.

Hundreds of other equally exciting apples are not sold widely due to their poor shipping qualities or less-than-standard appearance. As the trend toward standardization continues, these "heirloom varieties" become more rare and might disappear altogether were it not for the efforts of a small, scattered, but dedicated group of seed savers and cultivators who aim to keep the gene stocks going. In *The Heirloom Gardener* (Sierra Club Books, 1984), Carolyn Jabs writes, "At the turn of the century, a scientist compiled a list of 8,000 apple varieties available in the United States. In 1981, when the U.S. Department of Agriculture prepared a new list, only 1,000 of those varieties could be found."

Waverley Root, in his encyclopedic work entitled *Food* (Simon and Schuster, 1980), does not have a kind word for the modern Red Delicious: "It is sad to be obliged to report that its taste has been reduced to the lowest common denominator, which has been discovered to be productive of the largest number of sales." But the legendary Calville (called "the empress of desserts"), Root says, has a "hint of raspberry in its taste." He describes the Cox's Orange Pippin, originally from England, as leaving "an aftertaste like ice cream on the tongue," and says it has been called "the greatest apple of this age." Other apples that are difficult to find but whose praises have been sung include the Red Astrachan, Smokehouse, Lady, Black Gilliflower, Red Canada, and Seek-no-further. The names themselves evoke a wide range of subtle tastes, textures, and appearances.

Apples grow just about everywhere, but the popular Red Delicious come mainly from Washington, America's biggest apple-producing state. In 1981 Washington produced 2.76 billion pounds of apples. New York was second with .8 billion. Other leading U.S. producers include California, Michigan, North Carolina, Pennsylvania, and Virginia.

The best eating apples are Red Delicious, McIntosh, Golden Delicious, Jonathan, Winesap, and Stayman. For cooking, McIntosh, Golden Delicious, Rome Beauty, Jonathan, York, and Stayman are all acceptable, but the green Newton Pippins are reputed to be the best.

Season: Apples are available year-round. Rarely, however, are any sold fresh between late November and June—they're pulled from cold storage. You take your chances with a May apple. Most apple harvesting begins in August or early September, sometimes a little later.

Selection: Avoid soft, bruised, or shriveled apples. Some varieties, like the Newton Pippin, are fully green at maturity and others, such as Gravensteins, may be slightly green in spots. However, most green color is a sign of immaturity to be avoided.

Many apples are waxed to appear shinier. Though synthetic waxes are sometimes employed, carnauba wax, taken from the young leaves of the Brazilian wax palm tree, is frequently used. It is, by most accounts, harmless for human consumption. Doubtful purchasers can look for unwaxed apples, which seem to be in fairly good supply. The naturally occurring wax on apples sometimes resembles artificially applied wax. However, apples with only the natural wax can generally be brought to a greater shine, while artificially waxed apples have a fairly high gloss to begin with.

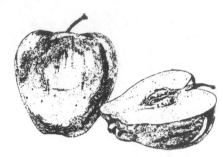

Storage: Refrigerated, apples keep for weeks, and most varieties are perfect for root-cellar storage.

Nutrition: It will be hard for the "an apple a day keeps the doctor away" crowd to swallow this, but nutritionally apples are not all they're shined up to be. Even the vitamin C content—4 milligrams in a fresh medium-sized apple—is not high and, from stored apples, it is gone completely.

Apricots

Origin: This delightfully creamy fruit comes from China, where it probably grew wild 4,000 years ago. Apricots were introduced to North America in the 17th century. There are at most a half-dozen varieties sold commercially, almost all of which come from California.

Season: Apricots are in season from mid-May to August.

Selection: Pick golden-yellow, nearly orange fruits. They should feel a little soft. Avoid a light yellow or greenish color. Apricots will ripen at room temperature after picking, but the flavor of tree-ripened apricots is superior.

Storage: Once apricots are ripe, refrigerate them. Enjoy this perishable fruit soon after it ripens.

Nutrition: Apricots contain potassium and considerable vitamin A.

Blackberries

Origin: Blackberries are one of the many berries found growing wild throughout the world. The raspberry is related to the blackberry. Loganberries and boysenberries are hybrids, crosses between the two. Trailing relatives of blackberries are called dewberries. If you make it to the arctic areas of our planet, you'll possibly find another relation, a golden cloudberry, growing there. The wild blackberry grows easily, quickly, and with claws, so hunt for it with gloves. Thornless types are cultivated for the market. Blackberries are marketed from many states.

Season: They are available May to August.

Selection: Look for bright color and dry, clean appearance. Avoid runny berries, and check the bottom of the container for any wet or moldy spots.

Storage: As they are highly perishable, blackberries should be refrigerated and eaten soon. Keep them dry until just before use.

Nutrition: Blackberries contain vitamin C.

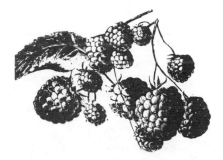

Blueberries

Origin: Many varieties of blueberries can be found growing wild around the world. The Inuit rely on blueberries native to their climate. Bilberries, also known as whortleberries, look like blueberries but are not as sweet. Huckleberries, often mistaken for blueberries, have larger seeds and grow only as wild berries. The wild blueberry has a superior flavor, although it is smaller than the commercial types that have been cultivated since 1909, when botanists began hybridizing the wild berries. In the United States, commercial blueberries are grown mainly in New Jersey, Michigan, Maine, North Carolina, Washington, and Oregon.

Season: Blueberries are on the market from May to September.

Selection: Choose full, fresh, well-colored berries free of running juices.

Storage: Refrigerate blueberries; they keep well only a few days. Frozen blueberries store nicely in an airtight plastic bag.

Avoiding the Chemical Feast

Many measures are employed to serve the public a year-round supply of handsome fruits. They are stimulated with hormones, colored with chemicals, shined with waxes, and protected with fumigants. Pesticides have also long played a major role in the fruit industry. At the turn of the century arsenic and lead residues on fruit were a problem. The Federal Food and Drug Act of 1906 established a tolerance of .01 grain of arsenic per pound of foodstuff. When the fruit industry was unable to comply, the solution was simply to increase the tolerance level, which by 1932 had reached .025 grain, or 2.5 times the original limit.

The use of toxic sprays has not abated in the 1980s. In 1983 the discovery of larvae on Florida's citrus crop unleashed the dumping of thirteen tons of EDB just before the toxic substance was banned, and little meaningful debate was allowed in California before widespread malathion spraying was begun to combat a threatened invasion of the Mediterranean fruit fly.

To avoid some of the worst transgressions, ask two basic questions about the fruit you buy: "Is it fresh?" and "Has it been grown organically?" The answers will seldom be clear-cut. "Fresh" ideally would be the time needed to pull the fruit from the tree, wipe it across your shirt, and sink your teeth into it—maybe six seconds. At the farmers' market where local farmers bring fruit they've picked in the previous day or two, "fresh" can mean twenty-four hours. At the supermarket, where the displayed fruit has enjoyed a long-distance truck ride, "fresh" may mean a week. And sometimes, for fruit pulled out of storage, "fresh" will mean six months. Generally speaking, time is an opponent of flavor and nutrition. The closer you get to a tree-ripened fruit, the more satisfying it will be. (The banana seems to be an exception.)

A similar array of definitions for "organic" awaits the consumer. Even health and natural foods stores can be reckless with the "organic-natural" labels, especially in states that have no legal definition for organic produce.

Wayne Ferrari is an organic apple grower in central California. Ferrari says, "We do use a spray, a natural product called rotenone." Rotenone is derived from the roots of tropical plants such as derris, a woody vine of Asia, and cube, a tropical American shrub. Though it is a poison and must be handled with care, rotenone nevertheless comes from a plant and breaks down into a harmless substance within a couple of days after use, leaving no poisonous residues.

Ferrari laments the need to use any spray, citing the decline of "beneficials" (insects that fit advantageously into the ecology). But in all other respects, the Ferrari apples are raised much differently than most commercial ones. Ferrari says that a commercial apple tree may be fed a growth hormone (so that it will bear fruit every year), growth regulators to elongate the apples, chemical fungicides to control scab (the brown patches), coloring agents, and a load of chemical fertilizers. Fred Lape in *Apples & Man* (Van Nostrand Reinhold, 1979) speaks of a menu of chemicals that a typical apple orchard might be fed: dieldrin, parathion, a fungicide such as dodine, Elgetol to abort flowering ovaries, Guthion for codlin moths, captan to fight bull's-eye rot, Thiodan for aphids, 2,4-D to kill herbage after an early spraying of simazine or paraquat, Ethrel spray to promote red color, and NAA (1-naphthaleneacetic acid) to prevent dropping before the apples are ripe. The apples are then rushed to cold storage, and since some store poorly they may be dipped completely in a diphenylamine solution beforehand. Ferrari avoids all these practices and stands on his organic claim, believing that the natural sprays are ecologically tolerable.

Ferrari and other organic farmers must survive financially. They all point to the high costs of organic practices. Ferrari says his organic sprays are much more expensive and time-consuming to apply than the petroleum-based, toxic kinds. A spokesperson from the 400-acre Twin Hill orchards in Sebastopol, California, says they have opted for synthetic chemicals because the cost of organic practice is too steep and the demand insufficient.

Most farmers echo the Twin Hill attitude, but they avow a willingness to farm as organically as the public demands. If the demand is there, and they can sell the product, they'll do it. This simply means that you, the consumer, are deciding the future of organic farming. This is not to minimize the effect of "politics" nor the activity of the massive agri-chemical industry, but consumer pressure *has* directed considerable change in the marketplace and it will undoubtedly continue to do so if an ecology- and health-minded public uses it effectively.

Your options for finding fresh and organic produce are several. If circumstances allow, it's most desirable to plant your own fruit trees or shrubs. The benefits are substantial, in terms of flavor, nutrition, economy, and ecology. You can also forage. Wonderful edible berries can be found buried in the snow in Alaska and hanging from the majestic saguaro cacti in the Arizona desert. Excellent guidebooks, such as Fielder's *Wild Fruits*, are available from most libraries. (Be careful to identify the fruit correctly and to avoid unsafe varieties.)

You can also locate organic growers in your area, visit them, ask about their methods, and make arrangements to purchase some of their produce. The farmers' markets offer another option where freshness at least is bound to be higher than in store-bought produce (although some farmers sell apples from storage). When you do buy fruit from a store, try to patronize one that claims its produce is organic *and* makes a disclosure of the fruit's origins and the methods by which it was grown.

In selecting fruit, eye appeal is the "state-of-the-art" criterion for choosing the best. Consumers have been conditioned to choose the bigger, more colorful, blemish-free fruits. Appearance can aid in selecting fruit, but there is no known relationship between the appearance standards of today's highly graded apples, for example—fat and shiny—and quality. A sullen-looking crabapple with unsightly cleavages might explode with juice when you bite into it and taste like heaven. On the other hand, a huge, red, unblemished and juicy-looking Red Delicious is often as insipid as a slice of white bread.

All thin-skinned fruits should be thoroughly washed right before eating (not earlier). Wash even those grown organically. You may rinse them with a mild soap solution (such as Dr. Bronner's) which helps break down oil-based sprays and waxes. Though washing will remove most sprays from the surface of fruits, sprays and fumigants do penetrate the skins and remain inside the fleshy pulp. Even the thick skin of oranges fails to stop the absorption of certain pesticides and fumigants.

Nancy Frost, Chief of the Pesticide Section of the Environmental Protection Agency (EPA), says the extent of penetration varies considerably. It depends on the chemical, the amount used, the way it is applied, and the weather. Frost says, "Some chemicals on a sunny day will break down quickly on contact and not be absorbed to a great degree. A cold wet day, however, may retard the breakdown process, allowing the absorption to continue." Frost explains that for every chemical used there is an established maximum amount that can be applied while keeping the levels that build up in the pulp of the fruit within tolerance limits. In other words, we are consuming pesticide sprays when we eat fresh, nonorganic fruits—even well-washed—but the amount we consume, according to present EPA standards, is safe. Consumers who believe their food should be free of any chemical residue will restrict their purchase to organically grown fruits.

Cherries

Origin: The cherry tree is native to many parts of the world from the Arctic Circle to the Tropic of Cancer. The commercial cherries sold today, like many other fruits, are hybrids of European varieties. Sour cherries used for baking include the Montmorency, Early Richmond, and English Morello varieties, while the Bing is the preeminent sweet cherry. The Royal Ann, a sweet cherry, has a distinctively light yellow-red color. Michigan, New York, and Wisconsin sell most of the sours, and California, Idaho, Oregon, and Washington produce most of the sweet cherries sold in the United States.

Season: Sour cherries appear from June to August and sweets from late April through August.

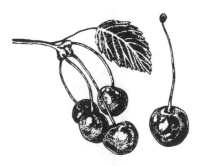

Selection: Find full, shiny, colorful cherries, firm but not hard. Avoid the ones with dark-colored stems.

Storage: Refrigerate cherries and eat them soon.

Cranberries

Origin: The cranberry is one of the few fruits sold mostly in its wild unhybridized form. Small, compact, not-too-sweet, it is typical of a wild temperate fruit that has been relied upon for thousands of years. The cowberry, also known as foxberry, mountain cranberry, and lingonberry, is in the same genus but of a different species; it is very popular in Scandinavia. Native Americans made pemmican from a mixture of cranberries and dried deer meat that was pulverized, shaped into patties, and dried in the sun. According to produce expert Joe Carcione, cranberry farmers are very ecologically conscientious, often using geese and swallows instead of synthetic chemical sprays to control weeds and insects. Most commercial cranberries today are raised in Massachusetts.

Season: The cranberry season is from September to December.

Selection: Cranberries are usually sold in bags and generally any bad berries have been removed by the packager. The berries should appear full and of bright color, never shriveled, soft, or yellow.

Storage: Cranberries keep four to eight weeks under refrigeration, longer in the freezer. Moisture will quickly spoil them.

Grapes

Origin: The first European visitors to North America found such an abundance of native grapes they named the place "Vinland." Many varieties are indigenous to the North American continent, but most sold in the United States today are varieties or hybrids of European stock. The cultivation of grapes, or "viticulture," is almost as old as agriculture. Different varieties are grown for table use, for wine, and for raisins, though the divisions often overlap. In overall U.S. production, grapes rank right behind oranges. A few popular varieties are the blackish-purple Concords and Ribiers, red Tokays and Emperors, and the commonly available yellow-green Thompson Seedless, which account for half of all vineyard acreage and from which most raisins come. Most grapes are grown in California and New York.

Season: The peak season is September to November, but some grapes are harvested as early as July or as late as the middle of winter. A few, stored under controlled atmosphere conditions, may be sold until May.

Selection: Pick bright-colored, plump grapes. If possible find those with "bloom," the powdery surface on very fresh grapes that older, heavily handled grapes have lost. Check the stems, which should be green and firm. If they are dry, brown, or black, the grapes may not be very flavorful.

Storage: Remove any bad grapes from the bunch and refrigerate the rest quickly. They will keep up to two weeks, but eat them as soon as possible for best flavor.

Nutrition: Grapes are high in simple sugars.

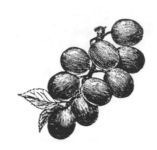

Melons

Origin and Varieties: Melon terminology is like the definition of fruits—confusing. The United Fresh Fruit and Vegetable Association states that "cantaloupe" refers to all netted muskmelons, so named for their distinctive musky aroma. Included among these are what we commonly call the "cantaloupe" as well as Persian melon, a very aromatic melon with a deep orange to salmon color. (There is also a "true" cantaloupe, named for Cantalupu, a former papal village near Rome, where it was first cultivated. This melon, however, lacks the netting for which the muskmelons are noted, and is about the size of a tennis ball.) Cantaloupes are harvested earlier than other muskmelons, and the latter are therefore sometimes called "winter melons." Honeydews, casabas, and crenshaws are the more popular winter melons. The crenshaw is a hybrid of Persian and casaba varieties developed in the 1940s.

Cantaloupes are originally from Persia or possibly central Africa. Christopher Columbus brought them to North America in 1492. In the off-season, many cantaloupes come from Mexico, but overall, California and the southwest states are the leading suppliers of melons in the U.S.

Watermelons, aptly named for their 92 percent water content, grow wild in Africa. They require a hot climate for growth. In the United States, watermelons are raised in many southern states and in California. In the off-season, the U.S. imports some from Mexico. Botanically, these melons are unrelated to muskmelons.

Season: *Cantaloupe* is available from May to September, *casaba* from July to November, *crenshaw* from July to October, *honeydew* from July to October, and *watermelon* from June to August.

Selection: Muskmelons should be a little springy, and neither too soft nor overly odorous. Avoid immature melons, as they lack sugar, and melon's sugar content doesn't increase after picking. Melons will, however, ripen, soften,

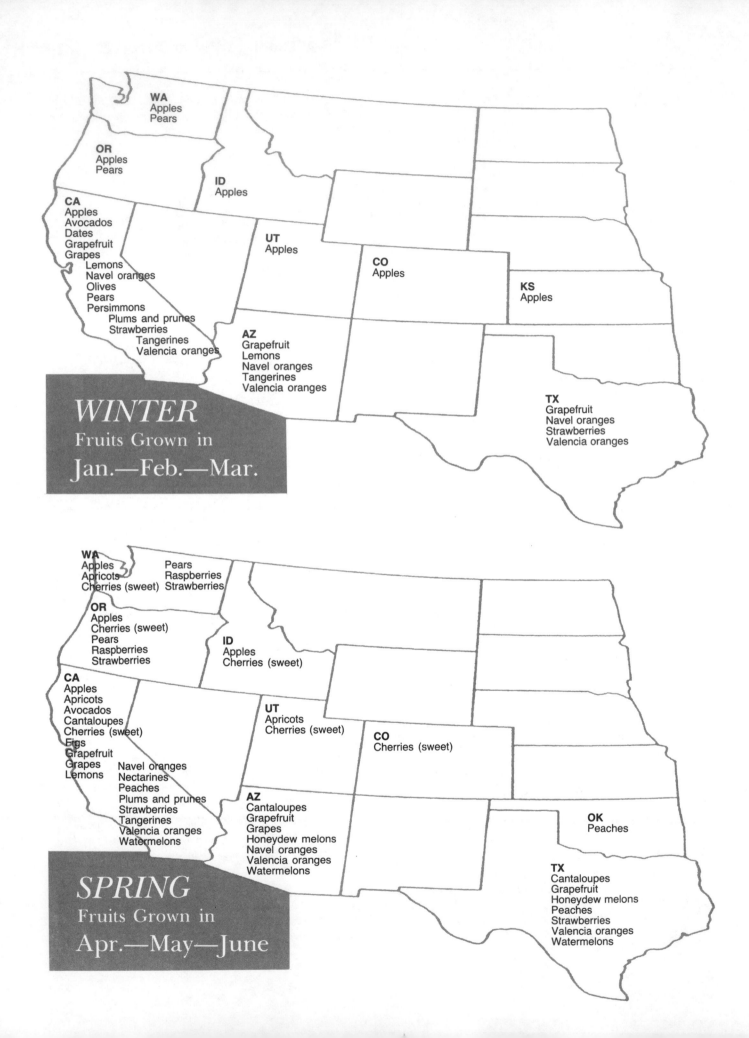

WA
Apples
Pears

OR
Apples
Pears

ID
Apples

CA
Apples
Avocados
Dates
Grapefruit
Grapes
Lemons
Navel oranges
Olives
Pears
Persimmons
Plums and prunes
Strawberries
Tangerines
Valencia oranges

UT
Apples

CO
Apples

KS
Apples

AZ
Grapefruit
Lemons
Navel oranges
Tangerines
Valencia oranges

TX
Grapefruit
Navel oranges
Strawberries
Valencia oranges

WINTER
Fruits Grown in
Jan.—Feb.—Mar.

WA
Apples   Pears
Apricots   Raspberries
Cherries (sweet) Strawberries

OR
Apples
Cherries (sweet)
Pears
Raspberries
Strawberries

ID
Apples
Cherries (sweet)

CA
Apples
Apricots
Avocados
Cantaloupes
Cherries (sweet)
Figs
Grapefruit
Grapes
Lemons
Navel oranges
Nectarines
Peaches
Plums and prunes
Strawberries
Tangerines
Valencia oranges
Watermelons

UT
Apricots
Cherries (sweet)

CO
Cherries (sweet)

AZ
Cantaloupes
Grapefruit
Grapes
Honeydew melons
Navel oranges
Valencia oranges
Watermelons

OK
Peaches

TX
Cantaloupes
Grapefruit
Honeydew melons
Peaches
Strawberries
Valencia oranges
Watermelons

SPRING
Fruits Grown in
Apr.—May—June

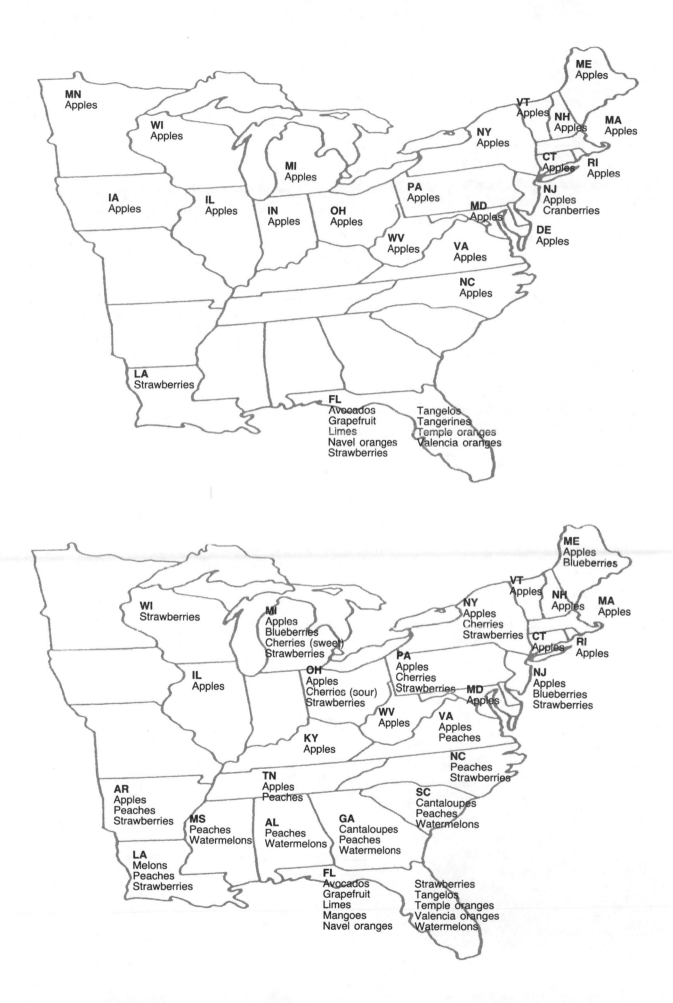

Map 1 (top)

MN
Apples

WI
Apples

MI
Apples

IA
Apples

IL
Apples

IN
Apples

OH
Apples

PA
Apples

NY
Apples

VT
Apples

ME
Apples

NH
Apples

MA
Apples

CT
Apples

RI
Apples

NJ
Apples
Cranberries

MD
Apples

DE
Apples

WV
Apples

VA
Apples

NC
Apples

LA
Strawberries

FL
Avocados
Grapefruit
Limes
Navel oranges
Strawberries

Tangelos
Tangerines
Temple oranges
Valencia oranges

Map 2 (bottom)

WI
Strawberries

MI
Apples
Blueberries
Cherries (sweet)
Strawberries

IL
Apples

OH
Apples
Cherries (sour)
Strawberries

KY
Apples

PA
Apples
Cherries
Strawberries

NY
Apples
Cherries
Strawberries

VT
Apples

ME
Apples
Blueberries

NH
Apples

MA
Apples

CT
Apples

RI
Apples

NJ
Apples
Blueberries
Strawberries

MD
Apples

WV
Apples

VA
Apples
Peaches

NC
Peaches
Strawberries

TN
Apples
Peaches

SC
Cantaloupes
Peaches
Watermelons

AR
Apples
Peaches
Strawberries

MS
Peaches
Watermelons

AL
Peaches
Watermelons

GA
Cantaloupes
Peaches
Watermelons

LA
Melons
Peaches
Strawberries

FL
Avocados
Grapefruit
Limes
Mangoes
Navel oranges

Strawberries
Tangelos
Temple oranges
Valencia oranges
Watermelons

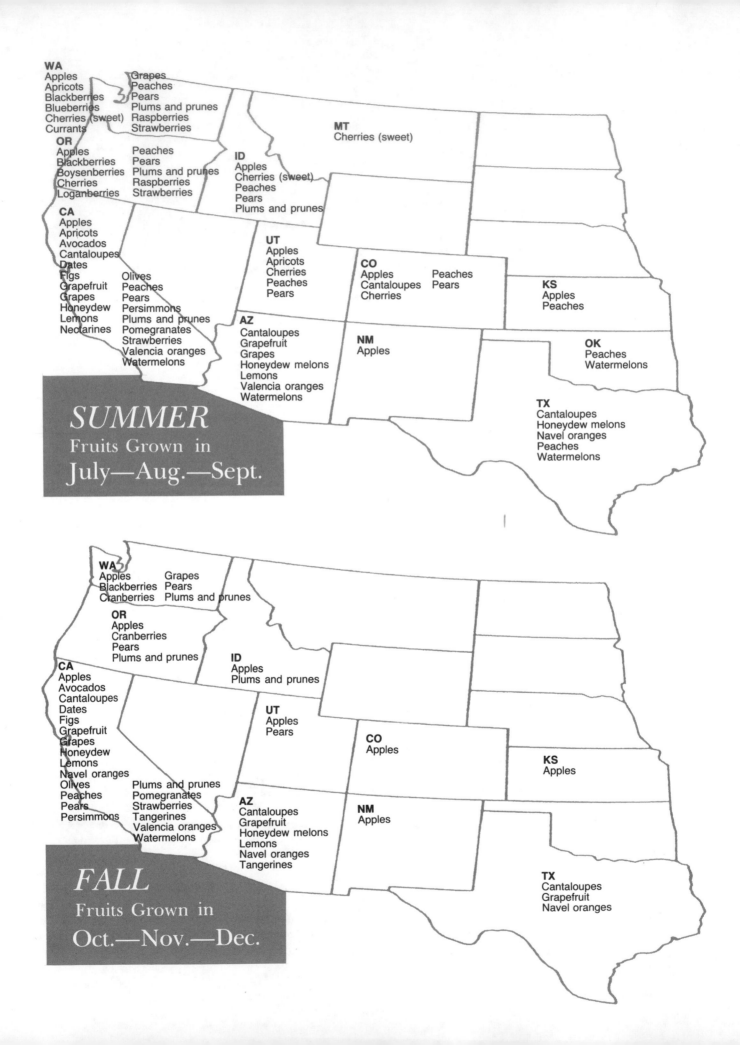

WA
Apples
Apricots
Blackberries
Blueberries
Cherries (sweet)
Currants
Grapes
Peaches
Pears
Plums and prunes
Raspberries
Strawberries

OR
Apples
Blackberries
Boysenberries
Cherries
Loganberries
Peaches
Pears
Plums and prunes
Raspberries
Strawberries

MT
Cherries (sweet)

ID
Apples
Cherries (sweet)
Peaches
Pears
Plums and prunes

CA
Apples
Apricots
Avocados
Cantaloupes
Dates
Figs
Grapefruit
Grapes
Honeydew
Lemons
Nectarines
Olives
Peaches
Pears
Persimmons
Plums and prunes
Pomegranates
Strawberries
Valencia oranges
Watermelons

UT
Apples
Apricots
Cherries
Peaches
Pears

CO
Apples
Cantaloupes
Cherries
Peaches
Pears

KS
Apples
Peaches

AZ
Cantaloupes
Grapefruit
Grapes
Honeydew melons
Lemons
Valencia oranges
Watermelons

NM
Apples

OK
Peaches
Watermelons

TX
Cantaloupes
Honeydew melons
Navel oranges
Peaches
Watermelons

SUMMER
Fruits Grown in
July—Aug.—Sept.

WA
Apples
Blackberries
Cranberries
Grapes
Pears
Plums and prunes

OR
Apples
Cranberries
Pears
Plums and prunes

ID
Apples
Plums and prunes

CA
Apples
Avocados
Cantaloupes
Dates
Figs
Grapefruit
Grapes
Honeydew
Lemons
Navel oranges
Olives
Peaches
Pears
Persimmons
Plums and prunes
Pomegranates
Strawberries
Tangerines
Valencia oranges
Watermelons

UT
Apples
Pears

CO
Apples

KS
Apples

AZ
Cantaloupes
Grapefruit
Honeydew melons
Lemons
Navel oranges
Tangerines

NM
Apples

TX
Cantaloupes
Grapefruit
Navel oranges

FALL
Fruits Grown in
Oct.—Nov.—Dec.

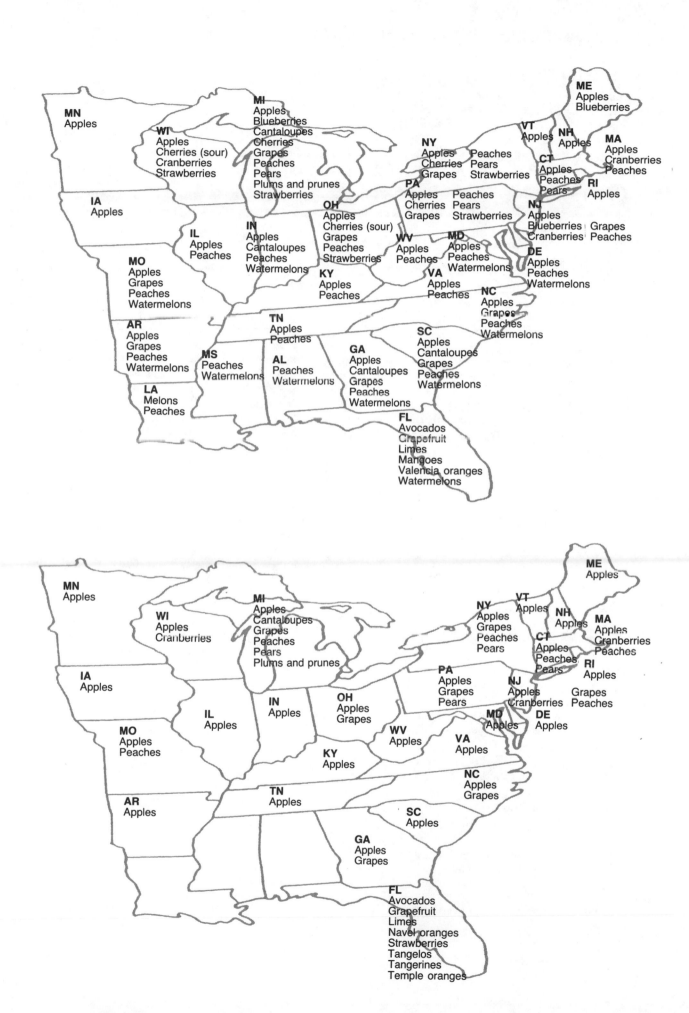

MN
Apples

MI
Apples
Blueberries
Cantaloupes
Cherries
Grapes
Peaches
Pears
Plums and prunes
Strawberries

WI
Apples
Cherries (sour)
Cranberries
Strawberries

ME
Apples
Blueberries

VT
Apples

NH
Apples

MA
Apples
Cranberries
Peaches

NY
Apples
Cherries
Grapes

Peaches
Pears
Strawberries

CT
Apples
Peaches
Pears

RI
Apples

IA
Apples

PA
Apples
Cherries
Grapes

Peaches
Pears
Strawberries

NJ
Apples
Blueberries
Cranberries

Grapes
Peaches

OH
Apples
Cherries (sour)
Grapes
Peaches
Strawberries

IL
Apples
Peaches

IN
Apples
Cantaloupes
Peaches
Watermelons

WV
Apples
Peaches

MD
Apples
Peaches
Watermelons

DE
Apples
Peaches
Watermelons

MO
Apples
Grapes
Peaches
Watermelons

KY
Apples
Peaches

VA
Apples
Peaches

NC
Apples
Grapes
Peaches
Watermelons

AR
Apples
Grapes
Peaches
Watermelons

TN
Apples
Peaches

SC
Apples
Cantaloupes
Grapes
Peaches
Watermelons

MS
Peaches
Watermelons

AL
Peaches
Watermelons

GA
Apples
Cantaloupes
Grapes
Peaches
Watermelons

LA
Melons
Peaches

FL
Avocados
Grapefruit
Limes
Mangoes
Valencia oranges
Watermelons

MN
Apples

MI
Apples
Cantaloupes
Grapes
Peaches
Pears
Plums and prunes

WI
Apples
Cranberries

ME
Apples

VT
Apples

NH
Apples

MA
Apples
Cranberries
Peaches

NY
Apples
Grapes
Peaches
Pears

CT
Apples
Peaches
Pears

RI
Apples

IA
Apples

PA
Apples
Grapes
Pears

NJ
Apples
Cranberries

Grapes
Peaches

IN
Apples

OH
Apples
Grapes

MD
Apples

DE
Apples

IL
Apples

WV
Apples

MO
Apples
Peaches

KY
Apples

VA
Apples

NC
Apples
Grapes

AR
Apples

TN
Apples

SC
Apples

GA
Apples
Grapes

FL
Avocados
Grapefruit
Limes
Navel oranges
Strawberries
Tangelos
Tangerines
Temple oranges

A Shopper's Guide to Jams and Jellies

Most people use the word "jam" to refer to that broad category of fruit spreads that we so eagerly apply on toast, muffins, pancakes, sandwiches, and crackers. If the $800 million yearly sales of their commercial counterparts is any indication, the potential for natural jams is almost unlimited. "The category is expanding dramatically because the consumer wants a better product," says Carol Pressman, national sales manager of Sorrell Ridge, a leading natural jam producer. Pressman estimates that natural jams account for about 2 percent or $16 million of the total market. Consumers are attracted to natural jams because they are free of refined sugar, artificial ingredients, and colorings. Although natural jams are more expensive than conventional products, many consumers are happy to pay the extra price for quality ingredients.

Natural jams are marketed under a variety of confusing terminology. Finding jars variously labeled jam, jelly, preserve, spread, fruit butter, and conserve, the differences are not readily apparent to the consumer. But these terms do describe somewhat different products. The following are some working definitions.

The term *jelly* commonly refers to the clear, wiggly product made from the strained juice of various fruits. *Jams* and *preserves* are now considered to be identical products and the terms are used interchangeably. They are the thick, opaque, gelled sauce of cooked whole fruit. However, old-timers recall that preserves once contained the seeds, while in jams they were strained out. A *fruit butter* is whole fruit that has been cooked down until it becomes smooth and thick and like a puree. It is less sweet and gelatinous than either jam or jelly. The word *spread* is applied to a wide variety of fruit, nut, and dairy products and is used to describe those concoctions that don't fall under the common Food and Drug Administration (FDA) standards of identity.

The FDA definitions of jams and preserves, jellies, and fruit butters specify minimum ratios of fruit to sweetener, and a minimum level of total sugar concentration, which may be achieved by the addition of natural sweeteners (such as honey or fruit concentrates) and commercial sweeteners (sugar, corn sweeteners).

Several natural jam manufacturers are unable to use the term jam or preserve on their labels because they prefer to produce products that have less sweetener, or ingredients in different combination, than what is required under the FDA specifications for the use of those terms. So natural jam makers have adopted the term conserve, which is not defined and regulated. Whether it is legal to use this undefined term on the label is being debated within the FDA and the commercial jam industry. Many feel that its use is not legal and such products should be labeled as spreads. But it appears not to be a high-priority issue within the FDA and it is doubtful that any action will be taken against manufacturers who use the term. In the meantime, shoppers can expect to see the word conserve applied to a variety of jam-, jelly-, and spread-like products.

Eden Foods of Clinton, Michigan, is well known for their organic commodities, soymilk, and macrobiotic imports. But they also market a rich, Pennsylvania-Dutch-style unsweetened apple butter and a line of seven fruit jams. Eden jams are made with real whole fruit (not concentrates), honey, and pectin. They are thick, farm-style jams and not too sweet, the honey being barely detectable beneath

---

and mellow after harvest. *Cantaloupes* should be cream-colored and covered with netting. Smooth spots spell trouble, as does a jagged stem end. There should be a depressed scar at the stem, called "full slip." *Persian* melons also should be without smooth spots and should give a little when pressed. A light greyish-green color beneath the netting is normal when the fruit is ripe. In a *casaba* melon, look for a golden-yellow color and some give at the stem end. The *crenshaw* is ripe when its rind, or skin, has softened (especially at the large end) and it has a golden skin and sweet smell. *Honeydew* melons with a white or greenish-white rind were picked too early. The skin of a ripe honeydew is green; it feels a little sticky or velvety and the rind is somewhat soft if pressed. Finding a sweet *watermelon* is not easy, even for the experts. Avoid shiny skins and greenish or white "ground spots" (these should be yellow or amber).

Storage: Refrigerate melons when they're ripe, but only for a few days. Watermelons keep a week if refrigerated.

Nutrition: Melons contain vitamins C and A. The darker orange melons have more vitamin A.

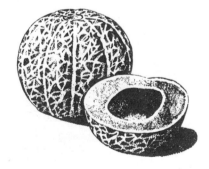

Nectarines

Origin: A native of the Orient, the nectarine is like a peach, only smoother-skinned and somewhat sweeter. Pre-World-War-II varieties were white-fleshed and reportedly of excellent taste, but they shipped poorly. Today, although

their full fruit flavor.

Cascadian Farm of Rockport, Washington, grows and markets organic berries that find their way into Cascadian's wonderful line of eight organic conserves. That they have a way with berries is evident in the variety they present, which includes huckleberry, blueberry, blackberry, and loganberry. The conserves are mildly sweetened with honey and gelled with pectin to provide a light texture. The texture varies slightly with the differing consistencies of the organic fruit from batch to batch.

Poiret is a one-of-a-kind Belgian pear spread imported by Lifetone International of Boca Raton, Florida. Poiret's only ingredients are pears and other fruits. Entire whole fruits are cooked down in a century-old process that produces a dense, viscous spread that looks and acts more like an extra-thick barley malt than a jam or jelly. They have eight flavors made from a 50-50 combination of pears with such fruits as apple, black cherry, lemon, and passion fruit.

Somerset Farms is a line of English preserves, made from fruit, grape juice, and pectin, imported by Signature Foods of Hunt Valley, Maryland. While the use of grape juice (concentrate) is preferred by many consumers over honey, in these preserves it simply overpowers the fruit flavors with sweetness and renders them tasteless. Somerset's appearance and texture is clear and more jelly-like than that of many other preserves. This is an odd line of jams that seems to be poorly defined, and distinguishable by little other than its intense sweetness.

Sorrell Ridge, produced by the Allied Old English Co. of Reading, New Jersey, is a line of fifteen fruit-sweetened conserves which includes grape (very jelly-like), cranberry, apple cider, and seedless red raspberry along with more standard flavors. Sorrell Ridge conserves used to be sweetened with honey but now are all made with fruit juice (grape, apple, and lemon concentrates). Their labeling is inconsistent between flavors. They claim to be "unsweetened—fruit only" on one flavor, "unsweetened—no sugar added" on another, and "sweetened with natural fruit juice concentrates" on another. Since they all contain variations on the basic formula of fruit, fruit concentrates, and pectin, this is confusing, especially since the fruit concentrates are definitely there to add sweetness. But surprisingly, the line is not overly sweet. It is flavorful, and nicely textured with pieces of whole fruit.

Westbrae of Emeryville, California, has two lines of natural jams. Their five flavors of butter-like, unsweetened fruit spreads contain only fruit, apple puree, and agar (to provide consistent gelling). Their fruit-sweetened conserve line has five flavors, including a grape jelly; these are made from fruit, grape juice concentrate, lemon juice, and citrus pectin. The fruit spreads have a vivid fruit taste and are mildly sweet, just like fresh fruit itself. The conserves are dense and opaque with a good flavor but are of looser texture than traditional style preserves. They have a nice, balanced sweetness which is noticeably less sweet than most other brands.

Whole Earth from London, England (also imported by Lifetone), is one of the original fruit-sweetened spreads and is available in nine varieties. They are sweet but not as sweet as you would expect from a product that lists the sweetener, apple juice concentrate, as its first ingredient. Other ingredients are fruit and pectin. Whole Earth spreads are a loosely gelled and sometimes inconsistent product that can be quite runny at times. But the flavor is clean and fruity and the variety delightful. Flavors include hedgerow fruits, Seville orange, and black currant.

many varieties are sold, there are two basic kinds—clingstone and freestone. Clingstones are named for the way the flesh stubbornly clings to the pit. California supplies most nectarines in the United States.

Season: Nectarines are available from late March to September.

Selection: The sugar content of nectarines does not increase after picking, so avoid purchasing green, immature fruits. Select ones that are firm with a slight softening along the seam. The skin should have a breath of red in a yellow or yellow-orange setting. Avoid very hard and/or dull-colored nectarines.

Storage: Firm fruit will soften at room temperature in a few days, after which it should be eaten or refrigerated for, at most, a few days.

Peaches

Origin: Peaches originated in China, but the juicy sweet varieties sold today don't even resemble the small, hard, bitter ones from the Far East. The peach wended its way through the Near East, and southern Europe, and finally arrived in the Western Hemisphere in the 17th century. Most peaches sold fresh are of freestone varieties, which are softer and more delicate than clingstones. Today peaches are raised commercially in at least thirty-five states, but California is responsible for the canning of nearly all the cling peaches. California's peach-canning industry is the largest fruit-packing business in the world.

Season: Peaches are available from early May to September. July and August are the peak months.

Selection: As with nectarines, the sugar content of peaches does not increase after picking. Avoid selecting immature, green fruits, which are disappointingly dry and flavorless. However, brilliant pink or red colors do not necessarily guarantee the best flavor. Choose a soft yellow fruit that gives a little when pressed. If the fruit is fresh and locally grown, there is less chance that it was picked when immature. If you find fuzz on peaches, chances are they've escaped the standard commercial bathhouse that washes, de-fuzzes, and sometimes waxes the fruit. And fuzzy peaches are less likely to have been sprayed. Fuzz is fine to eat, but if a peach has been sprayed, it's possible the spray will adhere to the fuzz and dissolve less easily.

Storage: Refrigeration keeps a ripened peach for about two weeks.

Nutrition: Peaches are a source of vitamin A.

Pears

Origin: A fruit cultivated by the ancient Greeks and Romans as well as by the Chinese, the pear was brought to North America by colonists in the early 17th century. Thousands of varieties are recorded, none native to North America. Principal commercial varieties are the Bartlett (yellow), Anjou (green to yellow-green), and Bosc (goose-necked shape, yellow-brown to cinnamon). Others include Comices and Winter Nelises. Some, such as the Bartlett, are soft and juicy when ripe, and others, like the Bosc, can be enjoyed for their sweetness even before they soften. Certain grainy or sandy varieties such as the Seckel are originally from China. Pears sold in the United States come from California, Oregon, and Washington.

Season: The availability of pears depends on their variety. Bartlett is a summer fruit, available from July to November. The Seckel is available in the early autumn months. The Anjou arrives in October and is around till May.

Selection: Most pears are sold unripened, but two to three days at home will do it. A slight softness means they are ready. Some, especially Bartletts, bruise easily, but can be enjoyed even when they look a little beat up. Still, choose pears with as few cuts and dark spots as possible.

Storage: After pears ripen, refrigerate them and eat them soon. Before ripening, pears will keep several weeks under refrigeration.

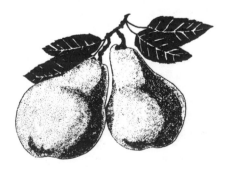

Persimmons

Origin: Though persimmons belong to the tropical ebony family, native North American varieties were found growing wild in Virginia by Captain John Smith in the early 17th century. Wild varieties can still be found in the southeastern United States. The persimmon has become hard to find, however, as the acreage of persimmon trees in this country has fallen more than 90 percent in the last half century. (The wood is quite valuable and the trees have been heavily lumbered.) The persimmons sold commercially today in the United States have an Oriental heritage, probably Chinese. California produces nearly all the commercial crop. Though they grow well in warm areas, persimmons exhibit a cold tolerance of 3°–11° F for many continuous growing seasons.

Season: Persimmons are available from late September to mid-December.

Selection: Be careful! Biting into the flesh of a brilliant orange, slightly firm, apparently ripe persimmon is a mistake you will make only once in your lifetime. Some varieties of persimmons (usually identified as "Japanese") are ripe, edible, and sweet while still firm, but most domestic varieties only become sweet when they are mushy. Make that "sloshy," to be safe. Before then they can make your mouth pucker, due to the large tannin content that is present prior to sweetening. Frost does not, as is sometimes believed, cause the persimmon to lose its astringency but actually slows down ripening.

Choose full-bodied, colorful fruits, on the reddish side rather than light orange (a lighter-colored Japanese persimmon, however, may be perfectly ripe). And be sure to wait till they get very soft before opening them up. If you do, you will enjoy a delicious food that most people in the United States never have the opportunity to try.

Storage: Allow persimmons to ripen in a closed plastic bag. Refrigerate them for at most a few days.

Nutrition: The persimmon is not very high in iron, but contains more than any other fresh fruit, except for dates. It is rich in potassium and quite rich in vitamins C and A.

Plums

Origin: The family name of the Chinese philosopher Lao-tse is Li, which means plum tree. The plums sold in the United States today had their origin in China; their forebears were brought to California by Luther Burbank a century ago. There are native American plums, but none is commercially important. A wide selection of varieties is sold, including Santa Rosa (early season), El Dorado (mid-season), and Casselman (late season). Plums come in a rainbow of colors—greens, blues, reds, and yellows—and different shades of each. Most are grown in California.

Season: Plums are on the market from May to August.

Selection: Consult your produce seller because the signs of plum ripeness differ with variety. Some are ripe when firm and green, while others must be soft and dark red. Some do not ripen well off the tree. Others do. Ask and experiment.

Storage: When fully ripe, plums are perishable and should be refrigerated.

Nutrition: Plums supply potassium.

Pomegranates

Origin: One of the most unusual of fruits, the pomegranate is an imperfectly round shape with a bumpy rough surface and is about the size of an apple. Most varieties are red, but a few are yellow. Their insides abound in tiny glittering rubies, cell-like packages of seeds bathed in a delightfully tart juice. The main varieties in the United States are appropriately called Wonderful and Red Wonderful.

Pomegranates originated in the Near East, where religious significance surrounds them. The Prophet Mohammed declared, ''Eat the pomegranate, for it purges the system of envy and hatred.'' In Greek myth, Persephone, the daughter of the corn goddess, Demeter, was abducted by Hades to the underworld. Neglecting the corn, Demeter came looking for her daughter. But because she had eaten a pomegranate seed in the underworld, Persephone had to remain with Hades for a third of each year ever after. When Demeter and Persephone are together, the corn grows; when they are apart, the earth is barren.

Do not be like Persephone—use caution when eating. Pomegranate juice flies with great speed in all directions as you begin to pursue it. There are techniques for eating this fruit, but describing them would steal half the fun. Today's pomegranates are raised in California.

Season: Pomegranates are available from September to December. October is the peak month.

Selection: Look for good color and a skin free of cracks when you buy pomegranates.

Storage: Refrigerated, this fruit keeps at least several weeks.

Nutrition: Pomegranates supply potassium.

Raspberries

See Blackberries.

Strawberries

Origin: This fruit grows wild in many parts of the world and is native to North America. The commercial variety sold today is bred for its hardiness and is much different than some of the smaller, wild types. Nevertheless, it sometimes is quite sweet and tasty. In the United States, strawberries are raised primarily in California, but some crops are grown in Washington and Oregon.

Season: Strawberry season runs from February to November; the peak month is May.

Selection: Pick bright red, shiny, dry strawberries. Look at the bottom of the container for hidden moldy berries. Green caps should be attached and nicely colored. Big strawberries are no promise of flavor—small berries sometimes are the best.

Storage: Fresh strawberries must be kept aired out and cool; eat them soon. Frozen strawberries will keep.

Nutrition: Strawberries contain vitamin C.

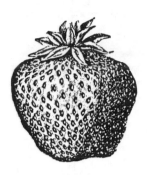

Subtropical Fruits
Citrus Fruits

Origin and Varieties: The U.S. citrus industry is a commercial phenomenon that has turned American consumers into citrus-lovers almost overnight. Through aggressive marketing—including strong nutritional claims for its products—this industry has led consumers in northern climates to believe that citrus is one of the surest cold preventives and one of the few reliable sources of vitamin C one can find. Both claims are grossly overstated, but they've served as the impetus for retail sales of $8 billion a year to the U.S public. Thus, fruits like the orange, which is native to southeastern Asia, are being eaten in large quantities in cultures never before familiar with them.

The citrus family has many members. The common sweet orange is a refreshing fruit with a spirited taste, as are its relatives, which include the mandarin orange (some varieties of which are called tangerines); the grapefruit; the Temple orange, which is a cross between the tangerine and the sweet orange; the tangelo, a cross between the tangerine and grapefruit; and the kumquat (not a true citrus but of a closely related species). The lemon and lime are useful as flavoring agents. The Seville or bitter orange is grown mostly in Spain and goes into sugary marmalades.

Season: The citrus industry applies strict quality-control measures to guarantee the best appearance of these fruits, and relies on a great number of nonorganic methods. Chemically farmed and treated citrus products are always available.

Selection: Citrus fruits are all extremely well-groomed for market and are available year-round. A handful of small-scale farmers sell organic citrus. If you can find them, they are the ones to choose.

Storage: Most citrus fruits are so heavily treated with chemical dips and fumigants that they can be stored without refrigeration for some time. In the refrigerator, they will keep a little while longer. Chemically treated citrus fruits spoil very slowly.

Nutrition: When the many overstated nutritional claims are discounted, the fact remains that fresh citrus fruits do have vitamin C and fair amounts of calcium.

Dates

Origin: The date palm is one of the oldest of cultivated plants, if not the oldest—the Babylonians were growing it 8,000 years ago. Muslims regard it as the Tree of Life. Islamic literature reveals that God commanded Adam to cut his hair and fingernails and bury the clippings in the ground. Immediately a palm tree sprang up, laden with ripe and tasty dates. As Adam fell to his knees and thanked God, the Archangel Gabriel appeared and said, "Thou art created of the same material as this tree which henceforth shall nourish you." Thus the date became a principal symbol of life and food for Islamic people. The Koran, which generally prohibits consumption of alcoholic beverages, makes an exception for a spirit beverage made from fermented dates and water.

Most of the world's 3-million-ton annual date production occurs in the Middle East, Iraq today being the leading producer. In this century, however, the date palm has been successfully raised in the dry, hot climates of southern California and Arizona. Deglet Noor and Medjool date trees grow in California's Coachella Valley.

Popular varieties of dates include the Khalasa—"quintessence"—and Barhee, named for the "barh" or hot winds of the desert. Also, Halawy, "the sweet," and Khadrawy, "the verdant," are popular Middle Eastern varieties. Deglet Noor is interpreted as "date of light" and Medjool means "the unknown." The latter is perhaps the richest-tasting of all the dates. A single Medjool is an ample dessert for all but the most sweet-toothed person.

Season: Dates are available year-round.

Selection: Choose those that look plump and soft. Dry or flaky dates should be avoided. They are not nearly as tasty as fully fresh ones.

Storage: Refrigerate dates after opening package. Keep loose dates well-wrapped to prevent drying. As dates

Upsetting the Apple Cart

While technology loads the fruit baskets of Americans with an unprecedented bounty, questions arise not only concerning production methods, but also regarding consumption habits and whether they have been unduly shaped by the fruit industry's marketing practices. Questioning something as wholesome as fruit-eating is risky business, but consumption patterns of North Americans have changed so markedly in this century that the effects are worth considering.

Though today we individually consume about the same quantity of fresh fruit as in 1909 (when the first reliable data were compiled), intake is up considerably from pre-industrial days due simply to the year-round availability of a world market of fruits made possible by refrigeration and better transportation. Furthermore, since the turn of the century, our choice of fruits has widened dramatically. Whereas we once consumed fruits indigenous to our temperate zone, today we emphasize those imported from outside our climatic belt. Per capita consumption of the apple, a fruit native to the temperate climates and once America's leading fruit, has been

overtaken by an array of domesticated subtropical and imported tropical fruits. Sunkist Growers reported United States per capita citrus consumption in 1980 to be 29 pounds per year, making citrus the leading category of fresh fruit consumed. Second was the banana, a tropical fruit, at 22 pounds, followed by apples at 21 pounds, peaches 6 pounds, and pears 4 pounds. Even though these figures exclude juices, of which much orange is consumed, they show that more subtropical citrus and tropical bananas are eaten than all the temperate fruits combined. U.S. production of apples fell from 3.4 million tons in 1919 to 2.6 million in 1960, while citrus production rose during that period from 1.4 million to 7.5 million tons.

Many will ask, "So what? Aren't oranges and bananas perfectly healthful foods full of valuable nutients?" Generally speaking, any fruit eaten in modest amounts in balance with an overall prudent diet promotes health. Fruit can be a natural, wholesome food. Tropical and subtropical fruits, however, as can be seen from the above figures, are becoming a major part of the North American diet,

and are eaten throughout the winter. An orange used to be a rare treat, found in a Christmas stocking. Never before have humans in temperate climates been able to indulge in these sweet, warm-weather foods in cold weather to the extent we do now.

Some health authorities are coming to question whether drinking large quantities of orange juice and eating bananas and papayas during a Minnesota winter impairs the body's ability to balance itself against the cold. Fruits have little fat, burn quickly, and provide scarce fuel reserves for warmth. Might consuming them out-of-season be physiologically unbalancing?

Another reservation about indiscriminate fruit-eating is the problem of sugar. In the United States, our intake of refined sugar has skyrocketed in this century. Annual per capita consumption jumped from 86 pounds in 1909 to 130 pounds in 1981. These figures do not include the sugar in fruits, but the demands made on the body in metabolizing the principal fruit sugars, fructose and sucrose, are similar to those for refined sugar. The apparent epidemic of hypoglycemic symptoms would suggest that all simple sugar consumption (including that of fruits) should be minimized by some people at least until blood-sugar regulating functions can be normalized.

Finally, there are political and economic considerations. For instance, countries where the banana industry exerts a strong influence on the lives of large numbers of people are known, derisively, as "banana republics." A political, economic, and social issue in countries such as Costa Rica, the Philippines, and Guatemala has been the continued growth of a banana industry that satisfies the profit goals of businesses and the sweet-tooth cravings of wealthier countries, but all too often robs peasant farmers of land and/or food. In the "banana republics," land that had once been devoted to staple grains and legumes serving the needs of the local population has often been converted to banana planting. Growers frequently abuse the rich soil by planting heavily, using large amounts of synthetic fertilizers, and never allowing the land to rest. Two U.S. corporations, United Fruit Company and Standard Fruit and Steamship Company, control 70 percent of the world's 37-million-ton-per-year banana production.

absorb odors, do not store them near onions, fish, or other strong-smelling foods.

Nutrition: The date is fairly well endowed with nutrients, but perhaps its outstanding characteristic is its complete lack of vitamin C, which makes it unique in the fruit kingdom. Dates, however, are rich in calcium, phosphorus, iron, and sodium. Their principal component is sugar. A fresh date is 20 percent water and about 65 percent sugar. Dried dates are 80 percent sugar. Date sugar is sold in many stores as an alternative to cane sugar.

Figs

Origin: Cultivation of the fig occurred 5,000 years ago. One reason for its ancient popularity may have been the ease with which the sun dries and preserves a fresh fig. All figs are delicious dried, but if you've never had a fresh one, you have something to look forward to. In their fresh state, the Mission is dark purple, the Kadota is yellow, and the Calimyrna (the California Smyrna) is yellowish-green. In the U.S., most figs are grown in California. The Bible includes numerous references to this fruit, such as Adam and Eve's sewing fig leaves together to cover their nakedness and Mary hiding the Christ child from Herod's soldiers in the trunk of a fig tree.

Today, from an agricultural standpoint, the most interesting aspect of the fig is the way the Smyrna fig tree is pollinated. Early American farmers had a rough time watching their Smyrna figs fall prematurely to the ground until they learned about the method of pollination called caprification. The Capri fig tree bears an inedible fruit that houses small wasps. These fruits are picked and hung in baskets on the Smyrna trees. The female wasp then attempts to enter the Smyrna fig to lay her eggs, leaving behind enough pollen from the Capri fig for fertilization to occur. This is an ancient practice still used in commercial fig orchards because it is the only way known to keep the Smyrna fig on the tree to maturity.

Season: Figs are available from June to October.

Selection: The riper, the sweeter. Size is not an indication of sweetness or flavor. A fig that has partially dried is quite acceptable, but may turn sour if the juice inside ferments.

Storage: The fig is a perishable fruit. Either eat figs soon after purchasing them, or keep them refrigerated for four to five days at most.

Mangoes

Origin: If you have ever been to India, you probably have fond memories of this delicate, perfume-scented fruit. Its flavors, aromas, and rainbow colors, as well as the texture of its flesh, fully capture the senses. In the U.S., the Hayden variety of Florida is the most popular. Others, out of season, come from the West Indies, Haiti, and Mexico.

Season: Mangoes are in season from May to September, with peak availability in June.

Selection: Select a mango that has some color other than green, as an all-green mango may never ripen. Pass over any mangoes that have black spots or are extremely soft.

Storage: If firm, the mango will ripen at room temperature in three to four days. After it's soft and ripe, it can be refrigerated for several days.

Nutrition: Mangoes contain vitamins C and A and potassium.

Tropical Fruits

Avocados

Origin: The avocado is a native of the Western Hemisphere. California and Florida are the two main U.S. producers.

Season: Avocados are available year-round, with a peak from January to May.

Selection: Avocados vary widely in size, shape, texture, color, and thickness of skin. They can be large or small, round or pear-shaped, smooth or pebbly, and green or dark purple. The dark purple Hass or Mexican variety is favored by many. Choose fruit that yields a bit to gentle pressure. Avoid both hard and mushy fruits as well as those that have dark spots or appear bruised.

Storage: Store avocados at room temperature. Under-ripe fruit can be ripened at room temperature (placing it in a paper bag will hasten the process). Do not cut avocados open until they are ripe. After cutting, brush them with lemon or lime juice to minimize browning. Wrap unused portions tightly and store them in the refrigerator.

Nutrition: Avocados provide thiamin, riboflavin, potassium, and vitamin A. They are rich in unsaturated oil, and are one of the few fruits to have significant levels of fat.

Bananas

Origin: As with citrus fruits, North Americans in this century have grown fond of bananas. We ate 4.5 billion pounds of them in 1980. Bananas have been a staple food in the diet of some tropical peoples for thousands of years. Before bananas ripen, they contain an appreciable amount of starch. Cooked green bananas can make a satisfying main carbohydrate dish. Plantains, which closely resemble the sweet bananas generally consumed in the United States, are frequently served this way throughout East Africa and Latin America. In a ripened sweet banana, on the other hand, the starch has been broken down into simple sugars. Ripe bananas are the highest in sugar of any fruit (other than dried fruits and possibly very ripe persimmons), and have become a candy-like treat in the U.S.

Bananas originated in southeast Asia before traveling like a forest fire around the world—to India, Arabia, the Canary Islands, Africa, the Caribbean Islands, and Mexico. They were introduced to the U.S. after the Civil War and remained a luxury item until the turn of the century when shipments from Latin America increased. Most bananas sold in the U.S. today come from Central America and Mexico. There are few varietal distinctions among commercial bananas, the two main ones being Cavendish and Gros Michel.

Season: Bananas are in year-round supply.

Selection: A fully green banana (full of starch) will sweeten and become soft after picking. Most bananas are picked very green; ripening is induced in air-controlled (ethylene-filled) rooms, and the bananas reach the stores in "green-tip" condition. The only bananas to avoid are ones with a cloudy look which may have suffered cold damage and be unable to ripen.

Storage: If you buy yellow bananas with green tips, they will ripen in three days at home, after which they can be refrigerated for a few days. Do *not* refrigerate bananas before they are ripe unless you want to stop the sugar-forming process. Refrigerating a ripe banana will darken its skin color but will not affect the flavor.

Nutrition: Bananas are a source of potassium. A fully ripe banana is about 21 percent sugar. About 13 percent of

this is sucrose, which is chemically equivalent to table sugar.

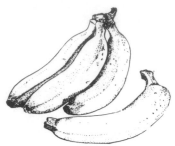

Papayas

Origin: Papayas are native to either Mexico or the West Indies and came with the pineapple to Hawaii, which is the commercial papaya center today.

Season: Papayas are available all year; peak season is May and June.

Selection: A fruity aroma and a little give to pressure signal a ripe papaya. They'll ripen at home in two to three days. Stay away from shriveled, bruised, broken, or very soft papayas.

Storage: Once ripe, papayas will keep refrigerated for a couple of days.

Nutrition: Papayas contain vitamins C and A. The papain enzyme is what papaya promoters talk about. It is said to aid in the digestion of protein and is used as a meat tenderizer. Health food stores sell papain pills for a host of digestive disorders, although the wisdom of using these supplements is uncertain. However, if papain is good for you, papayas have it.

Pineapples

Origin: This fruit was a rare and prized gift for anyone living outside the tropics—until air freight arrived. Now pineapples from Hawaii are sold in the continental U.S. all year long. Pineapples are probably indigenous to South America. The Carib Indians hung pineapples or their crowns over doorways to express welcome, and the fruit, or a depiction of it, still indicates hospitality. The Smooth Cayenne variety from the Hawaiian Islands is the biggest seller.

According to Waverly Root, "Pineapple became the most ruthlessly regimented of all cultivated fruits, living out its life in an artificial atmosphere of man-made chemicals and subjected completely to the manipulations of machines." He goes on to tell of fumigators and fertilizers, herbicides and pesticides, and hormones to make the fruits ripen to the same size at the same time. The roots of the trees pass through the center of the asphalted mulch paper and the trees are rigidly aligned. If a pineapple is too large or too small to be picked by the mechanical harvester, it is left to rot.

Season: Pineapples are available year-round.

Selection: The pineapple's failure to ripen after picking prevented its widespread distribution until recently. Much of the starch is stored in the stem instead of in the edible part. Therefore, early picking means a fruit with no starch for conversion to sugar. Before the fruit is picked, just before it ripens, the starch converts to sugar and travels to the edible fruit where the sweetness increases. Picked too early a pineapple can be hopelessly flat. How do you choose one that you know didn't suffer this fate? Some fruit authorities maintain that a yellow-amber outer color is the best indicator of flavor. Others contend that green pineapples can be sweet and tasty, or that a flavorful pineapple will exude a sweet, fruity aroma.

The booklet published by the Pineapple Growers Association of Hawaii states: "Ease in pulling the leaves out of a crown is not a sign of ripeness. That's just . . . 'an old wives' tale.' Forget it." Whatever other criteria you use in selecting a pineapple, it is a good idea to choose one that is plump and firm, with fresh green leaves.

Storage: Eat the sweet pineapple soon, or store it in a plastic bag (to retain moisture) for three to five days at most.

Nutrition: Pineapples supply vitamin C.

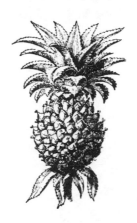

Dried Fruits: What to Look For

When people first discovered dried fruits, it must have been a landmark day ranking with the discovery of fire. Nature's harvest does not apportion itself to meet our every need. Fruits are borne mostly in the warmth of summer (which is the best time to eat them), and if not eaten quickly or preserved, they will spoil. The microorganisms responsible for spoilage require warmth, air, and moisture. When a certain amount of moisture is removed at the right time, however, the fruit will remain edible for weeks and even months at room temperature, longer if refrigerated.

Ounce for ounce, dried fruits usually have more vitamins and minerals than their fresh counterparts because the fruit is dehydrated and the nutrients are concentrated into a smaller volume. (For example, raisins are high in iron, providing 3.5 milligrams per 100 grams, whereas the comparable amount of grapes contains just .4 milligrams of this important mineral.) To get those concentrated nutrients, though, you must consume large amounts of sugar, which is the principal component of dried fruit. A grape is 82 percent water and 16 percent carbohydrate, while a raisin is 18 percent water and 77 percent carbohydrate—most of which is simple sugar. Also, some nutrients are lost in the drying process. A 100-gram portion of grapes contains 100 International Units (I.U.) of vitamin A; the same weight of raisins has only 20 I.U. Drying also destroys almost all of the ascorbic acid (vitamin C), a principal nutrient in many fruits.

Just about any fruit can be dried. Marco Polo in the 13th century wrote of sweet melons that were cut into sections and dried in the sun: "Thus dried, they were sweeter than honey." Fruits can be dried nicely in the sun in a hot, dry climate (temperature over 90° F and humidity under 60 percent), or in a 140° F oven, or in any of the number of dehydrators currently marketed for home use. Drying fruit is not a complicated task, and a little reading will tell you how to get good results.

Ninety-nine percent of the dried fruits sold in the supermarket (with the exception of raisins) is treated with a compound of sulfur that is used solely for cosmetic reasons—to lighten the color. Unless your penchant is for light-colored dried fruits, avoid it. Much commercial dried fruit is also blanched, which means the processor has dried a cooked instead of a fresh fruit. Blanching causes the loss of flavor and nutrients and the reason for doing it—to make the fruit easier to chew—does the consumer with healthy teeth no favor. Unsulfured peaches, apples, apricots, and pears from natural foods stores will be markedly darker in appearance than their bright, sulfured counterparts. Their flavor will also be truer to the undried fruit.

Raisins may well have been the first popular dried fruit. Raisin grapes were growing in 2,000 B.C. in Persia and Egypt, and records of a thriving raisin trade date to 400 B.C. Asia Minor at the time of Christ was the center of a raisin industry.

The raisin is still the world's most popular dried fruit. Today, California is the biggest world producer. Though raisins had been known for many centuries in Europe, it was not until the last half of the 19th century that they began to be produced in California. Tradition has it that in 1873 a devastating heat wave left California grape growers with a shriveled crop, some of which one farmer gathered and sold in San Francisco. The public quickly embraced this new sweet food.

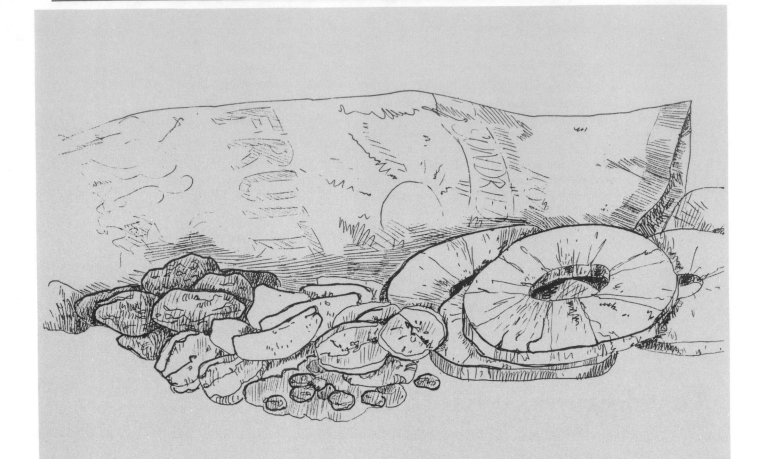

Several varieties of grapes make good raisins. The Thompson Seedless accounts for 95 percent of all raisins produced. Muscat grapes yield a delicious raisin that is larger and sweeter than the Thompson, and the seedless Black Corinth, sometimes called Zante, is grown for currants. Ronald Waltenspiel, who grows organic fruit and then dries it at Timber Crest Farms in Healdsburg, California, says that 90 percent of California's raisins are not treated either with sulfur or with pesticides.

Some raisins are dipped in hot water and mechanically dried (these have small checks in the skin and are of a lighter color); the package may indicate they have been sun-ripened, but it will not say "sun-dried." Others are sometimes covered with vegetable oil so they won't stick together, but you will usually find these treated raisins in baked goods or other store-bought products, not in packages or natural foods stores. The exception is the Golden Seedless or Golden raisin, commonly available in supermarkets, which is treated with sulfur dioxide to preserve its color. Imported raisins may be covered with mineral oil, or dried by means other than the sun.

The second most popular dried fruit is the prune. (The total dried fruit production in the United States in 1981 was 430,000 tons—258,000 of which were raisins and 121,000 prunes.) A prune is a dried plum, but not every dried plum becomes a prune. Only those varieties that can be sun-dried without fermenting while still containing the pit can be called prunes. This fruit originated in western Asia, but today three-quarters of the world's prunes come from California. Several varieties are sold, the most popular being the French. Whereas most raisins are dried in the sun, prunes are nearly all dehydrated mechanically. They are also pasteurized in boiling water.

The prune has long been noted for its laxative properties, a reputation that the prune industry has obviously profited from over the years. Prunes contain significant amounts of vitamin A and potassium, but as with all dried fruits, the nutrients come stored in a fairly sweet package.

Pineapple, which is naturally not as sweet as other fruits when dried, is usually glaceed—soaked in a sugar solution, which it absorbs. Most dried pineapple is sugared, though Ronald Waltenspiel distributes a dried-pineapple product that has been soaked in pineapple juice instead of in a sugar solution. A high-sugar dried pineapple piece is white, while Waltenspiel's are yellow.

8. SEEDS & NUTS

Along with peanuts or ground nuts, tree nuts such as walnuts, almonds, and pecans have enjoyed a renaissance recently, as shoppers have begun looking for healthful, economical alternatives to processed foods. The popularity of pumpkin, sesame, and sunflower seeds has also grown. Many consumers have realized that seeds and nuts are relatively high in protein and, especially if eaten unsalted, make for tasty, nutritious snacks.

Seeds and nuts are also versatile—they can be crushed or ground and then sprinkled on salads, vegetables, and grains. Another of their attractions is that most can be stored in their shells for months at a time. (A cool, dry, dark place is recommended.) Best of all, raw or roasted, salted or plain, whole or in pieces, seeds and nuts are crunchy and delicious.

In the following pages, we will take a look at a dozen seeds and nuts, providing information on their natural history, where and how they're grown, and what to look for in shopping for them. There is also a handy nutritional chart that compares the calories, fat, protein, and selected nutrients contained in these seeds and nuts.

One disadvantage to nuts is that eating them can entail some work, in the form of time-consuming shelling. This chapter is rounded out by a short guide to cracking some of the tougher nuts and a discussion of natural nut butters, in the hope that you'll be able to spend less time struggling with, and more time eating, these delicious foods.

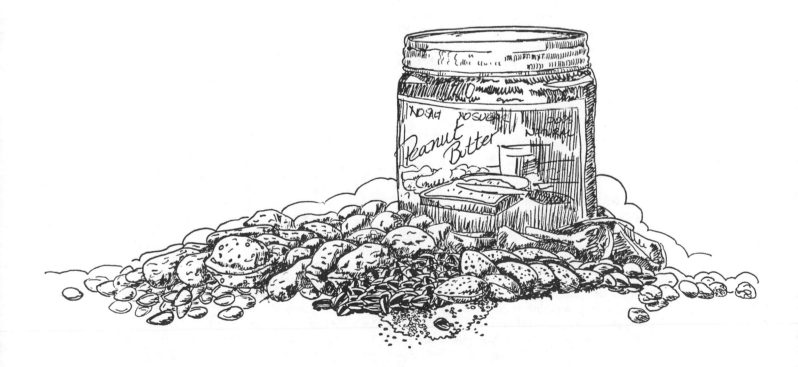

A Guide to Seeds & Nuts

A seed is the complete embryo of a young plant. Before seeds developed 350 million years ago, the dominant land plants were ferns. Ferns reproduce by broadcasting spores with either male or female sex organs. The sperm from the male plant makes its way through the water or earth to the female to create a seed embryo. This reproductive pattern worked especially well in a warm, moist environment, but as the land mass continued to rise the climate became drier. The atmosphere cleared, allowing the sun to further reduce the shaded moist habitat of the ferns. This drier land offered a great opportunity for those plants that could adapt.

A new type of plant began to develop in these higher, drier areas. The coniferous, or cone-bearing, plant has both male and female organs (cones) on the same plant. Fertilization takes place above the ground, the wind bearing millions of pollen grains from the male to the female cone. The fertilization of the female cone results in a naked seed embryo, which is cast forth as a fully developed young plant embryo with its own food source.

The conifers created the first true seeds, but these seeds are not a major modern food source because, for one thing, they must be pollinated by the wind. To ensure success the male cone must produce enormous amounts of pollen. In addition, the seed produced is usually naked—it has no hard outer covering—and once the cone opens the seed is unprotected.

About 130 million years ago, as the earth continued to cool, new plants developed more compact and efficient reproductive structures. The angiosperms, or flowering plants, contain the male and female organs on the inside. This development meant that while fertilization could still be accomplished by the wind, it could now be carried out even more efficiently by insects who, attracted to a flower's nectar, color, or scent, would directly carry the pollen from flower to flower. These angiosperms also enclosed their seeds in a hard protective vessel, called a seed coat.

Although sea vegetables and mushrooms comprise a small part of our diet, almost all of our vegetable food is derived from the flowering plants. Not only do they provide us with seeds such as grains, beans, and nuts, but we also eat their flowers, leaves, stems, and roots.

There is growing evidence indicating that seeds and nuts were the major staples of early humans. Archeological excavations lead one to believe that prehistoric men and women frequently used the seeds and nuts of a wide variety of wild plants, especially in the northern climates. The season during which food could be gathered was short, and as seeds and nuts are easily storable they were no doubt a more stable and convenient food source than roaming bands of reindeer or mammoths. Today, the cereal grains have replaced nuts as a staple food. Although they contain vitamin E and minerals, and are high in protein, nuts are also high in saturated fat, so eat them with moderation.

The following seeds and nuts are commonly found in the natural foods store. These stores may also stock flavorful butters made only from the unhydrogenated, unsweetened seed or nut (salt may be added). You can also make them yourself at home with the help of a hand mill. In addition, keep your eyes open for local favorites—hickory nuts, black walnuts, and butternuts are sometimes sold in the autumn by enterprising food foragers—or you can gather them yourself.

Seeds

Pumpkin Seeds

The commonly available pumpkin seeds do not come from the Halloween-type pumpkin but rather from a gourd-like variety grown specifically for its seeds in Central America. The highly nutritious seed contains up to 29 percent protein and played an important part in the diets of both North and South American Indians. Sometimes pumpkin seeds are called pepitas (*pepita* is the Spanish word for seed); they may be flat and oval or cylindrical.

Sesame Seeds

Sesame is the oldest known herb grown for its seeds. Used throughout prehistory, the seeds were an important food of the early Mediterranean and Eastern civilizations and continue to be to this day. Sesame seeds are extremely nutritious and highly versatile. The expression "Open Sesame" signifies an entrance into splendor and abundance. The Near East created two famous sesame dishes, hummus and halvah (made with tahini, or sesame paste). Greek and

Turkish soldiers carried the seeds at all times like K-rations. Five thousand years ago the Chinese burned sesame oil to make soot for ink blocking. The Egyptians milled sesame seeds to make a flour used in bread and other dishes. The Romans ground them into a paste to spread on bread.

Nutritionally the sesame seed is a powerhouse. It contains over 35 percent protein and has twice as much cal-cium as milk. Rich in phosphorus, niacin, and thiamine, sesame seeds also have as much iron as liver. In addition, the seeds are composed of 40 to 60 percent oil, an oil which is prized for its flavor and also for its stability since it resists oxidation and rancidity. In addition to its use in cooking, sesame oil is utilized in making fine lubricants and cosmetics.

Nutritional Content of Nuts and Seeds

Variety & Portion Size	Cal-ories	Protein (g)	Fat (g)	Fiber (g)	Vit C (mg)	Vit B₁ (mg)	Vit B₂ (mg)	Niacin (mg)	Potassium (mg)	Calcium (mg)	Iron (mg)
Almonds 12–15 nuts	90	2.8	8.1	na	tr	.04	.10	0.7	104	38	0.70
Brazil nuts 4 medium	97	2.2	9.9	0.3	0	.13	na	na	100	28	0.50
Cashews, roasted 6–8 nuts	84	2.6	6.9	0.2	na	.06	.04	0.3	70	6	0.60
Chestnuts, fresh 3 small	29	0.4	0.2	na	na	.03	.03	0.1	62	4	0.30
Filberts (hazelnuts) 10–12 nuts	97	1.6	9.5	2.3	1	.07	.08	0.8	71	38	0.50
Peanuts, raw 20–24 nuts	80	3.8	6.6	0.3	tr	.12	.03	2.7	na	7	0.45
Pecans 12 halves	104	1.4	11.0	na	tr	.11	.02	0.1	63	11	0.40
Pignolia nuts 2 tablespoons	84	4.7	7.3	na	na	na	na	na	na	na	na
Pistachios 30 nuts	88	2.9	8.0	0.3	na	na	na	na	na	na	na
Walnuts, black 8–10 halves	94	2.7	8.7	na	0	na	na	na	na	na	0.90
Walnuts, English 8–15 halves	98	2.3	9.7	0.3	tr	.07	.02	0.2	68	12	0.30
Pumpkin seeds (15 g)	83	4.4	7.0	0.3	11	.04	.03	0.4	na	8	1.70
Sesame seeds (15 g)	84	2.8	7.4	0.9	0	.15	.04	0.8	108	174	1.60
Sunflower seeds (15 g)	84	3.6	7.1	0.6	na	.29	.03	0.8	138	18	1.10

g: grams; mg: milligrams; na: data not available; tr: trace

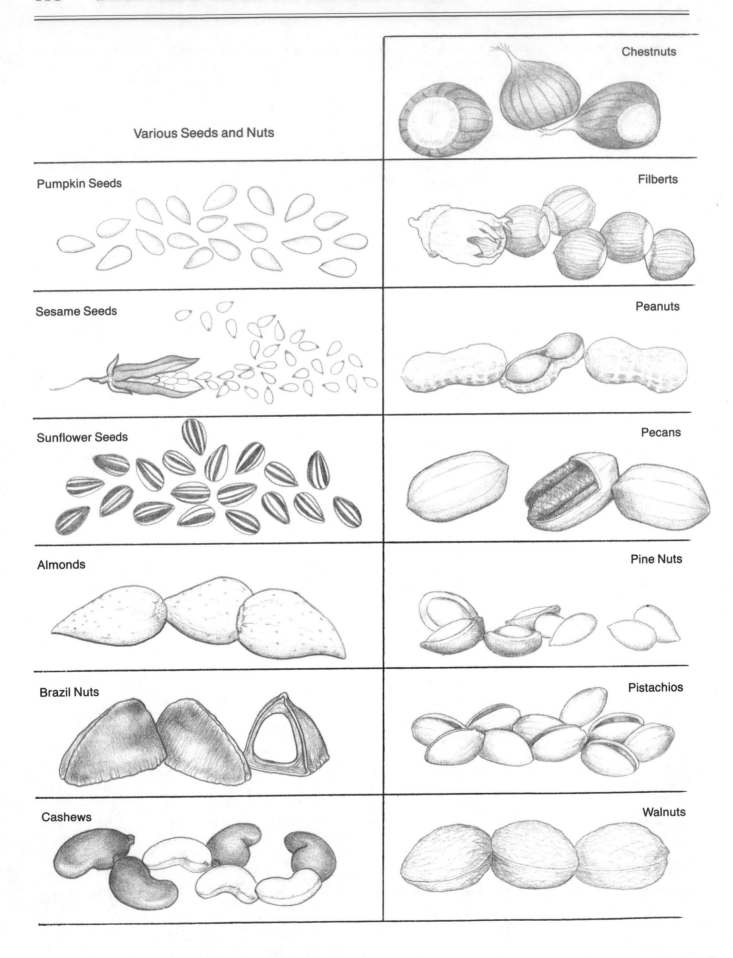

Various Seeds and Nuts

Chestnuts

Pumpkin Seeds

Filberts

Sesame Seeds

Peanuts

Sunflower Seeds

Pecans

Almonds

Pine Nuts

Brazil Nuts

Pistachios

Cashews

Walnuts

There are many varieties of the sesame plant, which grows anywhere from eighteen inches to nine feet tall. The plants are slim and have one to three flowers on each leaf axil. When dry the seed pods open and shatter. Usually much hand labor is needed when harvesting to prevent loss. Most of the seeds used in the natural foods market come from Central America: Mexico, Nicaragua, and Guatemala supply the bulk. California and Arizona grow a small amount and make an attempt to produce a few organic ones. The vast majority of the seeds sold are the natural brown and unhulled seeds.

Many Japanese cooks prefer to use black sesame seeds in their food preparation, claiming that the black seeds have a slightly stronger flavor. The oil content of black and brown sesame seeds is practically identical, although black seeds are slightly higher in polyunsaturated oils. Black sesame seeds are also somewhat lower in protein than the brown. Beneath the outer coating of the seeds, both black and brown sesame seeds are white.

Because sesame seeds are so tiny, a fine mesh strainer is necessary to clean them. Insect eggs and other small foreign matter can be problems. Although most stores carry only highly cleaned seeds, lightly toasting them before use is a good idea. Fortunately, most people think they taste better toasted.

Sesame seeds are currently at the center of a natural foods controversy due to the fact that the hull of brown sesame contains calcium oxalate crystals. Calcium oxalate forms when oxalic acid—which is commonly found in green leafy vegetables such as spinach, Swiss chard, beet greens, and rhubarb, as well as in sesame seeds—reacts with calcium. The calcium in this compound is so tightly bound that it is insoluble and cannot be absorbed by the body. Some scientists have presented evidence suggesting that eating calcium oxalates may be harmful to health and produce such reactions as gastrointestinal irritation, mineral depletion, kidney stones, and even arthritis. Opponents of this evidence maintain that the experiments use purified crystalline oxalic acid in concentrations unobtainable naturally except by ingesting enormous amounts of certain vegetables. Most nutritionists agree it is unlikely that anyone would develop calcium deficiency or other symptoms due to oxalate binding except where foods containing calcium oxalate constitute a large or exclusive part of the diet. For most natural foods eaters, who obtain plenty of calcium in their diets from grains, sprouts, sea vegetables, and vegetables—especially the *brassicas* (especially broccoli, turnip greens, bok choy, collards, rutabagas, and kale)—the oxalic acid content in some vegetables or in sesame seeds presents no problem.

Natural foods stores originally stocked only the brown unhulled sesame because commercial hulling methods used caustic chemicals, lye, bleaching agents, and excessively high drying temperatures. Hulling also deprives the seeds of 80 percent of their iron and thiamine, half of their riboflavin, and all of their potassium and vitamin A. In addition, it damages the quality of their oil and protein. Since unhulled sesame seeds are normally not eaten in quantities large enough to make their calcium oxalate content bothersome, and are certainly more nutritious, they naturally became the preferred form. However, one company, International Protein Industries of Smithtown, New York, has developed a chemical-free hulling process and supplies a very high-quality line of hulled sesame seed, called Protein-Aide, which is now carried by most natural foods stores.

Sunflower Seeds

The sunflower is native to North America. Its seeds were used extensively as a food source by Native Americans—made into bread, ground into meal, blended in drinks, and mixed with fat or grease and made into cakes. After the Spanish introduced sunflower seeds to Europe in the 16th century, Peter the Great of Russia is said to have brought them to his country in the 18th century. Sunflower seeds are now prized in Russia, where in some areas they are a major food crop. In the U.S. today they are grown in North Dakota and the Midwest as well as California.

Sunflower seeds are pressed to yield a high-caliber cooking oil (see page 172). The roots of a plant closely related to the sunflower produce an edible tuber known as sunchokes or Jerusalem artichokes (see page 48).

Sunflower seeds are nutritionally similar to sesame seeds but are even higher in protein and phosphorus, although they have much less calcium. They also contain a trace of fluorine, which may be one reason that the Russians claim they are good for the teeth. Another may be that they are high in vitamins D, E, and B-complex.

Sunflower seeds can be purchased hulled or unhulled, but hulled seeds are the most popular. Hulling is a simple mechanical process and the seeds keep well even when they are hulled. As with sesame seeds, the important thing to check for is cleanliness. There should be few shell fragments and broken seeds. Sunflower seeds should be firm, neither rubbery nor too dried-out and hard. Toast these seeds for a snack, or use them as an ingredient in bread or vegetable dishes.

Nuts

Almonds

One of the oldest and most widely grown nuts is the almond, which was probably native to North Africa and Western Asia, but was also cultivated throughout the Mediterranean from earliest times. The almond is versatile and will grow in all warm temperate climates. A member of the rose family, it is closely related to the peach. There are two basic types of almonds: the sweet type, which is edible, and the bitter, which is as inedible as a peach pit, though it does serve a purpose in cosmetics and scented oils.

The fruit of the almond tree resembles a flat dwarf green

peach, and the unshelled almond nut looks like a peach pit. When the fruit ripens it dries and splits open, revealing the nut in its shell. Almond trees are small, generally twenty to thirty feet tall with small pink or white flowers that appear before the leaves. The Spanish brought almonds from the Mediterranean to California during the establishment of missions. Most of the almonds used in the U.S. are grown in California, where they claim the third-largest acreage of all fruit and nut crops. Italy and Spain are also major almond producers.

Almonds are grown under conditions similar to those of walnuts, and organic almonds are rarely sold outside of California. Unlike walnuts, most almonds are sold shelled and whole. One reason for this is that the tough brown skin on the seed that remains after shelling is not only edible, but provides some protection against oxidation and rancidity. Almond pieces, and especially sliced almonds, tend to spoil more quickly and need to be refrigerated. Of course the price of broken or split nuts should be low.

Good almonds should have a smooth and even shape, not unlike the bottom of a steam iron. The skin of shelled almonds should be intact and unmarked, although usually a few scratches appear as the result of the shelling process. Almonds can be eaten raw but are more flavorful after roasting. Store-bought blanched almonds—those with their skins removed—are best avoided. Blanching can be done at home by pouring boiling water over the nuts.

Brazil Nuts

Brazil nuts are never cultivated. They grow wild only in the dense South American forest, mostly in Brazil and Venezuela, the trees towering up to 150 feet. The nuts are contained in a pod, similar in shape to a coconut, which holds eight to twenty-four nuts. When ripe, the pods fall with such force they can bury themselves in the ground. The nuts are removed from the pod, dried to reduce their high moisture content, and put through a heavy brushing process to remove the rough brown skin. Brazil nuts, though tasty and nutritious, are not especially popular, and in a bowl of mixed nuts they are usually the ones left on the bottom.

Cashews

The cashew is the fruit of a tropical and subtropical evergreen, a species related to American poison ivy and sumac. Originally from Brazil, the plant is now grown in almost all tropical areas; the world's leading producers are India, east Africa, Brazil, and China. The evergreen grows to about forty feet and bears clusters of pear-shaped fruits called cashew apples, which are used locally in beverages, jams, and jellies. Below this fruit hangs the crescent-shaped cashew nut. The kernel has two shells, an outer one that is thin, flexible, and somewhat leathery, and an inner one that is hard, like most nuts, and must be cracked. Between these two shells is a brown oil that is so toxic it can blister the skin. This oil must be burned off before the second shell can

be removed.

Traditionally the fruits were picked by hand and the nuts removed and dried in the sun. They were then placed among burning logs where the heat would crack open the outer shells and expose the oil. This oil would then catch fire quickly, giving off fumes equally hazardous to eyes and skin. Nowadays the nuts are roasted in perforated drums where the oil drains into containers below, to be saved for industrial uses. Cracking the inner shell is a delicate task, and until 1960 was done almost solely by hand by women in India, the world's supplier at that time. With the development of mechanical crackers other countries have made strong inroads into India's market.

After shelling, the nuts are heated again to remove the skins and make them fit for consumption and shipment. Cashews are always sold shelled. They are kidney-shaped, white, and have a soft texture.

The difference in price between whole cashews and pieces has become so great that buying whole cashews is seldom justified. Cashews come to the stores via large importers who buy from many countries. The nuts are shipped in twenty-five-pound vacuum-packed cans, and if it's important to know, you can ask someone in the store to look on the can and see where they came from, although there really isn't much difference among Brazilian, Indian, and Chinese cashews. Cashews often seem stale—top-quality nuts that are crisp and solid are rarely available. One reason for this may be their 45 percent fat content, which is not good as far as storage is concerned. Nevertheless, many people find cashews quite tasty. Dry-roasted shoyu-flavored cashews (sometimes referred to as ''tamari-flavored'' cashews), are becoming increasingly popular.

Chestnuts

Known in ancient times among the Greeks, Chinese, and Japanese for their food value, chestnuts have been called the greatest tree-food crop in the world. In Japan chestnuts symbolize both success and hard times. To the early Christians they symbolized chastity.

The American chestnut tree had a tragic history. Where vast forests of chestnuts once grew there are now none. A blight appeared in 1904, and over the next forty years destroyed them all. The trees now grown in the eastern U.S. are crossbreeds of Japanese and Chinese species. The few commercial chestnuts the United States produces come from a Spanish chestnut grown on the west coast. Practically speaking, all chestnuts are supplied from Europe. The horse chestnut of North America is unrelated and inedible.

The chestnut is a magnificent tree, growing from 70 to 90 feet tall, with a broad spread. Some trees have been known to reach 2,000 years of age. The nuts grow two or three together in a spiny burr about the size of a baseball. When ripe, the burr opens and the nuts are removed. Chestnuts are lower in calories, protein, and fat but are higher in carbohydrates than other nuts.

Chestnuts can be eaten fresh or dried. Fresh chestnuts,

sold in their brown shells, are called roasting chestnuts. They should be a clear deep reddish brown with silky smooth shells. If the shells are dry or brittle, it means that the chestnuts are old. Roasting chestnuts can be shelled and cooked, or baked or roasted in the shell. Chestnuts can also be bought already shelled and dried. These should be soaked first, or, for a slightly different flavor, they can be roasted, then cooked. The dried nuts seem to be sweeter and they are certainly more convenient, but they will be more expensive.

Filberts

Even though they are of different species, filberts and hazelnuts are so similar that their names are used interchangeably. Filberts have been the subject of many legends. Their ancient Roman name—*nux Phyllides*—came from a nymph who was turned into a nut tree. The Normans called them after Saint Philibert whose name-day coincides with the ripening of the trees. They are often used as symbols of love, though Circe used a hazel rod to turn Odysseus's men into swine. To the Celts, the hazel was the emblem of concentrated wisdom and its x-shaped branch was used for divining rods and dowsing.

Filberts grow wild on small shrubs or trees and are found all across the United States in woodlands and pastures, behind barns, and against fence rows. Most commercial filberts come from Turkey, Spain, or England, where they are the most common nut tree. Oregon and Washington produce all the filberts grown commercially in the U.S. Filberts have a pleasant taste, and their small round shape makes them easy and fun to eat. Ground or whole, they are perfect for cookies. In Europe, ground filbert butter is considered a real delicacy.

Peanuts

The peanut, ground nut, or goober pea, is not a nut, but a pea. After pollination its stalk becomes rootlike and sends down a shoot on which the pea develops underground. Peanuts are grown worldwide, mainly for their oil. In the United States, 50 percent of the crop goes into peanut butter, about 15 percent is crushed for oil, and the rest ends up in nut mixes.

Originating in South America, peanuts have been found in ancient Peruvian tombs. The Spanish first brought peanuts to Africa and they became a major source of food on slave ships. In colonial America they were used mainly as hog feed or grown as flowering shrubs much like sweet peas. They did not become popular in modern America until the 20th century, when George Washington Carver found over 300 uses for them.

Peanuts are high in vitamins, iron, protein, and calories. They are susceptible to the aflatoxin mold, one of the most powerful liver carcinogens known. Suppliers must test peanuts before they are shipped, and since roasting doesn't destroy the toxin, natural foods manufacturers re-test them before using in peanut butter or nut mixes. Write directly to distributors for the most current peanut-testing results.

Pecans

Pecans are a species of hickory nut native to the Mississippi River valley. Various Native American tribes prized them, and they were cultivated by Thomas Jefferson, who sent trees to George Washington at Mount Vernon. However, there was little commercial development of pecans until the 1850s, when a black slave known as Antoine developed the Centennial variety at a plantation in Louisiana. Today there are more than 300 named varieties of pecans, grown mostly in the South and Southwest of the United States.

The best pecans are oval-shaped, with smooth, light-brown shells. Some commercial sellers polish the shells. They may use a brown dye as well. Neither action should affect the pecans' meat, but if you are concerned, ask the store manager about the source if the pecans are sold in bulk and contact the seller directly if the pecans are packaged.

Pine Nuts

One common nut that does not come from a flowering plant is the pine nut or pignolia. Most commercial pignolias grow around the Mediterranean or in China, but the Mediterranean stone pine produces the most popular seeds. The umbrella-shaped tree is usually about eighty feet high at maturity. Its smooth cones have been harvested since prehistoric times in the dry southern European countries.

The pine cones are sun-dried to open them, after which each little nut is shelled by hand. This laborious process partially accounts for their high price—$6 to $8 per pound. The nuts are white or slightly gold in color, resembling elongated corn kernels. Italians feature pine nuts in a seasoning called pesto; they are delightful in any pasta recipe, although they have a definite piney taste and may take getting used to.

Native Americans in the West and in Mexico used pine nuts extensively. American pine nuts from the pinon tree are similar to the European variety, but their commercial production is still limited. Nuts grown in the United States are usually small, somewhere between the size of an apple seed and an orange pip. South American pine nuts may reach two inches in length, but are rarely found in natural foods stores.

Pine nuts are richer in protein than any other nut.

Pistachios

The pistachio, the seed of an evergreen believed to have originated in Syria, has been grown in the Mediterranean for over 5,000 years. It once grew wild in Russia, Turkey, and Afghanistan. Today Turkey, Iran, and Afghanistan are the principal producers, but North Americans are the principal consumers, eating almost 90 percent of the world's supply. California has recently started successful production and quickly sells all it can grow. Pistachio shells are naturally a greyish-beige color but are usually dyed white or red for eye appeal. Natural foods stores, however, don't find this treatment appealing and stock only the undyed ones. Being hard to open, pistachios are precracked by rolling under stone wheels. Pistachios are usually salted to enhance their flavor and aid in their preservation, though unsalted ones are sometimes available.

Walnuts

One of the most popular nuts in the natural foods store is the walnut. Its unique taste is compatible with a wide variety of grain, vegetable, and fruit dishes, and it is a favorite ingredient in desserts.

Almost without exception the walnuts sold in natural foods stores are identified as English walnuts. English trading ships first carried them worldwide, but their probable origin was in Persia; however, English walnuts have been under cultivation for so many centuries and in so many countries that their exact origin is unknown. Walnut trees are said in the Bible to have been prized by Solomon. The tree eventually spread to Rome, where its nuts were called Jupiter's acorns. Legend has it that while humanity ate acorns the gods feasted on walnuts.

Most of the world's English walnuts come from the United States, California supplying 90 percent. France is the largest foreign producer, followed by Italy and the People's Republic of China. In the U.S. the industry is encouraged by state and federal research agencies and motivated by a strongly organized cooperative. Commercial walnut production in California and on the Northwest coast utilizes chemical fertilization, insecticides, and fungicides. Organic walnuts are rare. They do grow wild in the Northeast, along with black walnuts and butternuts (both edible members of the same family). Until fairly recently, Americans never bought nuts in the store but rather gathered together every fall to go "nutting."

Like all nuts, walnuts are high in protein, fat, and oil.

Their high oil content makes them prone to rancidity once they are shelled, so the best way to buy them is in the shell. Look for shells that are well shaped, uncracked, and unbroken. Walnuts are naturally bumpy, but they should not have any big dents or stubby ends. To ensure uniform color and appearance, the nuts are usually washed and polished in a water and bleach solution, which lightens the shells to their familiar golden-tan color. The shells of organic walnuts therefore vary more in color and are darker overall. Nevertheless they should be clean and bright, not dirty or stained. The surest indication of a good walnut is its weight—a heavy nut is likely to have a full meaty kernel.

For the sake of convenience most stores sell walnuts already shelled and in various grades: halves, halves and pieces, and pieces. Naturally the halves are more expensive than the pieces. You will also notice that some walnuts are darker than others. The darker color develops in walnuts that grow on the side of the tree that receives the most sunshine. Although these darker nuts are richer and more flavorful, the light ones seem to be in more demand. But the outside color is not as important as its condition. The color inside should be white and clean, and the kernel should be firm, not rubbery. Rubbery kernels are an indication that the nuts are old and are probably going rancid. Also, if the inside of the kernel is turning from white to grey, the oil is coming out and rancidity is ready to begin.

In addition to the increased chance of rancidity, there is another price to pay for convenience. Shelled walnuts are much more processed than unshelled. Walnut shells are sometimes loosened by exposure to ethylene gas, and the shelled nuts are subjected to fumigants such as methyl bromide. To help remove their inner skins the nuts are blanched—dipped in hot dye or glycerine and sodium carbonate and rinsed in citric acid. Walnuts may also be bleached with chloride of lime and sodium carbonate to help even out their color.

Most natural foods stores buy a "lower" or "baking" grade of nut. These nuts, which have no need of perfect cosmetic appearance, are packed and shipped without excessive processing. Compare shelled walnuts from the bulk bins of natural foods stores with the ones plastic-bagged at the supermarket and you'll see the difference.

Cracking Nuts

Staying Sane When the World's Full of Nuts

Nut cracking, like gardening, is an exercise in delayed gratification. That doesn't mean it can't be fun. Nut lovers have devised a number of clever techniques to make shelling easier while keeping the nutmeat relatively intact. Otherwise, reckoning with such hard-shelled wonders as Brazils and black walnuts can bring new meaning to the word *angst*.

Pecans: Soaking pecans for eight to ten hours in a sinkful of water makes the meat flexible so it won't break during cracking. Some people achieve the same effect by spreading the pecans under a wet towel overnight or immersing them for twenty minutes in hot (145° F) water. Conditioning the nuts this way may brighten their color, and some people say it improves their flavor, too.

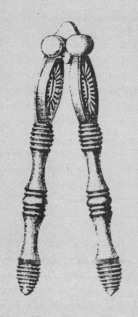

All nuts contain a fair amount of oil. To guard against rancidity, they should be stored like butter, in a refrigerator or freezer. Pecans that have been soaked need to be dried before storing. Oven-drying promotes rancidity; try blowing air over them on a dry day with a household fan. The drying process takes around fifteen hours.

Filberts (Hazelnuts): The easiest way to crack open a pile of filberts is to build a wooden grid or plywood stand with holes approximately an inch in diameter. The holes can vary slightly in size to accommodate different-sized nuts. Place a nut over an opening and hit it through with a hammer. The shell should crack apart, dropping the meat through the hole.

Brazil Nuts: Soak Brazil nuts in water for twenty-four hours, then immerse them in boiling water for three to five minutes. This softens the shell. In Brazil, where the nuts are grown and processed for export, workers use a hand-operated cracking machine that resembles a home bottle-capper. The nut is placed in a small cup, and the handle of the machine is pressed down carefully until the shell breaks.

Chestnuts: Chestnuts can be shelled by making a cut with a knife on the flat side and then immersing them in boiling water. Boil for twenty minutes, drain off water, and leave nuts in the pan to dry before shelling them with a small knife. They can also be shelled by roasting over a fire or in an oven. When roasting, make a cut through the shell to prevent bursting and use moderate heat (375° F).

But our favorite method for shelling chestnuts is "sand roasting." This technique comes from Dr. Jasper Woodroof's *Tree Nuts* (AVI Publishing Co., 1979), a definitive compendium on nut growing and cultivation that offers recipes for delicacies such as filbert taffy and "Imperial Pistachio Gourmet Pie." To sand roast chestnuts, half-fill a frying pan with sand and heat over a very hot fire. Add a handful of raw chestnuts: "If sand is real hot, it will require about 12 minutes to cook the chestnuts."

Black walnuts: Anyone who's dealt with black walnuts will tell you that this nut is probably responsible for more mental disorders than hard drugs and acid rock combined. The shell, a close relative of stone, has been known to yield to hammers and sledgehammers, but little else. Just getting to the shell can be an ordeal: each nut is encased in a soft, pale green outer shell that contains something resembling gooey coffee grounds. These "coffee grounds" will stain anything they come in contact with, so the trick is to get inside the walnut without touching them. Some enterprising souls have been known to wrap twenty-five to thirty nuts in a thick roll of newspaper, then compress the package under the wheels of a car. The soft coating

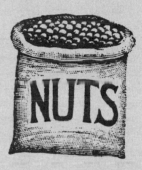

squishes away, leaving the hard nuts. After rinsing the nuts with a garden hose, let them season for thirty days so that the nutmeat has a chance to separate from the shell. This yields more unbroken pieces during cracking. As for the cracking itself, a hammer and a cement floor seem to be the most reliable tools.

Nut Butters

With the diverse array of wholesome, even exotic nut and seed butters available on the market today—including filbert, hazelnut, macadamia, pistachio, and cashew as well as the familiar peanut, sesame, and almond spreads—whole grain crackers and breads have never had it so good. *Whole Foods* magazine recently listed twenty-five nut butter producers with regional or national distribution, and there are probably another two dozen small-scale local nut butter makers as well. While statistics for national consumption of healthful nut butters are not available, one leading peanut butter creamer, Arrowhead Mills of Hereford, Texas, estimates its own annual output at about 820,000 pounds, worth $2 million in retail sales.

When making a decision about which of the many brands and flavors to choose, the natural foods consumer should also take into account quality considerations and product claims for each kind of nut or seed. Let's begin with peanut butter, by far the most popular and best-selling of the line.

Peanuts for butter are either blanched or left unblanched. Blanching, a steam-heat process, loosens the reddish seed coats, which are then removed by mechanical rollers. But also removed during this process is the peanut germ. Proponents of unblanched peanut butter point out that the skin and germ are integral parts of the peanut that add vitamins, minerals, and flavor, and that their removal is inconsistent with a whole foods philosophy. Others contend that their removal makes for a better product, because they find that the skins add a bitter taste, and the use of the germ increases the rate of rancidity. But the qualitative difference in nutrition or rate of rancidity is not sufficient enough to warrant the preference of one process over the other. Taste and one's personal approach to whole foods are the deciding factors.

Also a factor is the variety of peanut, often identified on the label, which influences both taste and quality. Valencia peanuts are grown in the dry areas of New Mexico and the Southwest, while Jumbos, grown in Virginia, and Runners, grown in Georgia, both thrive in moist environments. Valencia peanuts are naturally drier and less susceptible to aflatoxin mold, a known carcinogen. In addition, they have the advantage of being naturally sun-dried, which is convenient and economical in the desert environment. Valencia nut butter producers claim that slow sun-drying retains more peanut flavor than the more rapid (and expensive) process of forced hot air or oven-drying used on other varieties.

Another important consideration is whether the peanuts have been organically grown. In New Mexico, for example, unlike in the Southeast, peanuts are not alternately cropped with cotton, which is sprayed intensively for boll weevils. Several peanut butter producers, such as Arrowhead Mills and Westbrae, while not claiming "organic" come pretty close by guaranteeing the absence of herbicides and pesticides in the soil or on the crop. The industry organic standard is Section 26569 of the California Health and Safety Code, which stipulates acceptable conditions and parameters for labeling products in California as "organic." Some nut butters specifically state their compliance with this code on their labels.

When shopping for almond butter, two factors should be noted: the degree of oil separation and whether the almonds are organic. Many brands of almond butter show a dismaying pond of oil floating above the mass of nut butter in the jar. According to Gordon Bennett, president of Westbrae, oil separation in any nut butter is a function of product age, degree of nut grinding, and storage conditions. In general, the older the nut butter the more oil separation, but the storage and grinding can mitigate this considerably. A fine grind liberates more oil from the almond cells, whereas a coarser, rougher grind reduces oil separation. Moreover, a warm storage temperature seems to precipitate oil separation even from a coarse and freshly ground almond butter, whereas cooler temperatures keep the almond oil thick and emulsified.

Economic factors seem to determine the availability of organic almonds. The California Almond Growers Exchange, a farmer's brokerage house which enjoys over 50 percent of the almond market in California, has maintained commercial almond prices at $1.75 to $2.25 a pound, and organic almonds at up to $2.50 a pound, but offers almond butter stock (chipped almonds or almond pieces) for $.60 to $.80 a pound—obviously a considerable economic incentive for butter producers to buy commercial rather than organic almonds. However, almonds come inside a thick protective shell, and, Bennett says, extensive tests fail to show any herbicidal residue in the nonorganic almonds or almond butter.

There are two types of sesame seed butters: *tahini*, which is made from ground hulled sesame seeds; and *sesame butter*, which consists of toasted and ground unhulled sesame seeds. Sesame butter is thicker and more spreadable with a heavier and richer taste than tahini, which is lighter in appearance and taste. Most of the commercial production of sesame seeds is in Mexico and Guatemala. This makes organic growers both hard to find and difficult to monitor. Therefore, claims for organic sesame products must be weighed against the reputation of the supplier. One of the major issues in the production of tahini is the means of seed hulling. Most producers use the conventional means of soaking the seeds in caustic soda, lye, sodium hydroxide, or a brine solution to soften and remove the hulls. A more recent technique, which involves minimal steam heating and mechanical rolling and thus no caustic baths, is being promoted as being more natural. Another factor to take into account when buying tahini is whether the sesame seeds have been toasted or left raw. The toasting process breaks down the cell walls and releases more oil, thereby enriching the texture and adding a stronger sesame flavor. The raw sesame tahini taste is mild by comparison.

The nut butters reviewed below were obtained at stores in Boston and San Francisco, and do not necessarily reflect the best products, but rather the most readily available or interesting ones in those major markets. Since taste evaluations are highly subjective, the favored brand choices were determined on the basis of their quality ingredients.

Walnut Acres of Penn's Creek, Pennsylvania, makes a lovely, chunky-style roasted peanut butter. When the jar is first opened, an aroma of freshly roasted peanuts greets the senses. There is almost no oil separation and the taste is strong, clear, and inviting. However, after a few days the product has a tendency to dry out and thicken. Walnut Acres also produces flavorful honey-peanut, banana-peanut, and date-peanut spreads, as well as both almond and tahini butters.

Arrowhead Mills of Hereford, Texas, is the producer of a 100-percent-Valencia peanut butter. It is made from unblanched, roasted, sun-dried Valencia peanuts grown on "composted soil without herbicides and pesticides," and deserves commendation. Because of this product's wide distribution it is not unusual to find jars with considerable oil separation, which makes a great deal of stirring necessary. In addition, Arrowhead markets an organic, mechanically hulled sesame tahini that is ground creamy smooth without salt.

Maranatha is an energetic regional West Coast company located in Ashland, Oregon. They produce fifteen varieties of nut butters, many exotic, including macadamia, filbert, roasted pistachio, and cashew-peanut-date, among others. They are all packed in vacuum-sealed jars for freshness and several of their nut ingredients are California-certified organic.

Moonshine Trading Company of Winters, California, markets a line of gourmet nut butters elegantly labeled and packaged at a high price that is not justified by the actual product. There is so much oil separation that it takes fifteen minutes to stir it back in. The taste, however, is smooth and strong, and the resulting consistency appealing. Other butters include a nut crunch (almonds, cashews, filberts), cashew, and sesame.

N.S. Khalsa Company of Salem, Oregon, is the proud producer of a line of "roaster fresh" and made-daily nut butters. Their products include organic peanut butter, sunflower, hazelnut, and cashew butters. This line had the most oily almond butter sampled. But its taste was rich and insistent, quietly reminiscent of lightly sweetened chocolate.

International Protein Industries of Smithtown, New York, is the maker of Protein-Aide sesame tahini and sesame peanut butter. The first is made from unroasted, mechanically hulled seeds and is billed as the only spreadable tahini, which refers to its unique non-runny consistency. The second is made from the same type of seeds and fresh roasted peanuts. They are milled into a smooth, creamy texture with a unique taste.

Open Sesame of Santa Cruz, California, produces a toasted almond butter that uses California-certified organic almonds. They also turn out a line of tahini, cashew, hazelnut, and sunflower butters that are "still basically handmade." The almond butter has almost no oil separation and is easy to mix up. Its texture is light and chunky with a crisp taste.

The **Westbrae Company** from Emeryville, California, makes the samurai of nut butters. Their black sesame butter is as sharp as a flashing sword blade and as final as the unremitting downstroke. Made from an Eastern variety of sesame seed that has a black instead of brown seed coat, this sesame butter has a strong flavor that swaggers rather than spreads across crackers and bread. Westbrae also makes tahini, almond, peanut, and regular sesame butter.

9. BEANS

In a recent national survey of over 600 customers of natural foods stores, 85 percent said that they regularly purchase tofu, and 71 percent reported regularly purchasing miso. Only grains (purchased by 90 percent of the customers) outranked the popularity of these soybean products. In addition to bean products such as tofu and miso, most natural foods stores also carry bulk and packaged varieties of many other beans, such as azukis, chick peas, kidneys, lentils, limas, peas, and soybeans.

Especially for people who are looking for healthful ways to cut down or eliminate their consumption of meat, beans offer a number of attractions. They are low in cost yet high in nutritional value, providing vitamins and fiber. They are also high in protein, and the amino acids often found in beans are good complements to those found in grains, as David Wollner points out in the article that opens this section. Well before food scientists knew about such things as complementary proteins, traditional cultures found myriad ways to combine beans with grains. Rice and beans are popular in the Far East, rice and lentils in India, corn and beans in the Americas, soybeans and bulghur in the Middle East. The versatility of beans is also illustrated by the many ways they can be used in soups, casseroles, stews, and salads.

In addition to the opening story, with its tips on what to look for when buying dried beans in bulk, we will take a look at three soybean products that can add an exciting new dimension to a whole foods diet. Tofu and miso have become not only natural foods staples, but are increasingly being integrated into the eating habits of "mainstream America." Only ten years ago, the companies that made them in the West were small, unmechanized outfits reaching regional markets. As bigger and more high-tech-oriented companies enter the market, it is important for consumers to understand how tofu and miso are made and how different production approaches may affect the taste, texture, and nutrition of the final product. The other soybean product we'll look at, tempeh, is an Indonesian import that doesn't yet rival tofu or miso's popularity, but offers another tasty and nutritious way to incorporate beans into our daily diet.

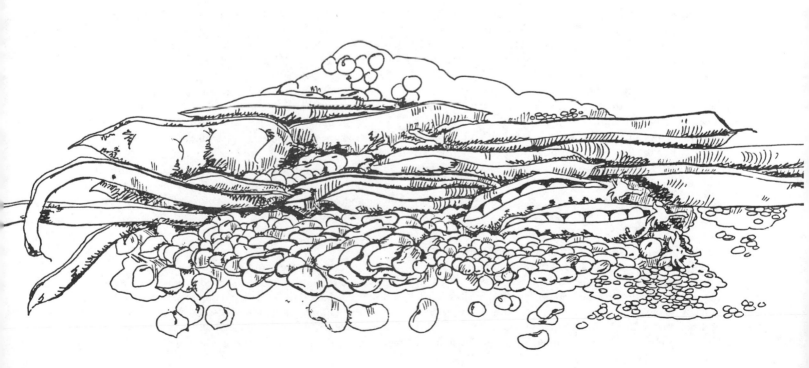

A Guide to Beans

Legumes, a large family of plants, are characterized by true pods enclosing seeds: carob trees, alfalfa, and clover are all legumes. Beans and peas are large-seeded legumes, usually reserved for culinary purposes.

Legumes are the products of a warm, dry period in the earth's past, a period that preceded the present, cooler epoch that has produced the grains. When a cooler climate settled over the earth, most legumes were limited to the tropical and subtropical regions. This explains why the majority of beans are considered to be indigenous to those climatic zones. Their warm-weather origins are exemplified by a higher proportion of protein and fat, a lower proportion of carbohydrate, and a considerably higher potassium content than that of the grains. The carbohydrate molecules in beans are also less complex and shorter than the highly evolved sugars found in grains.

Beans were a staple of Native Americans, who ate them to supplement their corn-based diets. The early European explorers found beans growing from South America to Canada and brought seed samples with them upon returning home. Europeans thus enriched their cuisines with beans from the Americas as well as with those they discovered in the Middle East and Northern Africa. They grew beans and dried them for use as winter provisions, grinding them into flour to make puddings and porridges. Beans became so popular in Europe that they gained an important place in winter rituals: for example, during New Year's celebrations, they were used as omens for the coming year. Meanwhile, in the East, different species of beans were consumed and also used medicinally.

The bean plant can be either a vine or a bush, while the beans themselves are the seeds that form in the pod. Usually, the plants are allowed to dry in the field and are then harvested and threshed much the same as grain. Sometimes, when the harvest is on a small scale, the mature seed pods are cut from the plant, and the seeds are stripped from the pod (shelled) and dried.

Shopping for Beans

Beans come in many different colors and sizes, so what exactly should you look for? As with most dried whole foods, appearance reveals quality. Regardless of color, shape, or size, the beans should appear vital, well-formed, of a consistent size and vibrant color. White beans should be white, not stained with grey. Beans should not be wrinkled or pitted, but smooth-skinned with round contours.

Fish-eyes (openings at the seams) indicate that the drying occurred too quickly and the starches, fats, and proteins of the inner bean have begun to oxidize. Checks (broken skin), splits (in two halves), and chips (surface pitting) are evidence of rough handling or an indication that the beans were harvested when too dry. These faults are unavoidable to a certain extent, but for a top-quality product, they should not affect more than 1 or 2 percent of the beans.

A test for quality can be made by biting into a bean. It should crackle and shatter. If this effort results in only a dent, then the bean has not been sufficiently dried. A refinement of this method is to split a bean in half. The inside of each half should be slightly concave. Because beans differ in degree of dryness, it is important not to mix one kind of bean with another, or even to combine different batches of the same bean—the drier the bean, the more cooking time it requires.

Both packaged beans and those purchased in bulk from a bin may contain some stones, so be certain to remove them and clean the beans carefully before cooking. Also, pick out those beans that have split; they are not good to eat. Beans that are whole, unchipped, and without fish-eyes can be sprouted. Bean sprouts are tasty, easy to digest, and provide abundant quantities of vitamin C. Dried beans are rich sources of calcium and contain vitamin A and several B vitamins. Soybeans and lentils are the highest sources of protein in the vegetable kingdom. Beans provide some of the essential amino acids, especially lysine, that are lacking or deficient in the cereal grains, and thus provide the perfect complement. Together, beans and grains are an ideal source of protein, as many traditional societies with a low intake of animal food can attest to. Falafel and pita bread, rice and miso soup, tortillas and refried beans are good examples of such complementary pairs.

The following dried beans are commonly found in natural foods stores and supermarkets. Experiment with other, local and/or heirloom varieties if you can find them—thousands still exist.

Azukis

Closely related to the common beans native to the Americas, these small, red, kidney-shaped beans were, until recently, available only as Oriental imports. While most azukis are still imported, good-quality domestic beans, mostly from a group of organic farmers in Ohio, have begun showing up in some natural foods stores and mail-order listings.

Ironically, even as the natural foods industry imports from Japan, conventionally grown azuki beans from Minnesota are being exported—to Japan. Azuki beans do not need presoaking before cooking.

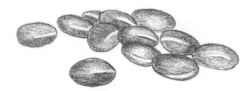

Chick Peas or Garbanzos

Chick peas, or garbanzos, are imported to this country primarily from the Middle East, although the state of Idaho is making a major effort to grow them. Chick peas are the primary ingredient of hummus and falafel. Italian-Americans will recognize them as the ceci that can be bought in Italian import stores. Chick peas need to be soaked overnight before cooking.

Kidneys and Pintos

Kidneys and pintos are members of the botanical group which includes Navy or pea beans, soldier beans, and black turtle beans. All are native to the Americas, and those you buy in the store are home-grown—probably from one of the northern states somewhere between Michigan and Maine. It was one of these varieties that the native North Americans ate along with their corn dishes. These beans all need to be soaked before cooking.

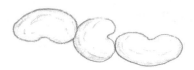

Lentils

Two varieties of lentils are sold in natural foods stores: green and red. The small, lens-shaped, greenish-brown "green" lentils are domestically produced, grown mostly in Idaho and Washington. They cook to a rich, earthy brown and are among the heartiest and most full-flavored of the legumes. Red lentils are imported, usually from the Middle East. These are actually "split lentils"—each piece is only half a lentil. Before splitting they have a brown seed coat and are slightly smaller than the domestic variety. Both flavor and color are lighter than those of the greens. Lentils do not require presoaking. Both varieties make a delicious soup and can also be pressure-cooked with rice before cooking.

Limas

Lima beans, also known as butter beans, are sold in three ways: as small baby Limas, which are also called sieva or Carolina beans; as large flat Limas, which are also known as Cape or Madagascar beans; and as potato Limas, which are as large as flat varieties, but rounder. Lima beans are native to South and Central America.

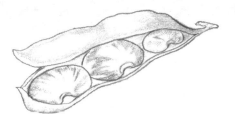

Peas

Peas are known to most of us as a fresh vegetable, but there are also a few varieties that are sold dried—either whole or split. Yellow and green varieties are nutritionally similar and are cooked in the same way. Whole peas require some soaking before cooking.

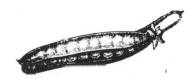

Soybeans

Virtually unknown in the United States at the turn of the century, soybeans have now joined corn and wheat as one of our major farm crops. Although most of our soybean crop is processed for oil and for animal feed, a growing portion is being used for human food. Prepared in many ways, soybeans have long been an important source of protein throughout the Far East. The following traditional soyfoods are becoming popular among natural foods shoppers in the United States: tofu, tempeh, miso, natural soy sauce (shoyu) and, to a lesser degree, natto.

Soybeans grown primarily for their oil content are, as a rule, smaller and more yellow than those varieties developed especially for food use. In addition, these beans often have a dark spot called the hilum. The "large-seeded" or "vegetable-type" soybeans are larger and have a lighter seed coat and nearly invisible hilum. They lack the strong bean-y taste of other soybeans and make especially mild and creamy tofu.

A variant, the black soybean, is becoming increasingly available, both from domestic and Far Eastern sources. Cooked with kombu, ginger, and root vegetables, it makes a delicious and striking side dish.

Tofu Fit For the Emperor

As recently as a decade ago, tofu could be found only in Oriental specialty shops, California supermarkets, and a very few natural foods stores. Today it is made in nearly every state, and sold in supermarkets from coast to coast. Tofu was once available only in unprocessed form or in a few traditional Japanese and Chinese preparations. Now tofu appears in many items, from frozen lasagna to imitation ice cream.

Tofu, still occasionally called "bean curd," is well appreciated by health-conscious consumers everywhere. Like other soyfoods, tofu is a good source of protein, and contains all the essential amino acids. Different types of fresh tofu range in protein content from 5.5 percent (silken) to 10.6 percent (firm Chinese-style). Regular soft tofu is just under 8 percent. Eight ounces of tofu provide the same amount of usable protein as 3½ ounces of steak or 5½ ounces of hamburger (a quarter-pounder plus three bites).

Although tofu contains all the essential amino acids, however, it is low in methionine and cysteine. When eaten with grains—which are high in these sulfur-containing amino acids—there is an increase in the usable amount of protein consumed. Tofu is 95 percent digestible, compared with the 65 percent digestibility of whole soybeans.

Calcium Content of Tofu

Curding Agent	Amount of Calcium (mg/100 g tofu)
Magnesium chloride	36
Natural nigari	42
Calcium sulfate	139
Glucono delta-lactone (used for some silken tofu)	14
Calcium chloride*	108

Source: Soyfoods Center, Lafayette, CA

*Northern Soy, Inc., Rochester, NY

Many calorie-conscious people have turned to tofu as an excellent diet food. Regular tofu contains only 147 calories per eight-ounce portion (that's one gram of usable protein for every eight calories). It is low in total fat (only 4.3 percent), especially low in saturated fat, and high in unsaturated fats. Like all vegetable-based foods, tofu contains no cholesterol.

Tofu is an excellent source of calcium (see table, below). If a calcium-based coagulant is used, the resulting tofu contains more of this important mineral than an equal amount of dairy milk. If nigari is used as a coagulant, the calcium content is roughly 40 percent of an equal weight of dairy milk. Tofu is a good source of other vitamins and minerals as well, including iron, phosphorus, potassium, B vitamins, and vitamin E.

Tofu is relatively easy to make. Whole soybeans are soaked overnight, then ground with water to a smooth puree and cooked with boiling water. The cooked puree is strained to separate the liquid (soymilk) from the fibrous pulp (okara). A coagulant is added to the hot soymilk, which then separates into curds and whey, similar to the process of making cheese from dairy milk. The curds are then transferred to cloth-lined, perforated settling containers, and pressed. The smooth white cakes that result are chilled and packed for immediate distribution.

Varieties

There are two basic types of tofu available in most natural foods stores and supermarkets: firm (sometimes called "Chinese-style") and soft. The main difference between these two products is in the degree of firmness. In some cases, the only difference in the manufacturing is the length of time the tofu is pressed in the settling containers. A soft tofu with a smooth, creamy texture requires more delicate handling and processing. Well-made, firm tofu should not be "grainy" or "chalky" but should have the same, smooth creaminess characteristic of the best soft tofu. Because the only difference between soft and firm tofu is in the amount of water left in the curd, firm tofu is, pound-for-pound, a better buy nutritionally. However, the difference is relatively small. Firm, Chinese-style tofu may have as much as 10.6 percent protein, while soft tofu has around 8 percent. Because of this slight difference, it may be better to base the texture of the tofu chosen on the recipe you are preparing or what tastes better rather than to always buy firm tofu because it's a better protein bargain. Soft tofu is ideal in miso soup, for creamy dips and dressings, and as a simple side dish or hors d'oeuvre with garnishes or dipping sauce. Firm tofu is better for deep-frying, grilling, and stir-frying. The firm texture also lends itself to slicing for sandwiches and simmering in stews.

A variety of extra-soft tofu, called silken tofu (*kinugoshi* in Japanese), is custard-like and extremely smooth (hence the name). Silken tofu is made differently from the two varieties described above. The soymilk from which it is made is much thicker and the coagulant (calcium sulfate or lactone) is mixed with the hot milk in the forming box, which has no draining holes. When the coagulant is added, the milk does not separate into curds and whey as with regular tofu but instead forms into a custard-like cake. Because no whey is drained off, silken tofu contains more water and less protein than soft tofu. When the whey is drained from regular tofu, some of the minerals from the coagulant are discarded with it. Because all of the curding agent remains in silken tofu, it contains 50 percent more calcium than dairy milk (if made with calcium sulfate). Its protein level is approximately 5.5 percent.

Chilled silken tofu is deliciously cooling, particularly during the summer. Its creamy texture and subtle sweetness give it an air of delicacy and refinement. Because of its extra soft texture, silken tofu cannot be pressed, and does not lend itself to frying or grilling. At its best, it is simmered briefly in light soups, or used as a component of smooth sauces and dressings. One Japanese company exports silken tofu in small cardboard cartons with a long, room-temperature shelf life. Some supermarkets and Japanese specialty shops also carry a domestically produced, fresh version.

Oriental food shops will also generally carry prepared, deep-fried tofu, or at least two basic varieties: *atsu-age* or "thick age" (tofu cutlets) and *aburage* or "age" (tofu pouches). Frying gives the tofu its chewy texture and rich flavor. Deep-fried tofu warms and satisfies when simmered in soups. Its hearty quality is welcomed by hardworking people and on cold winter days. Tofu pouches can be stuffed with any savory filling, and are a nice change from a sandwich lunch. Either type can be prepared at home from store-bought or homemade tofu.

Natural foods stores that specialize in Japanese products will often offer dried-frozen tofu (*koya dofu*). Dried-frozen tofu is not a modern "freeze-dried" backpacking food, although its light weight, high nutritional value, and long storage life would certainly qualify it for that use. *Koya dofu* was first made by Buddhist monks in a monastery near Mount Koya in northern Japan. The monks hung blocks of firm tofu outside under the eaves of the temple during the cold, snowy winter. The tofu would freeze at night and thaw during the day. This alternative freezing and thawing gradually expelled virtually all the water, leaving a non-perishable, sponge-like block.

This spongy texture is what makes dried-frozen tofu so appealing, even when fresh tofu is available. When simmered in savory sauces or broths, *koya dofu* soaks up flavors—much like a sponge. The freezing also alters its consistency, yielding a chewy, almost meat-like texture. Like deep-fried tofu, dried-frozen tofu can be easily prepared at home. You just place well-pressed slices of firm tofu in your freezer until they are completely frozen. Then thaw, squeeze out the extra water, and dry in a food drier or in the oven on very low heat. (More detailed instructions for preparing both *age* and *koya dofu* can be found in *The Book of Tofu*, by William Shurtleff and Akiko Aoyagi, Ballantine, 1979; Ten Speed Press, 1983.)

Coagulating Agents

Natural nigari is an alkaline mineral coagulant derived from the refining of natural sea salt. Although natural nigari yields the best-quality tofu—the best flavor and texture, true to tradition—some people are now questioning its use for reasons of purity. Pollutants are now present in the sea that weren't there when the traditional process was developing. Two other coagulants, however, can yield tofu with a taste and texture very similar to that made with natural nigari. These are "refined nigari" (magnesium chloride) and calcium chloride. Magnesium chloride is the primary constituent of natural nigari and is refined from the natural product. The calcium chloride used by a major Northeast tofu maker is a minimally refined product that is derived from a naturally occurring mineral found in ancient underground deposits. All three of these nigari-style coagulants yield tofu that is higher in protein than equal weights of tofu made with other common curding agents. Perhaps the most significant advantage of natural calcium chloride as a tofu coagulant is that it is a very rich source of dietary calcium, containing 23 percent more calcium than an equal weight of dairy milk.

Calcium sulfate (gypsum) is used, as we have seen, in making silken tofu. Today many tofu manufacturers use it either as the only coagulant in their tofu or in combination with one of the nigari-type curding agents. Used alone, it yields a soft, creamy tofu, since more water is incorporated as the curds form. The higher water content accounts for the lower percentage of protein, as well as for the soft texture. Used alone or with nigari, calcium sulfate (like calcium chloride) adds a significant amount of calcium to the tofu. The calcium sulfate used in making tofu is a minimally refined, mined product. In China, where tofu was first made, natural gypsum has long been the standard coagulant.

Kinugoshi, a type of silken tofu, is made using lactone as a curding agent. Glucono-delta lactone is an organic (from a biochemical point of view) acid that curdles soymilk in the same way that the lactic acid from Lactobacillus bacteria curdles dairy milk in the making of yogurt. Lactone incorporates even more water into the curd than gypsum, resulting in less protein and other nutrients per pound of tofu.

Because natural nigari contains a rich complex of naturally occurring sea minerals, it is still believed to yield the best tofu. The possibility of contamination from ocean pollutants, however, merits further investigation. And for those on dairy-free diets who are concerned that they are not getting sufficient dietary calcium from plant sources, tofu made with either of the calcium-based mineral coagulants (calcium chloride or calcium sulfate) is a reasonable choice.

The Emperor's Tofu

How do you choose the best tofu? Akiko Aoyagi and William Shurtleff, authors of the definitive *The Book of Tofu*, asked numerous tofu makers in Japan how they would go about making "tofu for the emperor." In their classic work, they write, "Our question allowed each craftsman to go directly to the heart and essence of his art leaving aside all consideration of cost, time, and economic profitability. Nearly all responded, 'To make the very best tofu we would use the traditional method.' " Let's make tofu worthy of the emperor's table our standard in discerning quality in the tofu we buy.

Just what is this "traditional method" that Japanese tofu makers from village shop to huge factory espouse as the source of "the very best tofu"? To begin with, the soybeans chosen are a large-seeded, Japanese-grown variety, soaked overnight in cold well water and ground slowly in a mill with natural stones. This puree (*go*) is boiled in a cast-iron cauldron heated by an oak fire. As the head of creamy white foam rises in the cauldron, the master stirs it back down with a split bamboo rod that has been dipped in a natural bubble extinguisher of vegetable oil mixed with natural limestone or wood ashes. After the foam rises and is stirred back down three times, the fire is damped and the puree allowed to simmer for five minutes. According to Shurtleff and Aoyagi's description, the puree is then ladled into a natural fiber straining sack. The steaming hot soymilk drains into a copper-hooped cedar barrel. The sack containing the fibrous pulp (okara) is then placed on a wooden rack, which is set across the mouth of the barrel. The remaining soymilk is extracted with a hand-operated press. The pulp is then returned to the cauldron and mixed with more boiling water, then returned to the sack and pressed again.

The master stirs a solution of natural nigari into the hot soymilk in three careful steps. Within twenty minutes buoyant, cloudlike curds appear in the pale yellow whey. After some of the whey is removed with a cloth-covered bamboo strainer and ladle, the curds are gently scooped into cloth-lined wooden settling boxes. The curds are covered with cloth, a bamboo mat, and a wooden pressing lid. The lid is topped with a weight. Twenty minutes later the master removes the lids, immerses the box in a sink full of ice-cold well water, and removes the wooden settling container. He then unwraps the cloth lining from the tofu and cuts it into small blocks. To be savored at its best, the tofu is served immediately with simple garnishes and the best shoyu dipping sauce.

The very best tofu, then, is made from large-seeded soybeans, ground in a stone mill, cooked in an iron cauldron over a hardwood fire, and processed with pure well water. The curding agent is natural nigari. Only handcrafted wooden and bamboo equipment and natural fiber cloths are used in making it. The process is a slow and careful one, performed by a master craftsperson. The best tofu is ideally eaten as fresh as possible—if not immediately, at least within a day of being made.

Obviously, tofu that meets all of these criteria is virtually impossible for the average North American natural foods shopper to find—and probably not much easier for the Japanese tofu connoisseur. Due primarily to sanitation factors, very few tofu makers in this country use wooden or bamboo equipment. Stainless steel is the order of the day. I know of only one local producer in Oregon who uses wood to fire his stainless, rather than cast-iron, cooker. Some tofu makers use only large-seeded soybeans, grown in the United States. (The tofu from these beans, which were especially developed for human food uses, is somewhat sweeter in flavor and has a creamier texture than that made with "standard" soybeans grown primarily for oil processing and animal feed.) A few producers use well water, and quite a few more use municipal water that is highly filtered. Only relatively small producers use stone mills to grind the soaked beans. Although natural nigari is widely recognized among U.S. makers as the best tofu coagulant, refined nigari and other coagulants have largely replaced it. Much of the tofu in this country is made in factories near large cities, packed in sealed plastic tubs or pouches, and stamped with a two-to-four-week shelf life before being shipped to the hinterlands.

How to Buy and Store Tofu

So what is the quality-conscious tofu buyer to do? Perhaps the single most important consideration in choosing tofu is its freshness. Several years ago, when visiting family in Kansas, my sister's friend asked if I would show her how to make tofu. She had been buying California-made tofu at the local supermarket and wanted to try making it herself. When she tasted the finished tofu, still warm, her first words were, "It isn't sour!" In those days, only a lucky few outside of the east and west coast areas had access to tofu that wasn't sour. Today, better distribution, better packing, more producers, better handling in the store, and a much faster turnover result in little tofu that is actually sour.

Unfortunately, just as little is truly fresh. The only way to be assured of fresh tofu is to buy from a local supplier—or to make your own.

Wherever your tofu is made, choose the freshest (check the last-sale date) package on the shelf. Because freshness is such an important factor, don't buy a packaged product without a ''pull date.'' Tofu should be found in your store's dairy section (not in the produce department, where there are much warmer temperatures). If it is located in the produce section, explain to the department manager that tofu is very perishable and requires the same low temperatures as dairy products. Avoid swollen packages, as this indicates spoilage. Some manufacturers now pasteurize their tofu, either immediately before or after packing, and follow this treatment with a quick chilling. If the tofu has to travel and may not reach the table for a week or more, this is probably the best approach. It does not harm the tofu in any way, and there is less impairment of flavor than if the tofu were to begin to spoil.

Tofu that has a slightly sour taste has begun to spoil but may still be used. Frying will both kill the souring microorganisms and mask the flavor. But if your tofu has a strong sour smell, feels slippery on the surface, and/or has a slight pink tinge, be sure to discard it.

Pasteurized tofu can be left in its package for a few days (theoretically until the last sale date). If it is opened, store any that you don't use in the refrigerator. Add enough cold water to the storage container so that the tofu is submerged. Change the water at least every day. Nonpasteurized tofu should be removed from the package and stored in fresh water immediately.

If the tofu you buy is made with organically grown soybeans, you are casting a vote for sustainable agriculture and a toxin-free environment. By choosing tofu from a small, local shop, you are encouraging craftsmanship and a strong local economy.

With all these considerations behind you, and your tofu in front of you in your soup bowl or on a shishkabob skewer, know that you're in good company. According to authors Shurtleff and Aoyagi, the Chinese believe that the enlightened sages, who subsist on ''the mists of heaven and the fresh morning dew, are particularly fond of tofu as their third choice.''

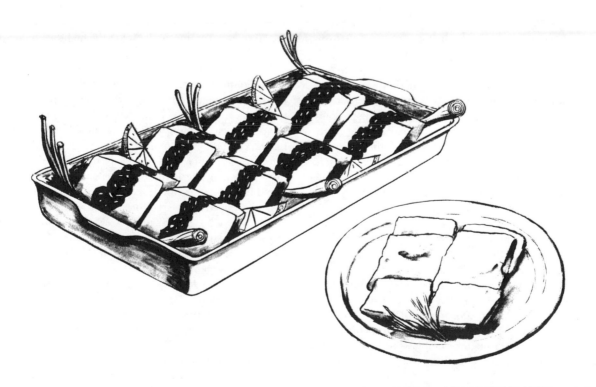

Tempted by Tempeh

This Indonesian Specialty Tantalizes Western Palates

Fragrant, delicious, and versatile, tempeh (pronounced tem-pay) has become one of the most important protein foods in America's move toward a meatless, natural, and nourishing diet. It joins such notables as Camembert, Brie, and Roquefort cheeses, classic Japanese misos, and naturally brewed soy sauce in the panoply of mold-cultured foods that have found acceptance in an evolving American cuisine. Made for centuries in Indonesia, this cultured soyfood is now produced in shops across the United States and Canada, and is available in most natural foods stores and even in some supermarkets.

Soybeans are notoriously difficult to digest when simply boiled or pressure-cooked. In Japan they are transformed into custard-like, creamy tofu and fermented to make shoyu, tamari, miso, and natto. In the U.S., livestock transform the protein-rich beans into meat and milk. In Indonesia, village craftspeople long ago developed a unique fermentation process to change soybeans into firm-textured, savory, quick-cooking, digestible and nourishing foods.

In a traditional Indonesian tempeh shop, whole soybeans are washed, covered with boiling water, and allowed to soak overnight. The beans are then hulled, partially cooked, cooled, and inoculated with a starter culture grown on hibiscus leaves. The inoculated beans are then wrapped in banana leaves and left in the naturally warm, humid environment until they are tightly bound by the firm white mycelium of the dominant mold of the starter culture, *Rhizopus oligosporous*.

The process used to make the tempeh sold in your local natural foods store probably varies from this traditional method in only a few details. The beans may be mechanically hulled before soaking. Perforated plastic bags are substituted for the banana leaf wrappers and the tempeh is incubated in a carefully controlled environment at 85 °F to 88 °F. After twenty-four to thirty-six hours the beans are bound by the mold into firm cakes. The cottony mycelium on freshly harvested tempeh resembles the nap of a new tennis ball. The aroma is delightful—a clean, fresh, mushroom-like smell.

The fermentation does much more than bind the beans together. It contributes to tempeh's flavor, which has been likened to that of chicken, fish, and sauteed mushrooms. Enzymes from the mold break down the complex proteins, fats, and carbohydrates of the soybeans, making them easier to digest and assimilate. Levels of certain vitamins are significantly increased.

Another important result of fermentation is greatly reduced cooking time, making tempeh both convenient and economical. Whole soybeans can take as long as six hours to cook. The cooking of the tempeh beans prior to fermentation requires less than an hour, and subsequent cooking of the finished tempeh takes about fifteen minutes, thus resulting in substantial savings in cooking fuel.

Tempeh is one of the richest vegetable sources of protein. According to William Shurtleff, co-author with Akiko Aoyagi of *The Book of Tempeh* (Harper and Row, 1979), "Tempeh contains 19.5 percent protein, or about as much as beef or chicken. Tempeh is a complete protein, containing all essential amino acids. It has the highest-quality protein found in any soyfood."

Tempeh is generally regarded as one of the few potentially significant vegetable sources of vitamin B_{12}, an essential nutrient abundant in many animal foods but almost totally lacking among plant foods. The source of B_{12} in tempeh is neither the soybeans nor the *Rhizopus* mold, but bacteria of the genus *Klebsiella*, which because of their ubiquitous nature often find their way into tempeh soybeans during their pre-fermentation preparation. In the traditional Indonesian method, the bacteria are also introduced with the mixed starter culture that is grown on hibiscus leaves. Virtually all U.S. shops use a pure culture *Rhizopus oligosporous* starter, and thus must rely on prefermentation "accidental inoculation" from environmental sources. Because some recent studies have revealed insignificant B_{12} levels for certain domestic tempeh samples, researchers are trying to develop a mixed culture tempeh starter that would, like the traditional hibiscus leaf culture, contain organisms that would assure high levels of B_{12} in the finished tempeh.

Tempeh is available in rectangular cakes, sausage-shaped cylinders, and burger-like patties, as well as in numerous pre-seasoned and precooked preparations. Choose tempeh in which the beans are tightly bound together by a dense, white mycelial growth. Gray or black spots are the result of natural sporulation of the *Rhizopus* mold and not indicative of spoilage. Some tempeh connoissseurs purposely let the mold growth progress to this stage, prizing the slightly stronger flavor that the lengthier aging gives the tempeh.

In addition to making regular soybean tempeh, tempeh producers may also combine the beans with grains such as rice, millet, and barley before inoculation and incubation.

Some processors steam-blanch their tempeh before shipment to arrest mold growth. Others ship the product frozen or vacuum-packed. Vacuum-packed, unblanched tempeh most nearly retains the taste and texture of fresh tempeh and therefore seems the best choice if fresh, locally made tempeh is not available. Tempeh will keep for an average of ten days in the refrigerator and for several months in the freezer.

Many people think that tempeh tastes best pan-fried. To pan fry, brush frying pan with unrefined oil and heat. Slice the tempeh in thin or thick slices—whichever you prefer—then place them in the pan. Brown for about eight minutes on each side. Natural soy sauce enhances tempeh's taste, as do herbs and other seasonings. Pan-fried tempeh prepared in this way is ready to eat; for a juicier texture, add water and simmer for another fifteen minutes.

There are several other ways to prepare this versatile food. For a rich flavor, marinate slices of tempeh for several hours in a marinade of water, shoyu, herbs, and rice vinegar; then simmer the water away. Tempeh can also be broiled, steamed, or deep-fried. It can be added to noodles or vegetable dishes, or served as hors d'oeuvres. *The Book of Tempeh* contains many recipes, as well as detailed instructions for making tempeh at home and a list of sources for tempeh starter.

Whether you make your own or purchase it from a natural foods store, tempeh is sure to become a favorite in your household. As you come to know its qualities of versatility and convenience, you may even begin to find it indispensable.

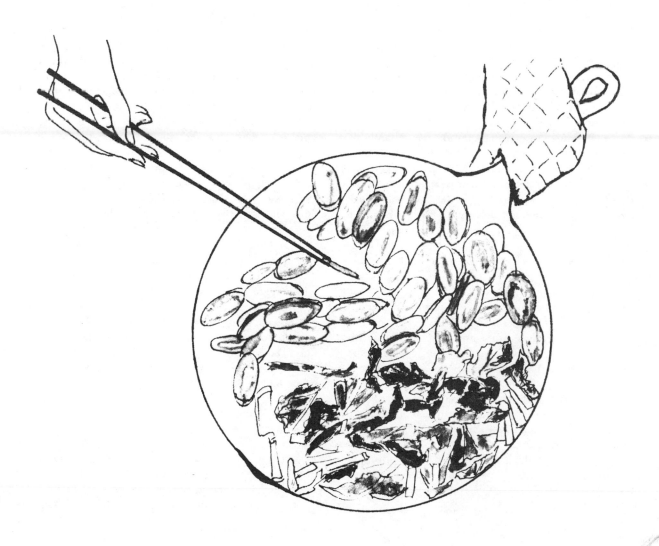

Miso: The ABC's of an Ageless Food

For centuries Japanese craftsmen, using natural fermentation, have transformed soybeans and grains into many types of *miso*, a rich, thick substance used for flavoring a wide variety of dishes. Each miso, like fine wine, has its own distinct flavor, color, and aroma. Throughout Japan even today each region has its own particular type of miso, and even though many Japanese are turning to Western cuisine, most still start their day with a hot, stimulating bowl of miso soup.

With the West's growing interest in natural foods and health, miso is steadily gaining in popularity. Many types are now available in America, most of these imported from Japan, but some made right here.

Miso is a source of essential amino acids, vitamin B_{12}, and minerals, and is low in calories and fat. The daily use of miso, which is considered a medicinal food by many Japanese, has been credited with numerous health benefits. It is said to break down and discharge cholesterol, help to neutralize the effects of smoking and environmental pollution, alkalinize the blood, and prevent radiation sickness. Like yogurt, unpasteurized miso is also abundant in lactic acid bacteria and enzymes, which aid digestion and food assimilation. Scientists studying Japanese populations have also discovered that those who regularly drink miso soup suffer significantly less from some forms of cancer and heart disease. Researchers at Japan's Tohoku University have recently isolated chemicals from miso that cancel out the effects of some carcinogens (cancer-causing substances).

Although methods used in making miso differ depending on the type of miso being made and the level of technology employed, the basic process dates back to preindustrial Japan. Cooked soybeans are mixed with *koji* (grain inoculated with *aspergillus* mold), salt, and water. This mixture is placed in a container to ferment. Gradually the enzymes supplied by the koji, along with microorganisms from the environment, break down the complex structure of beans and grains into readily digestible amino acids, fatty acids, and simple sugars.

Like most manufactured foods, quality varies depending on production methods and ingredients. Basically, there are three methods of miso manufacturing: temperature-controlled, naturally aged, and traditional (see sidebar on the next page).

The quality of miso used, particularly on a daily basis, may affect your health—and will definitely affect the taste of your food. Especially for children and those in a weakened condition, organic, unpasteurized, traditionally made miso is preferable. And in the preparation of uncooked foods such as dips and salad dressings, the fresh taste of unpasteurized miso is truly delicious.

For the busy cook who wants to add flavor and protein to standard American dishes such as soups, gravies, casseroles, and salad dressings, a little miso can be added like bouillon. This gives eleven grams of protein per tablespoon. For those people moving toward a more wholesome, natural way of eating, the meat-like quality of dark miso, and the dairy-like qualities of light, sweet miso can help ease the anxiety of that transition. For the experienced natural foods cook, Japanese cook, or gourmet cook, miso's possibilities are truly endless.

Although there are a few exceptions, for the purpose of food preparation miso can be divided into two groups based on color and taste. Sweet miso is usually light in color (white, yellow, or beige) and high in carbohydrates. It is marketed under such names as "mellow miso," "sweet miso," and "white miso." Because it is high in koji and low in salt, sweet miso ferments in just two to eight weeks, depending on the exact recipe and temperature of aging.

Miso with a higher salt content, lower koji content, and proportionately more soybeans is darker in color and saltier in taste than sweet light miso. It must be fermented for a longer period of time, usually at least one summer but as long as two to three years. This type of miso is marketed under such names as "red miso," "rice miso," "brown rice miso," and "barley miso."

It is important to understand that each miso has its own

recipe that determines the proper length of fermentation. White miso is not red miso aged for less time. Each type of miso has its own use in terms of both health maintenance and cooking. We will say more about cooking later, but in terms of health or food value, consider this: light, sweet miso is high in simple sugars and contains about twice the niacin and ten times the lactic acid bacteria as dark, saltier miso. Dark miso is higher in protein and, because of its larger proportion of soybeans, contains more fatty acids, which have been shown effective as anticarcinogenic agents. (Over-concern with miso's medicinal properties should not, however, eclipse the enjoyment of using this truly delicious food.)

The key to fine miso cookery is not to overpower dishes with a strong miso taste, but to integrate the more subtle aspects of miso's color and flavor in a gentle balance with other ingredients.

The light color, sweet taste, and creamy texture of sweet miso is suggestive of the ways it can be applied in American-style cooking. Sweet miso is an excellent dairy substitute. For example, try a little sweet miso instead of milk in mashed potatoes or creamed soups, and with tofu and lemon or rice vinegar in place of sour cream for dips and spreads.

To realize the full potential of sweet miso, explore its uses in salad dressings and sauces. Mellow white miso and good-quality rice vinegar create a delicate tartness that is both refreshing and cooling. Sweet miso and sake or mirin (rice wine) combine well in sauces for baked, broiled, or stir-fried vegetables or fish. Think of sweet miso for festive occasions and light summer cooking. In southern climates, mellow barley miso is excellent for year-round cooking.

The readily digestible amino acids, fatty acids, and simple sugars, and relatively low salt content of sweet miso make it ideal for the delicate constitutions of babies and young children. A very dilute mellow miso broth is readily accepted by children starting at age six to eight months.

In contrast, dark, saltier miso is excellent for basic winter cooking in cold climates. Its hearty quality combines nicely with beans, gravies, baked dishes, and vegetable stews and soups. Try dark miso in thick soups using root vegetables such as burdock, carrots, and daikon. A lentil loaf made with red miso warms the body and supplies a large amount of high-quality protein. Remember that dark miso is stronger in taste than sweet miso, so use it sparingly.

Any discussion of miso is incomplete without considering its use in miso soup. Miso soup and rice, with pickles and tea, constitute a meal by Japanese standards. In Japan, the dynamic flow of ingredients, texture, and color of miso soup reflects seasonal changes and geographic location. In the south, sweet barley miso, which gives miso soup a beautiful yellow to beige color, is preferred. In the

Making Miso: Methods Old and New

There are three basic methods of miso manufacturing: temperature-controlled, naturally aged, and traditional. Ingredients may be grown organically or using chemical fertilizers and insecticides.

Like much of today's beer, vinegar, and soy sauce, Japanese miso is usually made by a fast, completely automated, temperature-controlled process using chemically grown ingredients. For example, red miso (which must ferment one to two years at natural temperatures) can be made in just six weeks using the temperature-controlled process. The result, however, is a dark, often dry miso with a flat, and sometimes burnt, taste. Fortunately, very little of this type of miso is sold in American natural foods stores. Usually labeled in Japanese, it is the most common type sold in Oriental food markets. This miso is pasteurized to prevent further active fermentation so that it can be shipped in sealed plastic bags or other sealed containers. Temperature-controlled miso may also contain additives such as alcohol to retard bacterial growth.

With few exceptions, miso sold in natural foods stores is naturally aged. Although it is made by the same automated process, the fermentation is not temperature-controlled. A few large old factories that converted to automated, temperature-controlled production methods after World War II still set aside small volumes of miso in seasoned wooden vats each year for natural aging. This miso is then pasteurized and packaged for large natural foods distribution companies under each distributor's private label. The quality of ingredients varies widely.

In some homes and small shops in both Japan and America, a limited amount of traditional miso is still made by people concerned with flavor, health, and tradition. The traditional method dates back to 17th century Japan. It is characterized by the use of handmade koji, organic ingredients, slow cooking and cooling of soybeans, and long aging in wooden vats. Traditionally made miso should be kept refrigerated, and direct contact with air, which adversely affects its taste and color, should be avoided. Look for this fine variety of miso in the refrigerator section of natural foods stores in small tubs or in the recently introduced plastic bags that have a one-way valve prohibiting the entrance of air but allowing carbon dioxide, a natural byproduct of active fermentation, to escape.

The nature of the traditional process allows for the introduction of many types of "wild" microorganisms from the environment. Their contribution to fermentation adds the deep, rich taste and heady aroma of traditional miso. Fresh and unpasteurized, this type of miso has complex tones and subtle, balanced flavors that only great care, the highest-quality ingredients, and long natural aging can produce.

north, hearty red miso is favored, often in combination with carrots, burdock, and wakame, giving miso soup a very earthy color and flavor. Don't be afraid to experiment with the many possibilities of miso soup. However, since miso is the dominant taste here, be sure to use unpasteurized miso and to add it only at the very end of cooking (to prevent the miso from boiling).

For more information on the health benefits, use, and manufacture of miso, from the home-production level to modern factories, see *The Book of Miso*, by William Shurtleff and Akiko Aoyagi (1983, Ten Speed Press).

Recipes Using Miso

Kyoto-Style Miso Soup

Serves 4–6

> *4 cups cold water*
> *6-inch piece kombu*
> *1/4 cup bonito (dried fish) flakes*
> *1/4 cup mellow white miso*
> *1/4 block tofu (approximately 4 oz),*
> *   cut into 1/2-inch cubes*
> *1 scallion, sliced very thin*

Place kombu and water in saucepan and bring to a simmer, uncovered, over medium heat. Remove kombu as soon as the water begins to boil. (It may be reused to make soup stock or cooked with beans or vegetables.) Stir bonito flakes into simmering stock, then remove pan from heat and let sit for two minutes. Strain the broth, pressing all liquid from flakes with the back of a spoon. Return broth in pan to heat, add tofu and scallion, and simmer two minutes. Turn off heat. Remove a little broth and use it to soften the miso. Add to soup, and allow it to sit briefly before serving.

Although other vegetables may be added or substituted, simplicity and a flavorful stock are the keys to this authentic traditional miso soup.

Mellow Miso Dressing

Makes 1 cup

This dressing was adapted from a recipe that made at least one Miami restaurant famous. After tasting it, we think you'll agree it's easy to tell why.

> *1/4 cup unrefined safflower oil*
> *1/4 cup water*
> *1/4 cup mellow white miso*
> *1 1/2 tablespoons brown rice vinegar*
> *2 tablespoons rice malt*

> *1 rounded tablespoon chopped onion*
> *1/4 teaspoon dried mustard powder*
> *   (optional)*

Place all ingredients in blender and blend until smooth. For another delicious variation with an entirely different appearance and flavor, add several sprigs of fresh dill before blending.

When cooked, the flavor of this dressing changes and it becomes a wonderful sauce for broiled fish or tofu. Simply broil as usual and brush on sauce for the last minute of cooking. Garnish with paprika and parsley and serve hot.

Hearty Gravy

This gravy does as much for potatoes as Mom's did and is delicious over grains, especially bulghur and millet.

> *1 1/2 tablespoons olive oil*
> *1 onion, diced*
> *1–2 cloves garlic, minced*
> *3 tablespoons whole wheat or*
> *   unbleached flour*
> *3 tablespoons nutritional yeast*
> *1 2/3 cups water (approximately)*
> *3 tablespoons mellow barley miso*
> *1/4 teaspoon dried basil*
> *several sprigs fresh parsley (optional)*
> *1 tablespoon white wine or mirin*
> *   (optional)*

Heat oil in a medium-sized skillet, then add onion and garlic and saute over medium heat for three to five minutes. (Other vegetables such as sliced mushrooms or diced bell pepper may be added if desired.) Lower heat and add flour and nutritional yeast. Stir constantly for about one minute, then slowly add 1 1/2 cups water while stirring briskly to keep the flour from lumping. Stir frequently until gravy

begins to simmer and thicken. Combine the miso with two to three tablespoons of water, then add along with the basil and, if desired, parsley and wine or mirin. Gently simmer, uncovered, for about fifteen minutes, stirring occasionally. Keep gravy warm until serving. If gravy is too thick, add a *little* more water; if too thin, cook down to desired consistency or slowly stir in one tablespoon arrowroot flour dissolved in one tablespoon water.

Creamy Dill Dip

Here's a delicious and nutritious dip that you won't have to feel guilty about! It's high in protein and low in calories. Great for parties, snacks, or to satisfy hungry dinner guests.

> *8 ounces fresh tofu*
> *1/4 cup mellow barley miso*
> *2 tablespoons brown rice vinegar*
> *   or lemon juice*
> *2 tablespoons unrefined safflower oil*
> *1 or 2 cloves garlic*
> *several sprigs fresh dill*

Boil some water in a pot. Place tofu in boiling water. Remove from heat, cover, and let sit a few minutes. Then place the tofu in cold water for a couple of minutes. Remove, wrap in cheesecloth or porous cotton, and gently squeeze out excess water. Place all ingredients in a blender and blend until smooth. Let sit, refrigerated, at least two hours to allow flavors to heighten. (It is best not to attempt to adjust the seasoning before letting it sit.)

If you can't find fresh dill, substitute two tablespoons dried onion or three tablespoons fresh minced onion. Stir in onion after blending all other ingredients.

Savory Miso–Sunflower Spread

Makes 3 cups

This superb spread combines the concentrated nutrition of sunflower seeds, tofu, and miso.

> *1/2 cup sunflower seeds*
> *2 tablespoons lemon juice or rice vinegar*
> *2 tablespoons rice malt (brown rice syrup)*
> *2 cloves garlic*
> *2 tablespoons chopped onion*
> *water to blend (1/8–1/4 cup)*
> *3 tablespoons red miso (or any rice miso)*
> *1 tablespoon tahini (optional)*
> *1 block (approximately 1 pound) fresh tofu*

Roast the sunflower seeds in a dry skillet over medium heat, stirring constantly until golden brown and fragrant (about five minutes). Place roasted seeds in a blender. Blend briefly on "chop" or "crumb" until you obtain a fairly fine meal. Add next four ingredients and blend until well mixed. Add miso and tahini and blend. Crumble the tofu with your hands and add to blender, a third at a time. Blend until smooth. It may be necessary to stop from time to time, scraping the sides of the blender and pressing the mixture down to eliminate air pockets. If your tofu is very firm, you may have to add a *little* more water, but be careful not to overdo it or you'll end up with a dip instead of a spread. Serve on crackers, bread, or toast, or use with alfalfa sprouts in sandwiches.

Azuki Medley

Serves 5–6

This recipe brings out azukis' full flavor and sweetness. If possible, use organic squash—it is generally more flavorful.

> *1 cup azuki beans*
> *2 1/2 cups water*
> *1/2 bay leaf*
> *pinch of rosemary*
> *1 teaspoon unrefined vegetable oil*
> *1 large onion*
> *2 1/2 cups chopped winter squash (butternut, acorn, or buttercup)*
> *pinch sea salt*
> *2 tablespoons red miso*

Soak beans two to three hours; then discard water from soaking them. Place beans in pressure cooker with water to cover and bring to a boil, uncovered. Discard water (this removes azukis' slightly bitter taste). Add 2 1/2 cups fresh cold water and herbs. Bring to pressure, lower heat, and cook 45–50 minutes. Meanwhile, slice onion thinly and saute in the oil until translucent and limp. Add bite-sized chunks of squash and a small pinch of sea salt and saute briefly. Lower heat, cover, and cook until squash is somewhat softened but not completely tender (Check frequently and add a *little* water if necessary to prevent scorching.) Uncover and set aside.

Preheat oven to 375°F. In casserole dish, combine cooked beans, vegetables, and miso thinned in two tablespoons water. Cover and bake 30–40 minutes. Serve garnished with chopped parsley.

Lentil Loaf

Serves 6

> *1 cup green lentils*
> *4-inch piece kombu (optional)*
> *1/2 bay leaf*
> *3/4 teaspoon oregano*
> *1/2 cup bulghur*
> *2/3 cup oatmeal (uncooked)*
> *1/2 cup minced scallion*
> *2 cloves garlic, minced*
> *1/2 teaspoon basil*
> *1 tablespoon unrefined vegetable oil*
> *1 teaspoon lemon juice*
> *2 tablespoons barley miso thinned in 2 tablespoons water*
> *1/2 cup minced parsley (optional)*
> *water*

Wash the lentils and combine with kombu, bay leaf, 1/4 teaspoon of the oregano, and 3 cups water in a large saucepan. Bring to a boil, then lower to a slow simmer and cook with lid ajar for 30–40 minutes or until lentils are tender and most of the liquid is absorbed. Check frequently toward end of cooking time to avoid scorching. Meanwhile, bring 3/4 cup water to a boil in a small saucepan; add bulghur and a small pinch of sea salt. Stir and simmer one minute, then cover, remove from heat, and let sit at least 15–20 minutes.

When lentils are cooked, they should still be moist. If dry, add about 1/4 cup water or soup stock. Add oatmeal and mix. Add bulghur, 1/2 teaspoon oregano and all remaining ingredients and mix well. Press mixture into an oiled loaf pan, cover with foil, and bake at 350°F for 40–45 minutes. Remove foil for the last 10–15 minutes. Cool on a wire rack for 30 minutes if time permits. (This makes it easier to remove from pan.) To remove, run a knife or spatula around the sides of the loaf and invert over a serving plate. Slice, ladle a little Hearty Gravy (or another sauce) over the top, garnish with a sprig of parsley, and serve with additional gravy on the side.

This loaf is especially attractive surrounded by lightly steamed broccoli and/ or braised cherry tomatoes. A delicious, warming dish, Lentil Loaf is especially satisfying in the cooler months and it is at its best with Hearty Gravy or a miso-based tomato sauce. The combination of beans and grains provides an abundance of high-quality complete protein. Leftovers are good sliced and pan-fried, in sandwiches, or simply reheated.

10. BEVERAGES

Healthful beverages complement our daily meals. Whether we should drink before, during, or after eating may be a debated topic, but whether to drink at all is not even questioned. Our body is over 70 percent water and needs to be replenished daily. The types of liquids consumed need to be decided with as much caution as are all the foods we eat. And as we select our beverages from what is available in a natural foods store, it is wise to consider the merits of some of the less well-known items.

Herb teas have had a renaissance during the past decade. Reintroduced into the American diet through natural foods stores and companies like Celestial Seasonings, these healthful alternatives to caffeinated teas are now available in all types of food stores. Looking at the history and variety of teas, especially herbal teas, is a primary focus of this chapter.

We will also look at decaffeinated coffees, and decide how to determine their quality. Conventional caffeine-rich coffee is not commonly available in natural foods stores, but a few carefully grown organic coffees have recently been introduced to this market. If you are still addicted to this traditional food, you may find organic coffee if you search the market carefully.

Soymilk is the latest new beverage to appear in natural foods stores. In the Orient, consumption of soy beverages rivals that of soft drinks. For instance, in Hong Kong, VitaSoy, the largest soymilk manufacturer, has 40 percent of the soft drink market. But only since 1983 has there been an opportunity to find a truly palatable soymilk in the United States. Now with many natural foods companies processing their soy drinks in the U.S. rather than importing a Japanese product made with American soybeans, prices are coming down and soymilk can almost be thought of as an American food. Eden Foods of Clinton, Michigan was one of the pioneers in importing soymilk from Japan. They now have their own plant in Michigan and manufacture enough of this beverage to consider exporting it back to Japan! Our review of the soymilk boom is an important part of this chapter on beverages.

One of the most popular natural beverages is fruit juice. The natural juice lover has the pick of the world's best orchards and nature's range of fruits in the most exotic blends. The health-conscious consumer's selection of natural juices is done with an eye to the label, but most importantly with an appetite for thirst-quenching goodness. A review of some of the more interesting and delicious natural fruit juices wraps up this chapter.

Our thirst is insatiable. We simply need to know what are the most healthful drinks and how best to choose them.

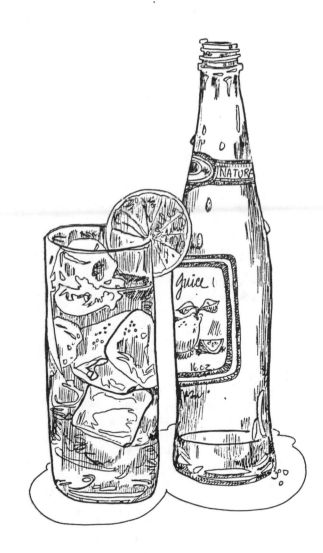

A Guide to Teas

When the philosopher Lao Tze was very old the burden of age lay heavily upon him. He sensed the imminent fall of his home kingdom of Chou. He saw that his teachings had failed to attract an audience or to gain acceptance. In a state of disillusionment he decided to leave China. Clambering atop a water buffalo, old Lao Tze rode west toward Han Pass, the mountains, and exile. But Lao Tze's journey had been foretold and another sage, Yin Hsi, the gate warden at Han Pass, awaited him. When Lao Tze appeared Yin Hsi recognized him and invited him to sit down to a cup of tea. They entered Yin Hsi's hut where Lao Tze, uplifted by the refreshment and persuaded by Yin Hsi's guileless talk, set to work writing the *Tao Te Ching*. Thus one of the world's great classics came about and the tradition of warm talk over hot tea became enshrined as a national pastime.

Tea drinking originated in China; the earliest documents mentioning it come from there. The ancient Chinese drank tea for the same reasons we drink it today—for comfort, for stimulation, and to satisfy thirst. They believed that tea was a gift bestowed by Heaven along with the other arts and technologies by which humankind had climbed from the abyss of barbarianism to the peaks of refinement and culture. Tea was a beverage to be drunk with each meal and also a strong medicine affecting health. It deserved respect. Physicians recorded the various effects of different tea concoctions and prescribed them to patients. The general public, with equal perspicacity, described a taciturn person as someone "with no tea," and an excitable person as someone "with too much tea," thus making the connection between the amount of tea consumed and subsequent behavior.

The English took up tea drinking in the 15th century, and through their involvement tea cultivation pushed beyond the borders of China. Cunning English merchants monopolized the China tea trade. Their promotional abilities at home made tea the most popular nonalcoholic beverage in England. But the polarity between East and West often brought about misunderstanding, and though the English and Chinese trading partners tempered their dealings with caution, in 1839 their partnership ended with war. Although the Chinese suffered a humiliating defeat, the English victory was equally joyless. They lost their monopoly of Chinese trade and had to look elsewhere to find tea. But where? At that time tea was cultivated only in China and Japan; China was now carved into spheres of influence and Japan's ports were still closed to the West.

The English took matters into their own hands. Finding wild tea bushes and transplanting Chinese bushes and expertise to those places, the English soon established huge plantations in Java (Indonesia), Ceylon (Sri Lanka), and India. Tea took its place as one of the world's first great cash crops.

Since that time, however, tea has experienced a dramatic turnabout—from Chinese medicine to American medical nemesis. Like other caffeinated drinks, it is considered to be a cause of excitability and high blood pressure and is suspected of being a possible carcinogen. As lifestyles and dietary factors have changed, so too have tea's effects. For the Chinese—living without central heating, dining simply from the bounty of the earth, and not confronting the complications of modern times—the stimulation of tea was a welcome addition. It warmed and animated them. As they collected tea leaves from wild bushes or grew the plants without adding synthetic chemicals, their teas contained the vigor of the untamed. Also, understanding tea as medicine, the Chinese imbibed it with respect.

Compared to that of the ancients, our modern lifestyle is fast, our food less simple, our existence farther removed from the earth. The quickening effect of tea, rather than adding a counterpoint to our lives, contributes to the overload. Maybe the physiologic effect is more severe in combination with the harmful foods and eating habits of our age.

All (non-herb) tea comes from the same plant, *Camellia sinensis,* which has three main varieties: China, Assam, and Cambodia. The tea bush is an evergreen capable of reaching heights of thirty feet. It does best in tropical and subtropical climates but will grow almost anywhere in temperate zones, although not well enough to be a profitable crop. Climate, soil, and altitude all affect the characteristics of the tea and its quality. Whether the tea is made from leaves, twigs, or stems, the time of year these parts of the plant are plucked, how much caffeine they thus contain, and the processing they undergo, are also factors that contribute to tea's taste and quality. Since the end of the 19th century, growers, exporters, and importers have graded tea according to these factors as well as by leaf size.

Six or more grades are produced, ranging in size from the unbroken orange pekoe to the smaller broken grades, fannings, and dust. Teas made from young leaves and buds, gathered from the first pluck, make the most stimulating cup (having the most caffeine, they receive the highest grade). The Chinese word *pekho*, meaning "white hair" or "down," refers to the "tip" in tea—the tiniest bud leaves, which are correlated with quality. Found in gour-

What Is Mu Tea?

The name of Mu tea is something of a paradox. People refer to this beverage as a full-bodied blend, but the word "Mu" is Japanese for "empty."

The paradox is easily resolved, however. "Mu" does mean "nothing" or "emptiness," but it also translates to "unique," a word that aptly suits this tea. Invented in 1963 by George Ohsawa, one of the pioneers of the macrobiotic movement, Mu tea was originally designed for the relief of menstrual cramps. The tea is also said to be good for weak stomachs, mucus-thick (as opposed to dry) coughs, and certain other digestive and respiratory discomforts. Healthy people drink Mu tea to relieve tiredness, as a weight loss aid, or simply as a refreshing, vitality-boosting tonic.

The taste is a real eye-opener. Mu tea comes in two rather pungent blends, #9 and #16. In a taste test, we found that both went down smoothly with faint spicy-sweet aftertastes of licorice and anise. In our batch, Mu #16 was milder than Mu #9. Some folks dab it with a little honey or rice syrup or apple juice, but we liked it straight.

The Mu blends are a showcase of ancient herbs. Mu #9 contains herbaceous peony root, hoelen, Japanese parsley root, cinnamon, licorice, peach kernels, ginger root, ginseng, and rehmannia. Mu #16 contains all of those plus mandarin orange peel, cnicus, atractylis, cypress, cloves, coptis, and moutan. Do you have friends who are proud of their discerning palates? Hand them a cup of Mu tea and ask them to name the ingredients.

Mu tea is generally available only at natural foods stores that carry macrobiotic items. It is imported from Japan by Great Eastern Sun Co. and Granum, Inc. under the Mitoku label, and by Erewhon, Inc. under its own label.

met shops, import stores, tea and coffee specialty shops, and larger whole foods stores, such teas are delicious, possessing flavor, lightness, aroma, and color unmatched by the more commercial blends in supermarkets. Twining's and Jackson's are two brand names of high-quality teas at affordable prices.

Tea is named after the country or region in which it is grown—China, India, Assam, Darjeeling, and so forth, and according to the processing it has undergone—black, green, oolong. The cut of the leaf is also included in the name.

All teas should be kept in airtight containers to prevent them from absorbing additional moisture and rotting. Kept airtight, a tea can be stored for about six months at home. After that time, it begins to deteriorate in quality and taste.

Bancha and Kukicha Teas

Bancha means "three tea," referring to the fact that the tea leaves and stems are at least three years old when harvested. Because of this, and also because it is picked late in the year, when the caffeine content of the leaves is at a minimum, bancha is considered to be the lowest grade of tea.

Before being packaged, bancha is roasted at least three times in cast-iron cauldrons to lessen the bitterness of the tea and, according to the producers, to bind the tea's tannin to the iron pot, thus reducing the level of tannic acid in the brewed tea. It therefore doesn't need to be roasted again at home.

Kukicha, meaning "twig tea," comes from the twigs of the same plant as bancha. The concentrations of caffeine are lower in the twigs than in the leaves of the tea plant. Kukicha, and not bancha, is really the type of tea recommended in macrobiotic literature, although it has also been said that when George Ohsawa recommended bancha tea, he was referring to a blend of leaves, stems, and twigs. In natural foods stores, kukicha is sold under the name Kukicha Twig Beverage.

Both bancha and kukicha work as buffer solutions to the stomach, neutralizing acidic or overly alkaline conditions; kukicha is soothing to the most sensitive stomach and can be enjoyed after every meal.

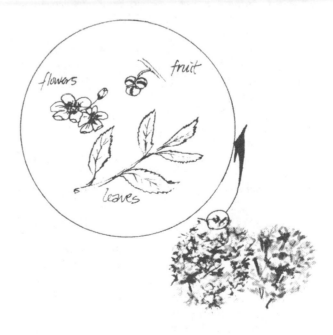

The dried stems, leaves, and twigs of the tea plant are used to make bancha tea.

Leaf Tea

What the connoisseur or tea taster looks for in tea is color, aroma, flavor, and astringency (liquor), placing tea drinking on a par with wine drinking in aesthetic complexity. The three major divisions of leaf tea are black, green, and oolong, and each refers to a different method of processing the leaf. Caffeine is the primary active ingredient in all three; caffeine's imprint is felt most strongly on the central nervous system, producing wakefulness, increased mental activity, heightened sensory perception, and quicker wit. A large dose extends the effects to the motor nerves and causes irritability. Caffeine when ingested also dominates the activity of the kidneys and heart, and in excess fatigues both of these organs. It raises blood pressure and accelerates the pulse. Initially caffeine inhibits the flow of urine, but eventually it acts as a diuretic and opens the floodgates. A five-minute infusion (normal brewing time) extracts about three-quarters of the caffeine. One pound of tea contains 210 grains of caffeine, of which 170 grains are extracted. Since a pound of tea makes approximately 150 cups, each cup averages about one grain of caffeine. (A pound of coffee, by comparison, has about 140 grains of caffeine, but makes only about 50 cups, yielding approximately 2.5 grains per cup.)

Black Tea

Black tea is sometimes referred to as red tea. Its infusion releases swirls of red fog which completely tint the water. The color comes from tannin, the astringent that also contributes pungency. As a free acid, tannin will coagulate protein, possibly disrupting digestion and the flow of digestive juices. However, the total amount in each cup is minimal—a five-minute infusion releases only about half the available tannin and of that only about 60 percent is a free acid.

Black tea is preferred by most people to green and oolong. Its processing is done in five steps: withering, rolling, roll breaking, fermenting, and firing. These steps are accomplished mechanically, except for the wither, which in some countries is still a natural process. In withering, just-picked leaves are thinly spread over racks and allowed to dry. Where the climate allows it, they are left in the sun. Indian teas are often withered naturally, while elsewhere high humidity makes indoor withering—under controlled conditions—imperative. Depending on the temperature and humidity, the tea leaves dry in eighteen to twenty-four hours. The wither is complete when 100 pounds of leaves have dehydrated to about 65 pounds.

Rolling breaks open the cells of the withered leaves and frees the concentrated juices and enzymes. Tea rolling, once done by hand, is now accomplished everywhere by machine. A tea roller, which compresses the leaves against a rotating surface, methodically grinds and breaks them apart while also giving them a gentle twist—a characteristic of fine tea. (When tea is brewed, some components infuse more rapidly than others—well-twisted tea has a more even rate of infusion.) After rolling, the leaves are placed into hoppers and mechanically beaten to get rid of the clumps that have formed. This step is known as roll breaking.

The leaves are next spread onto floors in fermenting rooms. There the chemical transitions begun with rolling—primarily oxidation of tannin—are completed. Temperature and air supply determine the rate of fermentation. The higher the temperature, the faster the rate, but the tea that results is not necessarily better. The optimum temperature falls in the range of 70° to 80° F. Air supply is largely determined by how thickly the leaves are spread. A thicker spread means less air can circulate to the bottom, and results in higher temperatures and faster fermentation.

Color, aroma, flavor, and astringency are determined by the process of fermentation. Fermentation is considered complete after one and a half to four and a half hours, and then the leaves are fired—exposed to blasts of dry hot air—to kill the fermenting enzymes. In addition to stopping fermentation, firing also reduces the moisture content of the leaves to a scant 3 percent. The leaves are left to sit until the moisture content returns to about 7 percent, and then the tea is packed. With this level of moisture the tea will mature in the package.

Black tea is sorted according to leaf size, size being one component of quality. Sifting machines separate leaf grades and broken-leaf grades. Flowery Orange Pekoe, Orange Pekoe, Pekoe, Pekoe Souchong, and Souchong are leaf grades, with Flowery Orange Pekoe and Orange Pekoe rated the top class and Souchong the bottom. Flowery Orange Pekoe and Orange Pekoe denote leaves that are well defined and closely twisted, and that contain many tips. Pekoe is small, tightly rolled, and has broader leaves. Souchong-grade leaves are the broadest and coarsest, usually from a later picking and from lower branches.

Broken-leaf grades are used in blends. From top to bottom they are Broken Orange Pekoe, Broken Pekoe, Broken, Fannings, and Dust. Broken Orange Pekoe contains some tips and therefore is the mainstay of quality tea blends. Broken Pekoe is from larger leaves, has no tips, and is used as a filler in blends. Broken is from still larger leaves and is used as a filler in cheaper blends. Fannings and Dust are pretty descriptive. These powdered leaves produce strong, unsubtle tea and quick color and are used as fillers in the worst blends of tea.

Green Tea

Green tea production seeks to retain the natural flavor of tea—while physical changes are encouraged and flavors intensified, chemical changes are held at bay. Green tea is unfermented. The first stage of manufacture is not the wither as with black tea, but rather steaming. The leaves are steamed—blasted with humid, hot air—immediately after picking to destroy enzymes and prevent fermentation. No moisture is removed, and the leaf becomes soft and pliable and ready for rolling.

The rolling process is the same as for black tea. Moisture is quickly expressed from the leaves, to prevent fermentation from beginning. Immediately after the roll, the leaves are fired. Firing is repeated several times and moisture content is brought down gradually. The final product contains about 3 percent moisture and is packaged immediately so that no other moisture is extracted from the air. The tea is not meant to mature after packaging, and at 3 percent moisture content it doesn't.

Chinese green tea is graded according to the age and style of the leaf. Gunpowder is in tiny balls, and is produced from young leaves; Young Hyson is long, thinly rolled, young leaf; Imperial is loosely balled, older leaf—the remains of Gunpowder. Hyson is older leaf in a mixture of styles, partly thinly rolled like Young Hyson and partly in loosely rolled balls like Imperial. Three other styles exist, made from the worst leaf: Twankay, which consists of old, open leaves; Hyson Skin, which is even poorer; and Dust, which is whatever is left.

Japanese green tea is classed differently: by method of production and leaf shape. Production names are: Pan Fired or Straight Leaf; Guri or Curled Leaf; Basket Fired; and Natural Leaf. Size gradings are from best to worst: Extra Choice, Choicest, Choice, Finest, Fine, Good-medium, Good-common, Nibs, Fannings, and Dust.

Green teas found in whole foods stores are from later season picking and contain less caffeine and tannin than choice leaves.

Oolong Tea

Oolong tea marries the qualities of black and green teas. Oolong is slightly withered, fermented, fired, rolled, refermented, and refired before packing. Almost all Oolong tea comes from Taiwan. Pouchong tea is Oolong mixed with gardenias or jasmines.

Herb Teas

Beverages made from flowers and herbs have been increasingly favored by an American public in search of non-caffeinated refreshment. In general, these "teas" originated in temperate zones and were used as infusions in those regions long before the introduction of coffee and tea. Like tea, these beverages bring us back to a time when food and medicine were one, and surviving knowledge of these flavorful beverages delineates their uses as remedies and tonics.

Both herbal teas consisting of the flower, leaf, or root of one plant and blends made from several plants are available. The emphasis of modern blending is on flavor and not medicine, which probably contributes more than anything else to their popularity.

Herb teas are sold in bags, loose packs, and bulk bins, but the best herbal teas are made from plants that you yourself pick and dry. Many herbs grow wild even in urban neighborhoods, and many others will grow in a garden plot or on a windowsill with minimal care. The quality of packaged herbs found in the store is usually good, but you will rarely come across any that are organic.

Unblended herbs can be infused for a daily beverage or blended with other herbs. They also permit one to concoct medicinal brews made to specific strengths and proportions.

Mugwort, like catnip, was popular in Europe before the advent of black tea. The upper leaves and the flowers can be used to make an infusion that helps eliminate fat deposits and soothes the lungs.

Mint tea is one of the thoroughbreds of herb folk tradition. Spearmint and peppermint are the most popular varieties. They also can be found in the wilds of city and country throughout most of the U.S. Used since earliest times, and part of the mythology of most ancient peoples, mint has been personified, deified, or just plain dried, by Hebrews, Greeks, Romans, and Arabs. Tea is made from the leaves after drying. Spearmint has a sharper taste than peppermint, while peppermint is more pungent and fruity. Some cultures looked to mint as a virility tonic, but today more herbalists recommend it as a remedy for poor circulation, lack of appetite, and upset stomach.

Raspberry leaf tea is thought a potent medicine for all discomforts connected with the female sexual cycles. The tea, made from the leaves, is aromatic and astringent.

Other plants that may be used to make good herbal teas include nettle, yarrow, chicory, wintergreen, sarsaparilla, birch, fennel, mullein, sweet goldenrod, dandelion, comfrey, clover, and alfalfa. Care must be taken to avoid poisonous plants and to not overdo the use of those having strong medicinal effects.

A final tip on tea buying: if the packages are dusty go elsewhere for your brew. A good rate of turnover is essential to ensure a fresh product. And at home, store herbals in sealed containers as you would regular tea. That way the tea will be equally as invigorating as the conversation you may share around it.

Chemical Coffee: The Dangers of Decaf

Are cancer-causing chemicals used to prepare decaffeinated coffee? Are some decaf blends to be shunned in favor of others? Yes, it's true: not all decaffeinated coffees are created equal. The first batch of decaf was prepared in 1908 by the son of a German coffee merchant who believed his father's premature death was hastened by caffeine overconsumption. The son steamed green coffee beans, then soaked them in a solvent such as benzene, which dissolved out the caffeine. The beans were steamed again to drive out the solvent, then dried and roasted. The coffee was called Sanka from the shortened French "sans [without] caffeine."

This original process—called the "direct contact method"—is still the most widely used commercial way of decaffeinating coffee beans. Which companies use it is a mystery: most firms consider their methods trade secrets. Over the years, the solvent of choice shifted from benzene, which is a carcinogen, to trichloroethylene. When this, too, was discovered to cause liver cancer in mice in 1975, the coffee industry voluntarily switched to methylene chloride. Recent evidence links this solvent with cancer as well, and that worries consumer advocates. The concern is that while steaming solvent-treated coffee beans does remove most of the solvent, certain oils in the beans can selectively combine with the solvent, making it impossible to remove completely.

Fortunately, there's more than one way to temper a bean:

•Indirect Method #1: Green coffee beans are soaked in near-boiling water, which over the course of several hours acts as a mild solvent and removes the caffeine plus certain aromatic oils. After draining, the *water* is treated with methylene chloride, which locks onto the caffeine. The solvent is evaporated with heat and the water is reunited with the beans, which absorb their original oils before they are dried and roasted. Coffee companies claim that with this process, the solvent never touches the coffee. But the FDA cautions that even though much of the solvent may evaporate, no such procedure is 100 percent efficient, which means that the water that washes over the beans may contain traces of methylene chloride. Methylene chloride is the solvent used by General Foods, which markets several brands of coffee: Maxwell House, Sanka, Brim, and Yuban.

•Indirect Method #2: This is the same as Indirect Method #1, but with a different, slower-acting solvent: ethyl acetate. Ethyl acetate is a natural constituent of coffee, bananas, and other fruits, and is considered safe. Procter and Gamble's decaffeinated instant coffees, High Point and Folger's Crystals, are processed in this way.

•Swiss Water Process: This uses no chemicals at all. The beans are soaked in hot water, which is passed through charcoal or activated carbon filters to remove the caffeine. Water and beans are then reunited.

The Swiss company Coffex uses the Swiss water process. Nestle Foods Corporation uses a water process method of decaffeination that they've developed and patented for use with their Nescafe and Taster's Choice decafs. They use only water and the natural oil extracted from coffee beans to remove caffeine. Some natural foods stores may sell other "water processed" or "European water processed" blends, but unless they're labeled "Swiss water processed," they were manufactured by one of the indirect methods.

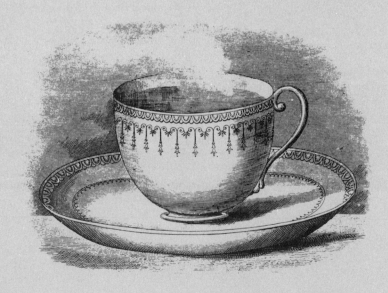

Soymilk—
Is it a Natural?

Soymilk is a jack-of-all-trades drink that has recently become perhaps the hottest selling item ever in natural foods stores. For the growing portion of the population that, for various reasons, is choosing to avoid dairy products, soymilk comes as the perfect alternative: it looks like milk and although it doesn't really taste like milk, it can be used in many of the same ways.

A cholesterol-free, low-fat, vegetable-based beverage, soymilk has distinct advantages over commercial dairy milk. Many individuals cannot tolerate lactose, the primary sugar in dairy milk—soymilk has none of this. Saturated fats, like those found in cow's milk, contribute to buildup of arterial plaque and lead to cardiovascular disease—soymilk contains mostly unsaturated and polyunsaturated fats. The antibiotics and other medicines that many modern dairy farmers regularly include in the rations of their animals can be passed on to the human consumer. In addition, environmental contaminants become concentrated as they work their way up the food chain and high levels are found in the fat of animals, including the butterfat in cow's milk. Soybeans, on the other hand, are generally grown with relatively small amounts of agricultural chemicals; those that are used are applied at such times that high levels of residues would not be found in the soybeans themselves.

The actual amounts of nutrients in a given variety of soymilk will vary according to the additional ingredients included in the formula and the amount of water used in the processing. But when prepared with the same amount of water as is present in dairy milk, and without added ingredients, soymilk has more protein, less fat, fewer calories, and more iron than cow's milk. It also contains significant quantities of several of the B vitamins, and no cholesterol. However, while soymilk is a relatively good source of calcium, it has only 18 percent of the calcium in cow's milk and just over half as much calcium as mother's milk. If soymilk is used as a direct substitute for either of these, it is important that adequate calcium be obtained from other dietary sources.

Nutritious, available in a wide variety of flavors and varying degrees of sweetness, able to keep for long periods of time in a single packet—is mild-mannered soymilk really a superdrink?

Yes and no. As it is currently manufactured and marketed, a number of reservations crop up. One consideration is the incredible energy expense involved in raising soybeans in the United States to be shipped to Japan to be processed and shipped back to the U.S. (with a lot of water added) to be sold to U.S. consumers. In addition, soymilks are considered by some to be just another example of "high-tech natural," a highly processed and slickly packaged food whose reputation for wholesomeness is largely undeserved.

For instance, would you buy—and consume— a food that has been vacuum de-aerated, vacuum deodorized, homogenized, centrifuged, hulled, and super-heated, and that has had its enzymes deactivated? What if this same item were then packaged in nylon-plastic-aluminum "flexible cans" and heated to 248° F to produce a sterile, shelf-stable product? And would you pay ten to fifteen times more for it than for its traditional counterpart, which you could make in your own kitchen? Not a chance, you say?

The fact is that in 1984 U.S. natural foods consumers spent more than $10 million for over a million gallons of various types of soymilk, and sales show no sign of a letup. Much of this money has gone to three reputable natural foods companies whose new products, and unique packages, are largely responsible for the soymilk boom. Eden's "Edensoy," Great Eastern Sun's "Ah Soy," and Westbrae's "Westsoy" and "Malteds," taking the natural foods industry by storm, are the hottest new products these companies have ever carried. For Eden, the new soymilk products are not just the hottest new introduction the company has ever made—the two original flavors of "Edensoy" have *each* accounted for more sales than any other Eden product. Led by "Edensoy," the three other similarly packaged best-selling products have been followed by other soymilks from local tofu shops, Chinese-American manufacturers and, most visibly, "Vitasoy" (imported from Hong Kong) and Health Valley's "SoyMoo."

While the current wave of soymilks are made by a recently developed process, soymilk, per se, is nothing new. References in ancient Chinese texts establish its origin sometime before the first century A.D. and its use in China as a hot breakfast drink and soup base continues to this day. In Japan, although soymilk has long been prepared as a

How to Make Your Own Soymilk

Considering the high cost of the popular soymilk beverages, I decided to see if I could make a rich, dairy-like soymilk in my own kitchen. The recipe that follows is a distillation of my own experiences, scientific research, and various published recipes for homemade soymilk, most notably those of Bill Shurtleff and Akiko Aoyagi found in both the Ballantine Books and Ten Speed Press editions of their classic *The Book of Tofu.*

The mild, relatively bland flavor of this homemade beverage results chiefly from the use of *hot* tap water in grinding the beans. This deactivates the enzyme responsible for the "bean-y" flavor that some people complain about in soymilk. While nearly any variety of soybeans will yield good-quality milk (assuming the beans are in good condition—not cracked, shriveled, or discolored—and not more than one year old), the sweetest, mildest-tasting, and creamiest soymilk comes from "large-seeded" or "vegetable type" strains such as Kanrich, Prize, and Vinton. Request these from your natural foods store. If they don't carry these types of soybean, suggest that they get them in stock.

Because of the relatively small amount of water in this recipe, the resulting rich soymilk contains over 80 percent more protein than dairy milk or "regular strength" soymilks and at least 60 percent more than even the Westbrae "Malteds."

Considering that the ingredient cost of six ounces of this soymilk is about $.04 (at $.40 per pound for soybeans), and that this recipe makes thirty ounces and takes no more than thirty minutes, including clean-up, you can pay yourself $6.50 an hour to make soymilk rather than buy retort-packed plain soymilks. The small amounts of sweeteners and flavors don't change the picture much. And there's nothing stopping you from doubling the recipe—all you need is larger pots—and "earning" $12 an hour (it does take marginally longer to boil more water and grind more beans, hence a dollar less than doubling the $6.50 rate for the smaller batch).

Homemade Soymilk

*1 cup soybeans, rinsed three times
    and soaked overnight*
4 cups (approx.) water

Equipment

*cooking pot (saucepan, 3-quart or
    larger)*
*pressing pot (saucepan or bowl,
    3-quart or larger)*
colander
cotton or linen dishtowel or bag
rubber spatula
wooden spoon
blender

Put 4 cups of water in the cooking pot and bring to a boil over a high flame.

While waiting for the water to boil, drain the soaked soybeans and cover with hot tap water. Preheat the blender by filling with hot tap water. If you use a glass blender, this also safeguards against possible cracking when you add the boiling water in the next step. (If the blender jar is not heat-resistant, use hot tap water for the next step instead of boiling water.)

Just as the water comes to a boil, drain the beans, empty the blender jar, and put the warm beans in the blender. Pour enough of the boiling water over the beans so that the water is at least two inches above the beans—more if you have room, as long as you leave at least an inch at the top of the blender. Put the pot with the remaining water back on the burner with heat reduced to low. Blend the beans until smooth. Heat the water in the pot to boiling. Pour the bean puree into the boiling water, cleaning the sides of the blender jar with the spatula, and return the heat to high. When the foam begins to rise (watch carefully or it'll be all over your stovetop!) lift the cooking pot from the flame, reduce the heat to a simmer, replace the pot, and simmer the puree for five minutes (keep an eye on the foam). During this time place the colander over the pressing pot and line it with the dishtowel or bag. Then pour the hot puree into the cloth-lined colander.

After pressing, the soymilk requires further cooking, so if you are using a bowl rather than another pot for a pressing pot, rinse the cooking pot quickly but thoroughly. Carefully twist the towel or bag closed, and press with a potato masher or the bottom of a strong jar. When no more liquid comes out, open the cloth and stir the okara (pulp) with a wooden spoon, fluffing it up. Sprinkle $1/2$ cup water over the okara, reclose the cloth, and press again to extract the last of the milk. Return the milk to the burner, bring back to a boil, and simmer for fifteen minutes. Et voila!—a quart of rich, creamy, dairy-like soymilk in less time than it would take to milk a goat. And for only seventeen cents' worth of soybeans.

This soymilk can be sweetened or otherwise flavored (sweet white or mellow barley miso is disarmingly delicious) and drunk as a beverage, hot or chilled. In Japanese tofu shops a favorite is fresh soymilk, still hot, seasoned with a drop or two of natural shoyu. Fresh soymilk is also ideal for use in cooking.

---

step in the tofu-making process, it has not become a part of the traditional cuisine; until recently, it was used only by a very small portion of the population, mostly the tofu makers and their families.

Neither is soymilk new to North America. From the beginning of the 20th century soymilk has been marketed both as infant formula and as a drink for adults. In 1935, auto manufacturer and soyfood advocate Henry Ford served a fourteen-course soyfoods dinner to the press at the Chicago World's Fair. Much early work to develop and popularize soymilk in America—as well as in Japan—was done by Seventh-day Adventists.

However, it was an Asian who came up with the idea of marketing soymilk as a soft drink and who set the stage for the boom that has accompanied the new generation of soymilk beverages in this country. In 1940, K.S. Lo's Hong

Kong Soya Bean Products Company began making "Vitamilk" (later renamed "Vitasoy"). After World War II, the vitamin-enriched bottled milk was sold through soft drink outlets and became a huge success.

With the modernization of the soymilk process, the "nutritional soft drink" marketing concept, and the development of packaging processes that could make soymilk a non-perishable product, in the 1970s there remained but one obstacle to selling soymilk to Americans—soymilk tastes, not surprisingly, like soybeans. And Americans (and the Japanese) expect milk (and milk-like drinks) to taste like milk. Consumers certainly don't want it to taste "bean-y." In 1966 researchers at Cornell University in Ithaca, New York, discovered that heat would inactivate the lipoxygenase enzymes that were responsible for producing the off-flavors naturally present in traditionally made soymilk. Subsequent research led to processes that involved hulling the beans before grinding them and using a vacuum pan to remove volatile off-flavors, further reducing the bean-y flavor.

In 1981, Marusan, Japan's second largest soymilk producer and the manufacturer of "Edensoy," introduced the stand-up retort pouch for its line of soymilk for the Japanese health food market. Retort pouches do not require hydrogen peroxide flushing before filling, as cardboard cartons do. They can be processed in a large pressure canner (a retort) at high temperatures after they are filled, thus yielding a virtually non-perishable product with no chemical used in the processing—a canned food in a lightweight, throw-away package. The stage thus set, soymilk was ready for the American natural foods market. If first year sales are any indication, the market was not only ready, but eagerly waiting.

What is the traditional process, used in tofu shops for centuries, from which the modern method used to make these products evolved? Basically, it's quite simple: soybeans are soaked and then ground with water in a stone mill. The resulting puree is mixed with hot water and cooked for a few minutes before it is strained through a cloth bag and pressed to remove as much of the creamy white liquid—soymilk—as possible. An extra rich, thick, and creamy version of this beverage continues to be made in many tofu shops where it is served hot with a dash of shoyu or a bit of sweetener. It's hard to imagine a simpler, more natural process than the making of this soymilk, which involves soaking, grinding, cooking, and filtering to separate solid from liquid. There are no artificial ingredients, and only minimal processing (restricted to cutting, grinding, drying or pulping, and the removal of inedible substances).

How does this traditional method differ from its high-tech counterpart that the natural foods industry has so keenly taken to? The three brands of retort-packed soymilk drinks currently available are made by two different Japanese manufacturers—Eden's "Edensoy" by Marusan, and Great Eastern Sun's "Ah Soy" and Westbrae's "Westsoy" and "Malteds" by the Saniku Food Company.

Although each of the three companies has its own formula, and each of the two processors has its own process, the techniques and technology used by all of the large soymilk manufacturers in Japan are basically the same. The most important difference between the traditional process and the modern one as practiced in Japan is the use of heat to deactivate the enzymes responsible for the formation of bean-y off-flavors.

Marusan and Saniku share similarities that are more important than their differences. Both use hot water to deactivate enzymes for the reduction of bean-y flavors. Both use vacuum pans to remove air and volatile off-flavors, and both include homogenization to prevent product separation. And both companies pack the finished soymilk in multi-layer, flexible cans, heat-treated at high temperature and pressure to ensure long shelf life without refrigeration.

The principal ingredients in soymilks are, of course, water and soybeans. Only "Ah Soy" offers the customer a choice of organic or conventionally grown soybeans, and then only in "original" (plain) and carob flavors. The three retort-packed products—"Edensoy," "Ah Soy," and the Westbrae line—are sweetened with barley malt, although this sweetener is listed at the end of the ingredient list on "Edensoy" and second only to soybeans on the Westbrae and Great Eastern Sun products. ("Edensoy" does taste less sweet.) "Edensoy" contains no added oil; both of the other brands include pressed corn oil for added richness and smoothness. The "Malteds" do not contain "pearl barley" (actually *hato mugi* or Job's tears), while both of the others do. In "Ah Soy" it is malted; in "Edensoy," unmalted. "Edensoy" does not list salt on the label, both others do. "Edensoy" lists kombu; neither of the others do. The flavor ingredients—carob, vanilla, chocolate, cranberry—vary from product to product.

Only the "plain" varieties can be considered as true milk substitutes for drinking or cooking (although some people have found that the carob varieties make delicious puddings). Eden promotes their soymilk product as a real food, not as just a tasty sensory treat. "Ah Soy" obviously is meant to appeal as a nutritious soft drink. And there's little doubt what message Westbrae is trying to get across with its 1950s soda fountain image: milkshakes without milk. This brings us to a significant difference between the "Malteds" and the other two products: thickness. Westbrae's "Malteds" contain significantly more "solids" than either of the other brands, and as a result are richer-tasting and creamier-feeling. They are also more highly sweetened and flavored, almost like liquid candy bars or soy ice cream. And they cost more.

There are other soymilk beverages on the market that are produced by processes dissimilar to the typical Japanese processing described here. They have not received the national distribution and media exposure of the retort-packed Japanese imports and do not have the immediate sensory appeal, nor do they include such selectively chosen ingredients as "Ah Soy," "Edensoy," and the Westbrae products. Most of these other soymilks are made by tofu shops or Chinese-American companies and are distributed only to limited areas or to ethnic markets.

Two other brands should be mentioned, Soy Moo and Vitasoy. "Soy Moo" is distributed by Health Valley Natural Foods of Montebello, California. There are actually two very different products being sold by Health Valley as "Soy Moo," one made in the U.S. and sold frozen in cartons, the other made in Belgium and packed in shelf-stable, aseptic "Brik Paks." Both products are offered in plain and carob flavors and are sweetened with honey. Although no significant source of sodium is listed as an ingredient, the nutritional analysis of both products indicates sodium levels as high as that in the Japanese products discussed above, and several times greater than the combined sodium levels of all listed ingredients.

The other widely distributed soymilk beverage is "Vitasoy," made in Hong Kong by Hong Kong Soya Bean Products. The "Vitasoy" being imported for sale within the health, natural and "non-Asian" consumer markets is sweetened with maple syrup, contains soy oil, and is decidedly thinner than the Japanese products. All flavors contain ingredients that health-conscious consumers will choose to avoid: potassium bicarbonate to balance excess acidity in the chocolate variety and carob gum in all flavors.

While industrially manufactured soymilk has been claimed by some to be more digestible than traditionally made soymilk, Bill Shurtleff, author of numerous books on soyfoods and director of the Soyfoods Center in Lafayette, California, maintains that the processing does not contribute to ease of digestibility and may, indeed, marginally decrease levels of some amino acids. Virtually all the processing developed by the Japanese soymilk industry has been brought forth in an attempt to make soymilk not taste like soymilk.

Soymilk is often regarded as an economical source of protein, and one would think that it would compare favorably with milk on a cost basis as well as nutritionally. However, anyone who has bought one of these six-ounce pouches knows that this stuff is anything but cheap. At approximately seventy-four cents per package it's over twelve cents per ounce and five times as expensive as cow's milk, four times the cost of Coca-Cola, and more than twice the price of Perrier. Definitely not the poor man's drink.

Why is something made from a lowly bean so expensive? With soybean market prices hovering around six dollars a bushel (sixty pounds), and only a handful of beans used in the making of each package of soymilk, the beans can hardly be blamed for the gourmet price that soymilk commands. Rather, it is logistic and processing factors that contribute to the high price. Most of the soybeans used to make all of these beverages are grown in America. They are shipped to Japan at about 13 percent moisture, processed, and returned, minus their fiber and at something over 86 percent water. Thus, U.S. consumers are paying to ship Japanese water across the Pacific and around the country. The processing is energy and capital intensive, and serves not to improve the product nutritionally, but to make it more marketable to a certain group of people for whom, evidently, money is no object. By the time you buy soymilk from the local store there are several markups on the finished product: the exporting company in Japan, the importer here, the distributor, and the retailer all have to get their share for handling the product.

Today the market for soymilk is growing, although its retail price indicates that it is popularly regarded not so much as an economical substitute for milk, but as an expensive, high-tech specialty food. Will this provide enough of a base to set the stage for domestic production, which in turn could lead to the introduction of reasonably priced soymilk, sold primarily for its nutritional benefits and not as a vehicle for flavors and sweeteners? The growing legion of people eating natural foods certainly hopes so.

Focus on Fruit Juice

With appealing choices like ambrosia, papaya nectar, Chenin Blanc grape juice, passion fruit delight, and boysenberry, the natural juice lover has virtually the pick of the world's best orchards and nature's range of fruits in the most exotic blends, all available on the grocer's shelf. Today, the natural fruit juice category is rich with both imaginative blends and sturdy single fruit flavors. Natural fruit juices are characterized by the absence of colorings, preservatives, and sweeteners, and the presence of high-quality juice that is relatively unfiltered.

Occasionally, natural fruit juices come with certified organically grown fruits. Most companies we contacted reported that the supply of organic fruit is too limited, expensive, or sporadic to meet their high production demands. Some juicers use organic fruits "sometimes," "now and then," or "selectively," as with Heinke's apple juice, Knudsen's concord grape, and with all three of Walnut Acres' juices. One juicer noted that the use of sprays on fruits relates more to length of the growing season and region of the country (and thus blossoming, fruiting, and ripening factors) than to warding off insects.

Minimal filtration of the juices is common, leaving a characteristic cloudy appearance and sediment at the bottom of the jar. This indicates a higher volume of "whole fruit" or "pure fruit" used versus concentrated filtered juice, which is another quality issue. With apple juice particularly, it seems that juicers may use a certain percentage of concentrate and added water rather than the whole fruit, without stating so on the label. A juice with a thicker texture and a richer, fuller taste tends to indicate a higher volume of whole fruit used.

R.W. Knudsen

A Rainbow of Flavors

R. W. Knudsen is the Campbell Soup Company of natural juices: they offer more varieties than any grocer could possibly stock, and it would take almost two months of different-drink-a-day-sampling to try them all. Fortunately, that's where the analogy between Knudsen and Campbell ends. Knudsen features fine natural ingredients in their single fruits, apple blends, exotic mixtures, special blends, herbal coolers, and frozen juice concentrates. Especially unique and appetizing is their line of seven grape juices made from varieties such as Riesling, Chardonnay, Ruby Cabernet, and French Colombard grapes. They also make Organically Grown Concord Grape Juice and an Organic Apple Juice. The four Knudsen Herbal Coolers (hibiscus, ginger, ginseng, and mint tea) are also welcome variations on the fruit juice theme. Knudsen & Sons, Inc., Speedway Ave., P.O. Box 369, Chico, CA 95927; (916) 891–1517.

Heinke's

Gold Medal Quality

The Heinke family has been making natural fruit juices since 1925, when the young California farmer Carl Heinke first dreamed of making "gold medal quality" fruit juice. The years of experience and personal commitment to quality show throughout the Heinke line. They offer two types of juice: 100% Pure Juice and 100% Juice Blends. There are twelve of the 100% pure juices (made without concentrates), including an organic apple, Concord and Zinfandel grape juices, and a unique Kiwi Apple Juice. They also make seventeen blends, which use concentrates and sometimes natural gum stabilizers for lighter, sweeter drinks, and grape concentrate added for sweetening. These range from Passion Fruit Mango Nectar to a simple Apple Cranberry. Heinke's says that in the past they used more organic fruits than today, but they anticipate a gradual return to organic ingredients as more become available. They raise their own grapes for the Concord Grape Juice. Heinke's, Inc., 5365 Clark Rd., Paradise, CA 95969; (916) 877–4847.

Eden

Nine from the Midwest

This Michigan-based natural foods producer and distributor markets nine natural juices under its well-known label. Eden juices are lightly filtered during pressing and, as much as is possible, are prepared from Midwest-grown fruits. Juice flavors include a pure Michigan Red Cherry, Apple, Apple-Apricot, Apple-Cranberry, Apple-Pineapple, Apple-Raspberry, All Natural Prune, and Michigan Concord Grape. They are sold by natural foods grocers primarily in the Midwest and on the east coast. Eden Foods, 701 Tecumseh Rd., Clinton, MI 49236; (517) 456-7424.

Lakewood
A Taste of the Tropics

Lakewood is a fifty-one-year-old family-run Florida juice company offering about three dozen blended juices that run the gamut in fruit mixtures. With the company's subtropical location, it is not surprising that they are particularly strong on exotic fruit blends, offering seven papaya drinks and other warm-weather favorites such as Pineapple-Coconut, Guava, and Mango. There's also a number of blends from apples, cranberries, and other berries that will appeal to northerners. The Three Berry, for instance, is made with apple juice, strawberry, raspberry, loganberry, and white grape juice from concentrate, as a sweetener. Lakewood Products, Box 420708, Miami, FL 33242; (305) 324-5932.

Walnut Acres
Choice of the Connoisseur

This is a small, modest juicer but one with high, reliable standards, delicious products, and little hyperbole. Their grape juice is vividly sweet and rich, containing a blend of pressed New York white grapes, organically grown under certification of the New York State Organic Growers Association and in close cooperation with local, small-scale orchardists. Walnut Acres also makes Cranberry Nectar, a 50/50 blend of unsprayed cranberries and untreated deep well water and honey, and a pure Organic Apple. The prices are on the high side, but the taste and agricultural ethics make them worthwhile. Walnut Acres has limited national distribution. Their apples are free from chemical sprays, are pressed and minimally filtered in stainless steel trays, and are lightly heat-treated. The company deserves more recognition for their high quality and product purity and is a common choice of the natural fruit juice connois-

seur. Walnut Acres, Penn's Creek, PA 17862; (717) 837-0601.

After The Fall
Taste of the Rural Orchard

After The Fall began as a shoestring operation in the woods of New York in 1972, and is now selling almost three million gallons of juices annually, mostly east of the Mississippi. They began using only organic apples, but now must use "the best available commercially grown apples." In 1984, After The Fall ended an eight-year association with Lincoln Foods, a packer that was processing and bottling ATF's juices. ATF founder and president Mark Panely says that unfulfilled quality expectations, and Lincoln's development of its own line (Winter Hill) in competition with ATF, caused the break. Apple blends are ATF's main juices (Apple Strawberry is their best seller), but they've recently added three tropicals—Acerola 'C,' Golden Passion Fruit Juice Nectar, and Orange Papaya. Now marketing fifteen juices in all, ATF's attempts to upgrade their quality are paying off. Their labels suggest the rural orchard and the small wood press, and their tastes and textures do not disappoint. After The Fall, Box 777, Brattleboro, VT 05301; (802) 257-4616.

Winter Hill
Cloudy and Flavorful

Winter Hill, a recent subsidiary of the fifty-year-old mainstream juicer Lincoln Foods, offers an attractive line of about twenty blended and pure fruit juices. A few of these include apple blends with strawberry, raspberry, blackberry, pineapple, and cherry concentrates. There are also more exotic mixtures like Cranberry Royale (Cape Cod cranberries with red and white grapes, Bartlett pears, and Hudson Valley apples), Kiwi Cooler, Passion Fruit Delight, and C-Plus-Acerola. Winter Hill stresses the cloudiness of its juices as an indication of minimal filtering and high fruit content and flavor. With their pretty pastel colors and rustic renditions of fruits and orchards, their labels are among the best in the juice field. The line is found in both supermarkets and natural foods grocers. Winter Hill Natural Juice Company, 1 Newbury St., Lawrence, MA 01842; (617) 685-9151.

11. CONDIMENTS

Condiments are the natural foods connoisseur's best source for additional healthful flavors. Herbs and spices can be used to season foods, but by using combinations of strongly flavored and concentrated foods, you not only can accentuate the tastes in your meal, but can also add to their healthful properties. In the past, many natural condiments were developed to help preserve foods through processes like pickling and fermenting. By using these types of foods in your diet, you can improve the digestibility of your meals, and benefit from enzymes and various microorganisms that can add to your overall health and well-being.

Vinegar is a perfect beginning to this chapter. Sharp and piquant, vinegar is hard to think of without experiencing the mouth-watering effects of its flavor. The difference between unrefined, naturally made vinegar and the standard supermarket product is as great as the difference between commercial white bread and homemade, naturally leavened whole grain bread. In this section, you can learn all the subtle nuances that distinguish different vinegars.

Salty condiments are the other major topic of this chapter. Regardless of the amount of salt you consume, it is an essential part of everyone's daily diet. The salty condiments described in this chapter are remarkable in the great contribution they make to the flavors and nutritional quality of daily meals. Many of these condiments were developed in Japan and are the culmination of generations of tried and tested tastes, guaranteed to make you wonder how you ever managed without them.

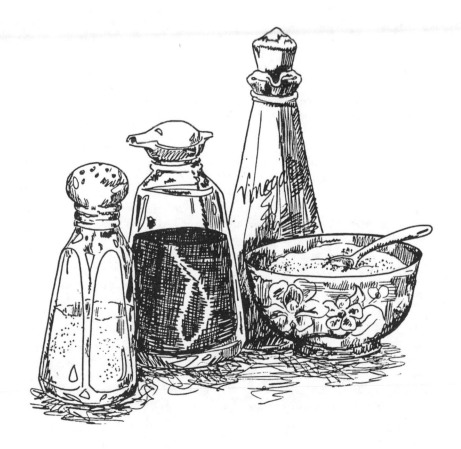

How to Distinguish Fine Vinegars

Ever since a batch of the first homemade wine turned sour, vinegar has played an important role in our cuisine and pharmacopoeia. It has been used by humankind since earliest times for flavoring and preserving. The ancient Greeks and Orientals also recognized its therapeutic value, and employed it in a variety of internal and external treatments. Today, we use it for streak-free window washing and for dying Easter eggs as well.

Although most references indicate that the literal translation of the French *vinaigre* is "sour wine," *-aigre* in Old French meant "eager," "sharp," or "biting." The French is derived from the Latin *acer,* also meaning "sharp." Vinegar, then, is not so much "sour" as it is "sharp" wine—and this more accurately describes the way a drop of it tastes on the tongue.

But vinegar is not limited to wine as its source. It can be made from any carbohydrate that has been fermented to produce ethyl alcohol. The end product is generally classified according to the source material. Wine vinegar is made from fermented grape juice, cider vinegar from hard apple cider—cider that has been fermented into alcohol.

Malt vinegar, made from an unhopped beer (gyle) produced by fermenting sprouted barley, is popular in the British Isles. It is, however, rare here. Even more uncommon is sugar vinegar, made from syrups of glucose, blackstrap molasses, or refiners' molasses. Rice vinegar, the result of a fermentation of rice by koji and a starter, is now available in most natural foods stores, and has long been popular in Japan (see sidebar).

Most vinegar is made in two steps. First, grapes or another carbohydrate food is fermented into ethyl alcohol (ethanol). This is then further fermented by a "mother culture" of acetobacter (bacteria that produce acetic acid). Partial exposure to the air results in an incomplete oxidation of the liquid. A mixture of acetic acid—the essential component of vinegar—water, and approximately .5 percent of alcohol make up the resulting vinegar.

Distilled vinegar is made from pure alcohol that has been distilled from the fermented wine, cider, or gyle before being turned into vinegar by the mother culture. As such, it carries few of the qualities (nutrients and flavor included) of its parent substance. Although alcohol from any source can be used to make distilled vinegar, in the U.S. it is generally made from grain. White, spirit, and grain vinegar are all names under which distilled vinegar is sold. Non-distilled vinegars are characterized by the distinctive flavors, aromas, and colors that are derived from the raw materials.

Three basic processes are used in making vinegar: the Orleans or French, the German or "generator," and the modern continuous process. The Orleans or French process is the oldest. In this process, fresh hard cider or wine is further fermented into vinegar in wooden barrels or small covered vats containing air vents in the top and upper sides of the vessel. A mother culture made from equal parts of nonpasteurized vinegar and fresh wine (or hard cider) is introduced into the barrel. Fermentation is allowed to continue until the acetobacter in the mother culture has converted the alcohol into acetic acid. Roughly three-quarters of the vinegar is drawn off and replaced with more fresh wine. This process is repeated as many times as necessary for a good vinegar to be obtained. Eventually, the mix of organisms becomes contaminated and the process has to be stopped. The barrel is then emptied, cleaned, and recharged with a new mother culture, and the process begins again. The Orleans process is slow and works only in small vessels, but the end product has a superior flavor and aroma due to the side reactions that the long, slow fermentation in the small container brings about.

In the 18th century a Dutchman, Hermann Boerhaave, developed a process that allowed more vinegar to be made in less time. By packing larger casks with grape pomace (the solid residue that remains when fruit is pressed for juice), more of the wine's surface area was exposed to the air and the rate of conversion to vinegar increased dramatically. In 1835, J.S. Schutzenbach further refined this process, reducing the process of fermentation from months to days. In his quick process, also known as the German or "generator" process, a large, two-chambered fermenting vessel (the generator) replaces the smaller barrels or casks of the earlier methods. The upper chamber contains a false bottom. It is filled to within eight inches of the top with a solid material, usually beechwood shavings, that has a large surface area (corncobs or other materials are sometimes used for cider or wine vinegars). The upper chamber is separated from the lower one by a screen. To speed up oxidation, air is blown up through the screen and packing material and is vented through the top of the generator. The fermenting liquid—wine, hard cider, or grain spirits—is sprinkled over the top of the packing, percolates through the mass, and re-collects in the lower chamber. It is then pumped back to the top and recirculated until the alcohol content is reduced to .5 percent—at which point it becomes vinegar. The vinegar is then drawn off and replaced with fresh alcohol. This process is repeated until residues cause poor circulation or until bacterial contamination reduces the yield of acetic acid. The generator is then cleaned and packed with fresh material. With cider or wine vinegar, this cleaning should usually be done twice a year; with distilled vinegar, the generator can operate for several years without a cleaning. Quick vinegar intended for table use is aged for several weeks, filtered, bottled, and pasteurized. Vinegar for pickling or further processing is not aged.

In the modern continuous process, the packing material is eliminated and replaced with a "cavitator," or turbine, which serves to incorporate air into the fermenting solution. Once the rate of fermentation has stabilized and the conversion to acetic acid is nearly complete, fresh alcohol is added to the fermenter at the same rate that vinegar is being drawn off. This process is fast and efficient, but yields a vinegar that has little body or character.

The traditional process used in Japan for making rice vinegar differs from the above processes. First of all, cider, wine, malt, and even distilled vinegar are produced in at least two distinct steps (malt vinegar requires four): the parent material is first fermented into alcohol, and then, in a separate step, the alcohol is inoculated with the mother culture and further fermented into vinegar. For the best traditional rice vinegar, these steps are combined into one: koji, cooked rice, water, and the mother culture are all put together into an earthenware jar. The koji enzymes convert the rice starch to sugars, yeasts (from koji and the mother culture) produce alcohol from the sugars, and acetobacter from the mother culture oxidizes the alcohol to produce acetic acid. A second difference is that, while the fermentation of most cider, wine, and malt vinegars utilizes only the liquids extracted from fruit pulps or grain mash, the grain itself is present throughout the fermentation process in the making of traditional rice vinegar. This accounts for the higher level of amino acids in traditionally made rice vinegars, as well as a more complex and balanced fermentation.

Buying Vinegar

The best-quality wine, cider, and malt vinegars are made by the Orleans or French process. Although few producers use this method on account of its slowness, better vinegar cannot be made by the quicker processes. The complexity of flavor and aroma of the traditionally made vinegar compares with that of the best wines. Unfortunately, few makers include the method of production on the label. Rich colors, fruity aromas, and smooth and gentle flavor are indicative of the mellowing that occurs only in the Orleans process. Some of these vinegars are unfiltered; the best are unpasteurized as well. Sediment occurs naturally in such vinegars.

"Pure malt vinegar" implies a natural product with no additives. Most commercially prepared varieties use caramel coloring to artificially produce a consistently dark color. Pure malt vinegar relies on the color of the malt and the oxidation that occurs during the vinegar fermentation for its rich, dark, clear brown color. The color may vary from batch to batch, but vinegar from several barrels is often blended for greater consistency.

Much of the vinegar that we consume is in prepared foods: salad dressings, sauces, mustard, pickles. If the list of ingredients simply says "vinegar," the Pure Food and Drug Act requires that the product include cider vinegar; unless further identified, this will be "quick process" vinegar (usually "non-aged"). A processor who is concerned enough about quality to pay a little more for good vinegar will probably indicate it on the label. "Grain vinegar," listed as an ingredient of some so-called natural pickles, is distilled vinegar and should be avoided. Look for "cider vinegar," "wine vinegar," "malt vinegar," and "rice vinegar" on ingredient lists; although these vinegars are often made by quick processes, they are still of much better quality than distilled vinegar. Again, a food processor who uses high-quality vinegar will tell you so. "Unpasteurized organic cider vinegar," "brown rice vinegar," and "pure malt vinegar" will appear on the labels of only the most conscientiously produced products.

Herb vinegars are made by steeping sprigs of herbs in vinegar, causing it to take on the flavor and aroma of the herb used. When buying herb vinegars, use the same criteria you would in choosing other vinegars. Is the vinegar identified by type or labeled simply "vinegar"? Of course, you can make your own herb vinegar easily: just place a sprig or two of a fresh herb in a bottle; fill with a good-quality, mild-flavored vinegar; cap the bottle and allow it to sit in a dark place for a few weeks.

Umeboshi vinegar, also known as "ume-su," is not—strictly speaking—a true vinegar. It is the product of a lactic fermentation of underripe ume (a Japanese fruit akin to our apricot) and salt, and not a bacterial fermentation of alcohol to acetic acid. Because of its high salt content, however, umeboshi vinegar tends to overpower other flavors. For this reason, it is best used sparingly.

The Superiority of Old-Fashioned Rice Vinegar

"The purpose of tradition is not merely to do things as they have been done for generations but, over the years, to improve that way . . . to make an even better product. . . ." Tetsuro Oyama's brother and father nodded in agreement as Steve Earle translated Tetsuro's Japanese for me. Then I nodded and smiled in return. In fact, we spent quite a lot of time nodding back and forth as Steve and I were given a tour of the traditional factory where genmisu (brown rice vinegar) is made—in Miyazaki on the southernmost island of Kyushu, in Japan.

The Oyamas' factory is nestled in the hills at the base of the beautiful Kyushu mountain range. Miyazaki itself is clean and picturesque. The surrounding rural land has not yet felt the sting of industry. The temperatures are higher here than anywhere else in Japan, but the seasons change slowly, and grass grows all year long. It is here and, as the Oyamas tell it, only here, where the traditional process of making brown rice vinegar is possible. The three essential factors in vinegar production—water, climate, and environment—exist at an optimal level in Miyazaki as in nowhere else in Japan.

The Oyamas' well yields water with a pH rating of 6.8; this near neutrality is necessary for making the best rice vinegar. (PH refers to the acidity or alkalinity of a solution. It represents the concentration of hydrogen ions, and literally means "the potential of hydrogen." A pH of 7.0 is neutral. A pH below 7.0 is acid; a pH above it is alkaline.) In addition, the water has been tested and found to be completely free of impurities. The land surrounding the vinegar plant, like so much of Japan, is covered with growing rice. But unlike most fields today, this land has never experienced chemical treatment of any sort. The air is equally clean and free of pollution.

The making of this vinegar is a seemingly simple process, as the only ingredients are whole brown rice, koji, vinegar

"seed," and water. However, the sense of timing and the amount of care needed to complete the process are far from simple.

Vinegar is made twice during the year: in the spring and in the fall (around mid-October). Because the process of fermentation takes place outside and there is exposure to the elements, the Oyamas complete the bulk of their work in the fall, thus avoiding the dangers that come with the summer rains.

The whole process begins with the making of the rice koji. Koji is a mold consisting of spores of *Aspergillus oryzae* growing on a grain host. In this case, the "host" is 70 percent whole rice, as the outer layers (the bran and germ) of whole brown rice present too much resistance for the mold to take hold. The koji used by the Oyamas is made for them by a traditional koji house and is the same as that used in making sake (Japanese rice wine). While the koji maker carefully watches his room of fermenting enzymes for three days and nights, the Oyamas begin cooking the rice that they have harvested themselves from their own fields.

The rice is cooked outside in an iron cauldron, which is heated by a wood fire in a pit beneath it. It literally takes the efforts of two people to remove the lid; this great weight on the pot creates an effect much like that of our present-day pressure cooker. When I asked Tetsuro why he didn't make use of simpler methods such as contemporary steam and steel cookers, he replied that he had tried this but the taste had suffered. He believes that the ancient way is best. The finished rice is a soft and watery porridge called kayu. When the koji arrives it is ready to be put into the vinegar jars, along with the kayu and water.

These "jars" are really large earthenware crocks (called *kame*), wide-mouthed with curving bottoms, that are sunk down into the earth and stand upright about waist high. By volume, they will hold about twenty-five gallons of liquid. The

Oyamas' crocks are more than two hundred years old; because the art of their manufacture has completely disappeared, they are irreplaceable. The crocks have the ability to "breathe" air and moisture by osmosis. Each one has its own unique quality of construction and thus imparts an individual taste to the vinegar within it. Because of this, the finished vinegars are left to age in large, glass-lined steel tanks, where their characters mix into subtle uniformity.

Into the jars go the rice kayu, the koji, enough water to fill the jars three-quarters full, and the vinegar "seed." This last ingredient—the seed—is comprised simply of some of the vinegar mash saved from the previous batch. Today, this seed has some of the essence of the first vinegar made by the Oyama family three generations ago.

Once the jars are filled, they are covered tightly with a layer of handmade rice paper. If there is even the smallest of pinholes in this paper covering, the crock will be empty except for a handful of tiny bits of hardened rice when it is opened after the four-to-six-month fermenting period.

Because the crocks cannot be opened for inspection, the traditional method of testing the vinegar's maturity—placing a copper five-yen coin on top of the paper—is used. The Oyamas know that it is ready by the bluish color of the oxidized copper coin, caused by the gases escaping from the vinegar mash. Both the paper and the coin are covered by a square of corrugated iron, which allows air to circulate over the paper while protecting the jar from rain and wind.

In the summer, when the temperature inside the crocks may reach as high as 86–96°F due to the natural heat of the fermenting vinegar, the grass around them is left to grow as protection against too much sun. If this heat was allowed to reach the jars, the action of the fermenting mash would cease. In the winter, however, the grass is cut quite close to the ground to allow the full impact of the sun's heat to affect the jars. The ability of the jars to breathe is most important when using brown rice, for the circulation of air allows the mash to thoroughly ferment the tougher, more substantial "skin" of whole grain rice.

As the days and nights pass and temperature and humidity constantly change, the action in the jars also changes. The mash, which becomes much like sake during the first two weeks, continues to acidify. The koji produces enzymes that break down proteins, starches, and fats into more digestible amino acids, simple sugars, and fatty acids. In four to six months (depending upon the weather, the kind of year, and the quality of the seasons), the color of the copper coin will tell the Oyamas when it is time to transfer the mash to the big glass-lined vats. Here the various characters of all the mashes will blend together for another month. Because the character of each jar is known, the Oyamas can mix stronger and weaker mashes together to achieve the proper balance.

When the mash is mature, it is put into large canvas sacks, which are placed in a solid cedar press (a huge old box mitred with wooden pegs). A massive wooden screw is tightened by hand, and the liquid vinegar is slowly squeezed out and collected in a jar sunk deep into the factory floor. The vinegar is then pumped through layers of pure cotton to filter out any remaining bits of mash and impurities. (The Oyama brothers used a synthetic filter once but found that it damaged the taste of the vinegar.)

Both bottling and pasteurization take place in the Oyamas' factory. Filled only part way up the necks in the bottles, the vinegar is heated very slowly to a temperature of 200°F. Both the vinegar and the glass bottles are quite fragile during this heating process, so great care must be taken. The heating expands the liquid up the necks of the bottles; because the bacterial action of the vinegaring process is stopped by the heat, the bottles are quickly capped to achieve a vacuum-like seal. The enzymes and organic and amino acids of the vinegar survive this "pasteurization" process. In fact, the vinegaring action is impossible to stop completely; if you leave brown rice vinegar on a shelf it will change dramatically over time. The Oyamas feel that the rich, opaque brown vinegar (which is the end result of all their vinegar if it is kept untouched for three years) is the finest of all vinegars in the world.

Rice vinegar came north to Japan from China. It has remained in Kyushu, as have many of the imported elements of Chinese culture. In Japan, there is a resurgence in the use of rice vinegar, but even this supposedly traditional product is not at all of the same quality as the brown rice vinegar made by the Oyamas of Miyazaki. These other vinegars are made from white rice with added enzymes; the jars are placed in a hothouse, similar to a nursery greenhouse, with controlled temperatures. Such modernization requires less time for making vinegar but further removes the product from the natural process that gives the Oyamas' brown rice vinegar its exceptional taste and quality.

The Oyamas' brown rice vinegar takes the usual approaches to making rice vinegar some steps further. It is organic and completely natural in its ingredients and method of production; hence, it possesses a quality superior to the majority of rice vinegars currently available. All you have to do to confirm this fact is to taste some vinegars and experience the vast difference between them and the Oyamas' product.

Brown rice vinegar has many practical uses. As a seasoning, it is gently tart and subtle. It is an excellent pickling agent, and its preserving ability will add days to the life of cooked grains and vegetables. This is an asset particularly in summer cooking. Brown rice vinegar may also be used as an external treatment to balance strong alkalines such as lye or caustic soda.

Tetsuro Oyama says that nostalgia alone—the remembrance of what good taste is—will sell his vinegar. I've tasted it, and I agree. While it is new to the American natural foods consumer and the supply of brown rice vinegar is still limited in the United States, interest in this versatile product is growing. In addition to the Oyama family, several other Japanese families who also produce traditional rice vinegar have begun to export their products through a variety of natural foods companies. The basic process is the same throughout, varying only in the nuances of individual family equipment and tradition.

What Is Real Tamari?

The product that many North Americans call "tamari" is actually natural shoyu, a soy sauce composed of soybeans and wheat, while original Japanese tamari is soy sauce containing little or no wheat.

The word "tamari" (but not real tamari itself) came to be widely used in the West through a linguistic quirk. In 1960 the Lima Foods Company in Belgium asked George Ohsawa, a leader of the international macrobiotic movement, what they should call their brand of shoyu to distinguish it from both regular commercial shoyu and from "chemical soy sauce," an inexpensive unfermented product made from hydrolyzed vegetable protein, caramel coloring, corn syrup, salt, and water (this product still accounts for more than half of all soy sauce sold in North America). Ohsawa suggested that Lima Foods name the new product "natural shoyu," since that was its name in Japan. Lima Foods thought that the word "shoyu" was somewhat difficult to pronounce in French and German and requested alternatives. Ohsawa mentioned that in Japan "tamari" and "murasaki" also referred to types of soy sauce. Lima Foods liked the word "tamari," finding it short, distinctive, and easy to pronounce, and decided to call their natural shoyu by that name. Ohsawa eventually came to use this terminology in his teaching and writing, and it was popularized by the macrobiotic movement, which played a key role in introducing the product to the West.

Little did anyone foresee the confusion that would result as people in the West became familiar with *both* natural shoyu and real tamari, and as distributors began to sell both these fine foods.

The Japanese word *tamari* comes from the verb *tamaru,* which means "to accumulate"—as, for example, water accumulates in ponds. The earliest tamari came from miso: a hollow was scooped out in the upper surface of a keg of fully matured miso, a deep bamboo colander was pressed into the hollow, and the liquid that then accumulated in it was ladled out and reserved for use as a seasoning.

Tamari was unquestionably Japan's most ancient type of soy sauce, just as "tamari" was the earliest word for soy sauce. The word *tamari* first appeared in a Japanese document of 775 A.D., and tamari itself was being produced commercially by 1290 A.D. (Modern shoyu was not developed until the early 1700s.) Real tamari is a direct descendant of Chinese-style soy sauce; both contain little or no wheat and are still made in essentially the same way.

While the word "tamari" has been known in North America for the past two decades, real tamari is just now becoming available. Unlike tamari, shoyu (including natural shoyu) is typically made with equal parts soybeans and cracked roasted wheat. Both products have roughly the same proportions of salt and water, although tamari has slightly less salt (16 percent vs. 17.5 percent).

The natural shoyu sold in North America (the shoyu which is often labeled tamari) is of generally high quality. North American natural foods distributors demand that their product be different from Japan's regular commercial shoyu in at least three ways: (1) it must be made from whole soybeans rather than from defatted soybean meal; (2) it must be fermented slowly and naturally at the temperature of the region rather than quickly in warm, temperature-controlled chambers; and (3) it must contain neither preservatives nor synthetic additives, which are found in most commercial shoyu. Most of the natural shoyu sold in North America is also made in traditional, well-aged cedar vats rather than in their modern stainless steel or epoxy-coated steel counterparts.

Compared with shoyu, real tamari has a slightly deeper flavor, darker brown color, and richer consistency. Since little or no wheat or other grains are used in its preparation, it lacks some of the subtle aroma and alcoholic bouquet that result from fermentation of the wheat in shoyu. However, when shoyu is heated during cooking, much of the delicate flavor and aroma from these volatile substances is lost. Tamari, however, gets its delectable flavor from amino acids in the fermentation of soy protein, and especially from glutamic acid, the natural form of monosodium glutamate; tamari contains 36 percent more of this natural flavoring ingredient than regular shoyu, and 40 percent more nitrogen. Since amino acids are not volatile, they remain to season the food, even after extended cooking. More than shoyu, tamari keeps simmered or sauteed foods tender during simmering. When brushed on the surface of baked goods such as rice crackers, it is known to produce the finest natural color and luster.

In Japan, real tamari is about 25 percent more expensive than a comparable grade of shoyu. This is partly because it is a considerably richer product and partly because it is often made by natural fermentation on a smaller scale. Now available in natural foods stores in this country, real tamari is waiting to find its rightful place along with natural shoyu as a fine seasoning in North America's emerging new cuisine.

Choosing the Best Sea Salt

Medical researchers who have concerned themselves with the issue of the high-salt diet in the United States have implicated this tasty condiment in the onset of many serious diseases. The sodium that makes up approximately 40 percent of salt (chloride comprises about 58 to 59 percent) has been linked to obesity, arthritis, kidney stones, high blood pressure, and an increased risk of cardiovascular disease. As a result, many persons are now on sodium-free or low-sodium diets, and the average consumer associates the terms "low-sodium" and "no-sodium" with a more healthful product.

Without adequate sodium, one may lose weight and suffer muscle cramping and general weakness. Sodium is essential to health. Individuals, however, vary greatly in their sodium requirements, and many do well with minimal levels over long periods of time. In fact, whole societies have been able to exist healthily on low-sodium diets. Sodium occurs in vegetables and other foods as well as being a component of salt. Celery and beets are two vegetables especially high in sodium.

The high levels of salt that are consumed in the typical North American diet, through the use of snack foods, fast and processed foods, soups, meats, and condiments—to say nothing of the salt that is added to foods when the salt shaker is dispensed with abandon—are unnecessary and probably detrimental to health. However, research scientists usually make no distinction among types of salt, nor do they take into consideration the composition of the rest of the diet. The connection between salt and disease might be less clear-cut if we looked at a low-fat, whole-foods, primarily vegetarian diet in conjunction with unrefined, natural sea salts, rather than at the conventional modern diet, which is high in saturated fats, refined foods, and refined and kiln-dried salts.

In addition, in a diet of whole foods the level of salt is often relatively low compared to the average modern diet—5,000 milligrams compared to 15,000 to 20,000 milligrams (three to four teaspoonfuls). The 1977 study *Dietary Goals,* of the U.S. Senate Select Committee on Nutrition and Human Needs, recommended 2,000 to 3,000 milligrams of sodium a day, and 5,000 milligrams of salt approximates this amount.

It is not known exactly how much salt is necessary to maintain health and vitality or if, unlike sodium, it is needed at all. But salt is a tasty and appetizing condiment that, when used in the right amounts, enhances the taste of foods. If you are able to, and choose to use it, what is the best kind to use?

Among commercial table salts two distinct types are available—mined land salt and refined sea salt. Both conform to the *Food Chemical Codex* which requires most salt to be not less than 97.5 percent pure sodium chloride. To make salt free-flowing, most large commercial processors, such as Morton's, add anti-caking agents and crystal modifiers such as sodium ferrocyanide and green ferric ammonium citrate, which coat the salt crystals and prevent them from attracting moisture. Iodized salt generally includes added potassium iodide (iodine), dextrose to stabilize the iodine, and sodium carbonate to stop the mixture from turning purple. For these evaporated, highly refined salts, most of the 2.5 percent that is not sodium chloride consists of these various additives. The *Codex* requires that "rock or solar salt [contain] not less than 97.5 percent of NaCl . . . the remainder consisting chiefly of minor amounts of naturally occurring components."

In addition to containing additives, commercial salt is also unnecessarily and excessively refined. It is comparable to white bread in that most nutrients are removed and then a few are artificially returned to create a semblance of healthfulness. The refined product, deprived of its naturally occurring balance of elements and nutrients, not only contributes little to health, but may actually deplete the body of the store of minerals necessary to neutralize and digest refined foods.

As a result, many health-conscious people have abandoned commercial table salt in favor of natural sea salt, believing it to be unprocessed and unrefined. It is also widely believed that sea salt has the added advantage of being high in naturally occurring minerals, including trace minerals (micronutrients which, though they occur in minute amounts, are essential for human health). Yet very little straightforward information exists regarding the amount of processing the natural sea salts themselves undergo and, indeed, how much refining, if any, is necessary to produce a salt without high concentrations of certain elements—such as lead, cadmium, arsenic, and mercury—that may be harmful. And no one really knows what percentage of trace elements occur in the sea salts. In order to explore these questions, *East West Journal* examined the claims of the suppliers of the most widely available sea salts while at the same time submitting their salts to a laboratory for analysis.

It was not possible to check for levels of all the possible elements, so we requested the levels of six major ones: sodium, chlorine, magnesium, calcium, sulfur (as sulfate), and potassium. We did not test directly for trace elements; however, their quantities, which fluctuate in proportion to the level of magnesium, can be inferred from the levels of that element.

We selected five salts available through natural foods outlets, both retail stores and mail-order houses. They are:

Arrowhead Mills: This sea salt is generally sold in thirty- or fifty-pound bags to natural foods distributors.

Muramoto's Sea Salt: One mail-order supplier describes this salt as "Hand-gathered, sun dried . . . up to 15 percent trace minerals." Muramoto's Sea Salt is also identified as "Balanced Minerals Sea Salt."

Lima Sea Salt (coarse):   Lima describes its product as a "100 percent natural and whole sea salt" that "has not been subjected to any chemical treatment and contains in a perfectly balanced composition all the mineral salts."

Erewhon Sea Salt: According to the label, Erewhon's salt is "sun-dried . . . , washed in sea water and dried again."

Maldon Sea Salt: This salt is described as "a healthy natural salt produced by the gentle evaporation of purified sea water, thereby retaining the same balance as occurs in sea water mineral salts."

The Composition of Sea Water

"Real salt is not sodium chloride—it is dehydrated ocean." This statement is commonly found throughout the literature on natural salt. The implication is that after removing the water from sea water true salt is left—salt that contains everything but the water itself, rich in trace minerals and other nutrients. Is this really what sea salt is?

About sixty elements occur in sea water (out of the 107 recognized by modern chemistry). After the water is removed from a gallon of sea water, about a quarter pound of minerals remains. Six major salts, which are compounds of only eight elements, account for 99.7 percent of these minerals. Only about 78 percent of the six major salts is sodium chloride—16 percent is comprised of magnesium compounds, and 5.7 percent is divided between potassium chloride and calcium sulfate. Most of the remaining .3 percent of the minerals is calcium carbonate, along with some fluoride, strontium, and boron. A minute percentage (0.003) consists of approximately fifty other elements, known as "trace elements," including gold, silver, and

platinum, lead, tin, arsenic, radium, and such truly rare elements as praseodymium and ytterbium (about 0.000024 parts per million of the latter). Do these elements occur in natural sea salt?

It's quite clear from our lab reports that none of the salts we tested could accurately be called "dehydrated ocean," which is about 78 percent sodium chloride. (See chart.) The Lima salt, at 97.51 percent sodium chloride and .416 percent magnesium, has the highest levels of trace minerals but is nowhere near the levels found in sea water. The Arrowhead Mills sample, if its added magnesium carbonate were removed, would be 99.56 percent sodium chloride, clearly a highly refined salt. The Erewhon sample is even more so. The Muramoto and Maldon samples fall somewhere between Lima and the other two.

Arrowhead Mills salt is supplied by the Leslie Salt Company, a large California producer of industrial, agricultural, and food grade salt. The Leslie company does not market any "sea salt" directly but, according to a company spokesperson, it does supply salt that is marketed by others as such. Any domestic sea salt labeled as containing .5 percent magnesium carbonate is probably a product of Leslie, since they add this compound to their salt. According to Leslie, this, and all Leslie salt destined for human consumption, is made from solar-evaporated, washed salt that is 99.4 percent pure sodium chloride. This salt is then further processed. It is "dissolved in pure drinking water. Chemicals are added to this brine to remove remaining traces of calcium and magnesium salts." The "purified" brine is re-evaporated in a series of vacuum pans and the last moisture is removed in a heated rotary filter. The result, Leslie states, is 99.95 percent pure sodium chloride. Our sample tested at 99.56 percent sodium chloride. The 0.227 percent magnesium is added as magnesium carbonate and does not indicate a high level of trace minerals. If your natural foods store sells sea salt in bulk, ask what their source is.

Noburo Muramoto's sea salt is processed by a small-scale method adapted from a traditional Japanese process. Muramoto developed his unique way of processing because his belief is that without good salt, good health cannot be attained. When he could find no salt that he considered suitable, he decided to make it himself. Muramoto located sun-evaporated salt on the west coast of the Baja peninsula in Mexico and now brings the unrefined salt into the U.S. He "cleans" it by re-dissolving, filtering, re-evaporating and crystallizing in enamel pans over gas flames. Muramoto has taught many students his technique over the years.

Various claims are made regarding the mineral content of the salt. Muramoto's only comment is, "My salt is good salt." The claim of "up to 15 percent trace minerals" by one mail-order company is exaggerated. Muramoto's salt tested at 98.19 percent sodium chloride and 0.209 percent magnesium.

It is difficult to get much information about the Lima salt, mostly because it is distributed by a Belgian company.

A booklet (in French) briefly describing Lima products states that its Atlantic salt comes from Brittany. Since the Lima brochure proclaims that "the only valuable salt . . . is that obtained by slow evaporation from the sea and which arrives at our table without having undergone any treatment except drying by air and grinding," one would hope that the salt they sell would fit that description. Lima's salt tested at 97.51 percent sodium chloride and 0.416 magnesium.

Erewhon's salt is from the Mediterranean coast of France. The supplier is Compagni de Salins du Midi, part of Codisel, a large commercial salt interest. The sodium chloride content of our sample of Erewhon salt was 99.63 percent, with 0.002 percent magnesium.

The Maldon salt, from the county of Essex on the southeast coast of England, is evaporated in large pans over fire, rather than by solar evaporation. As the crystals form they are raked from the pans by "salt masters," artisans of long training. The only further processing this salt undergoes is drying. According to the label, the "controlled heating and purifying methods are a family-kept secret" so we were unable to get detailed information, but the level of sodium chloride from our lab report was 98.49 percent. The magnesium level was 0.038 percent.

Why does salt prepared only by evaporation of sea water and subsequent drying not contain all of the minerals that were in the original sea water? And why do some salts contain smaller amounts than others?

In most solar-evaporated salt processes ocean water is not simply contained in a bed until all the water evaporates. Instead it is moved from one pan to another, becoming progressively more concentrated. Calcium carbonate and calcium sulfate crystallize first and settle onto the floor of the pans. Sodium chloride is next. Ideally, these salt crystals are removed from the pans before all of the water evaporates. The remaining "bittern" consists mostly of excess magnesium salts with some calcium chloride, as well as undesirable amounts of heavy metals such as arsenic and lead. The amount of refining at this point determines the percentage of sodium chloride, magnesium, and trace elements in the salt.

The harvested salt is stacked and, still moist, allowed to air-dry. As it sits in the stacks, the remaining bittern, now consisting of elements more soluble than the salt, drains to the bottom of the salt stack, leaving naturally refined sea salt in the upper portion.

The Presence of Minerals

Natural sea salt manufacturers try to distinguish their salt from commercial kinds mainly by claiming greater levels of trace minerals. There are higher levels of minerals in natural sea salt, but they comprise possibly 2 to 3 percent, with trace elements comprising a minute portion of the 2 to 3 percent. This is certainly not close to the 12 to 15 percent often claimed by suppliers, but it is higher than the 0.5 percent or less of commercial salts like Morton's or Leslic's.

How effective these infinitesimal amounts of trace elements are is open to question, yet we can be certain we are receiving some benefit. These minerals are called "trace" for a reason; for them to exist in a natural balance is probably more important than for them to exist in large quantities. (Sea vegetables and wild vegetables are more reliable sources of trace elements than sea salt, and it is not wise to rely solely on salt as a source of trace minerals.) Iodine, a volatile element, is not present in natural sea salt. The dextrose in commercial salt stabilizes the added iodine compound, potassium iodide. Sea vegetables and green vegetables grown in iodine-rich soil are good natural sources of that mineral.

Actually, salt that contains too much magnesium can lead to serious problems. According to some nutritional research, dark grey sea salt, containing high levels of mag-

The Compositions of Sea Salts

Component	Manufacturer				
	Arrowhead Mills	Erewhon	Lima	Maldon	Muramoto
Moisture, %	0.040	0.030	3.620	0.240	0.980
Sodium, %	38.850	39.280	36.980	38.660	38.260
Chlorine, %	60.090	60.420	57.400	59.780	59.350
Magnesium, %	0.227 *	0.002	0.416	0.038	0.209
Calcium, %	0.009	0.020	0.151	0.237	0.176
Sulfur as Sulfate, %	0.021	0.094	1.050	0.690	0.680
Potassium, %	0.007	0.024	0.254	0.036	0.192
Sodium Chloride, % (dry basis)	98.770	99.630	97.510	98.490	98.190

* Magnesium found in Arrowhead Mills salt was also calculated as magnesium carbonate, inasmuch as this was declared on the label. The magnesium calculated as magnesium carbonate is 0.79%.

nesium salts, has been linked to permanent skeletal damage. Salt that is too low in these same salts may contribute to kidney complications. Although there is little hard documentation precisely delineating the composition of salt that is best for enhancing human health, as far as magnesium goes, 2 percent is generally considered to be the highest acceptable level.

The Human Factor

Still another factor to be taken into consideration, perhaps one that natural sea salt suppliers should emphasize more than the issue of trace mineral levels, is how salt is produced and what level of consciousness goes into the manufacturing process.

The Maldon salt works have been in operation at the same location for generations; its artisans are masters of their craft. Similarly, *le paludier* of Brittany works in salt marshes that have been developed over hundreds of years, following with pride in the path of his forebears. Muramoto is not part of an established salt-making community, but his basic technique is rooted in a long Japanese tradition. On the other hand, the salt of Codisel (Erewhon) and Leslie (Arrowhead Mills) is handled not by men and women, but by machinery. In choosing your salt, do you choose to support a milieu that fosters human excellence through mastery of one's craft, one that encourages human labor in necessary tasks? Or do you favor the corporate manufac-

turer, always looking for ways to cut costs through labor-saving devices?

The method of refining the salt most probably plays some part in its overall quality as well. It is not clear how the subtle energies of crystalline minerals are affected by solar drying, kiln-drying, or other means of evaporation, yet these various methods certainly do affect the final product. It is our general opinion that a less industrialized method of processing does produce a more healthful food. This idea is subjective and not confirmed by laboratory analyses; some people, however, are able to detect differences in taste among types of salt. The common consensus is that the less industrially processed salts have a slightly sweeter and less salty taste than those which are more "pure."

Useful as they are in determining levels of nutrients and other measurable factors, it is important not to use laboratory analyses as our only guidelines in making choices about the food we eat. Any competent chemist could reconstruct a crystalline substance that would be virtually indistinguishable from a truly natural salt, but it wouldn't be natural salt. A food is more than the sum product of its nutrients. The place from which it came, the consciousness with which it was harvested and processed, and the means of processing, are all factors that contribute to its quality and healthfulness. Our choices determine not only the well-being of our bodies, but the health of our planet as well.

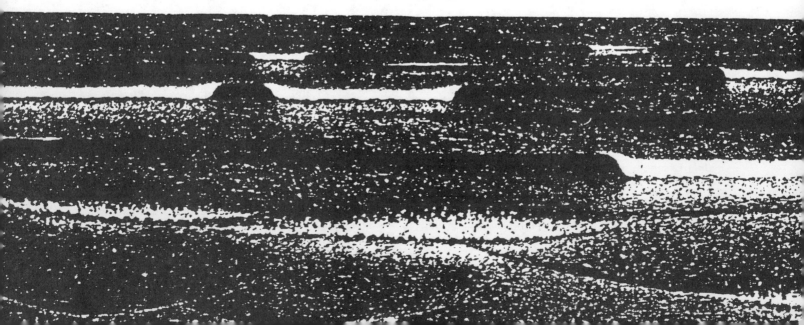

Umeboshi—Japan's Incredible Salt Plum

The tart sour flavor of the umeboshi or dried salt plum is a far cry from the sweet taste that most people expect of dried fruit. The effects of eating it, however, are quite soothing, and one grows accustomed to, and even fond of, its astringent qualities.

The *ume* or Japanese plum (*Prunus salicina*) is a sour green fruit resembling an unripe apricot. It was introduced to Japan at least 1,300 years ago from the Chinese mainland. The plum tree adapted readily to the Japanese soil and climate. Its fruit appealed to Japanese tastes even more than it had to Chinese ones, and it came to be used as a staple food.

Due to the wetness of the climate and the fertility of the soil, the plum tree in Japan has changed distinctively in shape and flavor from the plums currently growing in both mainland China and Taiwan. Japanese plums are plump and round, while Chinese plums are smaller, more egg-shaped, and have a protruding navel. The Japanese plums also contain far more citric acid, which is what makes the umeboshi both sour and medicinally effective.

The fruit matures just before the spring rains begin in mid-June. If left to ripen it will turn a light yellow, but umeboshi—and other plum products such as plum wine, plum candy, and plum concentrate or extract (*bainiku ekisu*)—are always made from green plums.

Umeboshi's origins reach far back into history. Until modern times, it was one of the many foods that was always prepared in the Japanese home. Umeboshi is made from plums, salt, and shiso leaves. In its preparation, freshly picked plums are washed, then packed into vats with crude salt. The salt draws out the juice by osmosis, so that the plums are soon covered by a run-off liquid conventionally called "plum vinegar" or *ume-su*. (Plum vinegar is available in natural foods stores and can be used in place of umeboshi to flavor many dishes. It is not real vinegar, which undergoes fermentation, and it is salty.)

Purple *shiso* leaves are added next. (Shiso, *Iresine herbistii*, is known in America as the beefsteak plant.) The freshly picked leaves are hand-rubbed and rolled to break open the cell structures. When they are placed in the vats, their color is quickly drawn out by the plum vinegar to make a deep red dye. This dye gives the umeboshi its color and contributes a tangy flavor that is compatible with the sourness of the plum. Shiso also contains a natural preservative, perilla-aldehyde, which is known to possess over one thousand times the preserving ability of synthetic preservatives.

In the hottest part of the summer—in mid-July, when the rains end abruptly, the skies clear, and the earth bakes in mid-summer heat—the plums are taken from the vats and laid out in the open to dry. After parching all day, they are returned to the vats to absorb more of the plum vinegar during the night. This cycle is repeated for three or four days.

The umeboshi owes both its flavor and its medicinal effectiveness not to the flesh of the plum but to the plum vinegar. This highly saline citric solution becomes more and more alkaline with age, its originally sharp acidity turning increasingly sour. The soft flesh of the umeboshi, soaked by night and dried again by day, absorbs and captures the essence of the potent brew. Umeboshi's citric acid aids in eliminating lactic acid, a common cause of fatigue, from the body. It alkalizes in digestion, soothing the stomach and strengthening the blood.

In home production the plums are stored for consumption once they have been dried, but modern manufacturers return them to the vats until they are sold. Prior to packaging, they are dried in the sun a final time.

Ume paste (not to be confused with ume extract or concentrate) is made by pitting the umeboshi plum and kneading it into a paste. Though it is equal to the whole plum for flavoring and cooking purposes, the latter is generally preferred for medicinal uses.

Ume extract or *concentrate (bainiku ekisu)* is made by reducing one kilogram (2.2 pounds) of fresh plums to 20 grams (less than 1 ounce) of thick, dark syrup. The concentrate, unlike umeboshi plums or paste, contains no salt. It is generally made into a drink used to relieve acidic conditions—a quarter teaspoon of extract is mixed in a cup of hot liquid. Because it is so concentrated and useful for all kinds of digestive upsets, ume extract is an excellent aid for travellers. It is now available, mixed with another ingredient, in the form of "plum balls."

This description of natural procedures applies to the manufacturing of the umeboshi sold by most natural foods companies. Much of the commercially produced umeboshi, however, is now made with both preservatives and artificial coloring agents.

One umeboshi goes a long way. Its sourness should be savored bit by bit. A piece of umeboshi at the center of a rice ball will keep the rice from spoiling for several days. Ume paste, spread across vegetables in sushi, is a tart and flavorful alternative to vinegar. Blended with oil and vinegar, either the plum or the paste creates a delightfully fresh-tasting salad dressing. When spread over corn on the cob, many people believe that umeboshi tastes even better than butter. *Ume-sho-bancha* ("plum-salt-tea"), a potent and effective remedy that alleviates indigestion, is made by combining one umeboshi (in pieces) and a teaspoon to a tablespoon of shoyu in a cup, then adding hot bancha or kukicha.

As a sour, tart, salty flavoring agent and as a soothing remedy, very few foods can rival the umeboshi. The versatile little plum is truly one of Japan's national treasures.

Plum Ball Master

Tofu hot dogs smothered with sauerkraut, reconstituted tempeh swimming in garlic sauce, soy ice cream in tiny honey-sweetened cones, and carob-covered lecithin candy bars—all the latest in natural convenience foods were served up for sampling at the 1983 National Nutritional Foods Association convention in Denver. To entice retailers to order these wares, manufacturer-exhibitors used the latest in high-tech gimmickry. The real star of the show, however, was a new food fashioned with antique technology. To the delight of a constant crowd of onlookers, ume (Japanese plum) balls were being made on a 100-year-old hand-operated wooden machine by Japanese artisan Shoichi Inagaki.

At work in the Eden Distributors booth, the fifty-six-year-old Inagaki enthralled crowds with his grace, precision, and speed in turning out the tiny black balls. He deftly kneaded a wad of "dough," pressed it through the copper dies of the card-table-sized machine, and sliced the twenty strands as they came through. Minutes later, after a few more deft movements, he had pressed 200 quarter-inch stumps onto a plate. Inagaki then rested another plate on top and, in a final dance-like swirl of motion, rotated it briefly to produce perfectly shaped plum spheres.

It looked effortless and, indeed, Inagaki stood there making plum balls hour after hour. Occasionally he would allow someone in the crowd a turn. Inevitably, the seemingly simple, easy steps would result in a series of misshapen, variously sized objects, bearing little similarity to Inagaki's perfect plum balls.

Ume's history is a long one. The fruit has been recognized as a powerful medicine in China for at least 4,000 years. In its salted and pickled form—umeboshi—its use in Japan goes back at least to the middle of the Heian Era, circa 950 A.D.

Claims for umeboshi's medicinal and nutritional properties are many and varied, and some of them have recently been confirmed by modern science. Among other things, umeboshi is said to be an aid for insomnia, an appetite booster, and a cure for diarrhea, worms, and malaria. The Japanese even have a saying that can be roughly translated as "An umeboshi a day keeps the doctor away."

It wasn't until the beginning of the 19th century that an even more useful form of the fruit—ume extract or concentrate (bainiku ekisu)—was first developed. Ume concentrate was first widely used in late 19th-century Japan because of its ability to combat dysentery. By the mid-1920s ume extract was being produced commercially.

The final development—a solid, concentrated form of ume—did not come until the 1960s, when ume concentrate was mixed with white rice flour to form small dry rectangles called plum granules.

It was at this point that Inagaki entered the scene. With his forty years of experience in making herbal medicines, he thought he could improve upon the hard-to-swallow granules. He also searched for a more healthful alternative to white rice flour. In 1977, he finally developed the combination he was looking for—50 percent ume and 50 percent jinenjo, a mountain potato known for its properties as a digestive aid. Adapting the 100-year-old herb granulating machine, he began to practice turning out the new plum balls. It took him four years to perfect his technique. Today, no one else in the world makes plum balls by hand.

Of course, the plum balls exported by the Muso Co. in Japan and distributed in the U.S. by Eden Foods are now made by machines—which were designed after consultation with Inagaki. As was demonstrated at the NNFA show, artistry and tradition still have as important a place as innovation in the natural foods business.

The Three Flavors of Japanese Cuisine

Dashi, Shoyu, and Mirin Are the Keys to This Ancient Culinary Tradition

Everyone knows the difference between food that is made and presented with care and that which is thrown together without much consideration. When care is taken to use only the freshest ingredients and to harmonize colors and textures, the cook is well on the way to creating a memorable experience. If seasonings are also harmoniously blended, not dominating the foods but serving to enhance natural flavors, a meal becomes deeply satisfying. Perhaps nowhere is the awareness of this harmony more highly developed than in Japan.

Dashi (stock), *shoyu* (Japanese soy sauce), and *mirin* (Japanese sweet rice cooking wine)—the omnipresent ingredients that provide the characteristic flavor of Japanese cuisine—are often called the three tastes of old Japan. Understanding how the Japanese skillfully blend these basic seasonings takes much of the mystery out of their culinary tradition and provides a valuable lesson in the marriage of flavors.

Properly combined, mirin's mild sweetness mellows shoyu's savory saltiness. Dashi rounds out both of them, to create a balanced, satisfying dish. Combined in various proportions, dashi, shoyu, and mirin are the bases of delicate clear soups, hearty noodle broths, and savory dips and sauces. These delicious seasonings, which by no means must be limited to Japanese fare, can be used to enhance all styles of cooking.

Ever since shoyu found its way into the royal kitchens of Louis XIV of France in the 17th century, it has gained international recognition as a versatile and delicious seasoning. High in glutamic acid, a natural form of monosodium glutamate (MSG), shoyu is an excellent flavor enhancer. It is used for marinating and pickling, as well as in soups, broths, and sauces, and in simmered or sauteed dishes.

High quality traditional shoyu accounts for less than 1 percent of Japan's shoyu production. Over 99 percent is made from defatted soybeans, fermented at elevated temperatures for 3–6 months, and often bottled with additives. When shopping for traditional shoyu read labels carefully. Look for a product that has been aged naturally for one to two years and that is composed only of wheat, soybeans, sea salt, and water. The best place to shop for high-quality shoyu is in natural foods stores. Asian markets usually sell only commercial soy sauces and Chinese soy sauce, which is a different, saltier product.

Shoyu should be added during the last few minutes of cooking. In longer cooking, its complex flavor and delicate bouquet are lost. When using shoyu to season soups or sauces, I often get the best results by adding a little sea salt early in the cooking to deepen the flavor of the ingredients, then adding shoyu to taste shortly before serving. Though tamari, a related seasoning that contains no wheat, can generally be substituted for shoyu, its cooking qualities are somewhat different. Tamari can be added early on in the cooking since its flavor is not volatile (see "What Is Real Tamari?" on page 158).

Mirin, the perfect complement to shoyu, is indispensable in Oriental cooking. Mirin was the traditional sweetening agent long before the arrival of white sugar. It is still commonly used in Japan to provide a balance for shoyu and other salty seasonings and to enhance the flavor of vinegared dishes. Before discovering mirin I usually seasoned soups, gravies, and stir-frys with only shoyu or miso, with the result that they usually tasted either overly salty or a little flat. While living in Japan I experienced the delicious difference that the addition of a small amount of mirin makes. Mirin's mild sweetness rounds out the flavor of many dishes, providing a satisfying, balanced taste and reducing the craving for strong sweets.

Though this sweet, golden liquid is one of Japan's most valued seasonings, in the U.S. today authentic natural mirin is as scarce and costly as it is delicious. Many brands of mirin, especially those sold in Oriental markets, are not naturally brewed and are sweetened with sugar or corn syrup. The sweetness of naturally made mirin is derived only from sweet rice and rice koji. When shopping for mirin, read labels carefully to see whether it was naturally fermented and check for purity of ingredients (sweet rice, rice koji, and water are the only ingredients in authentic mirin).

A related product, known as *aji no haha* in Japan, is sometimes marketed under the name "mirin" in this country. Though somewhat different in flavor, high-quality

aji no haha "mirin" can be used in place of authentic mirin with fine results. To determine quality, check the list of ingredients—the best will contain only rice, rice koji, water, and sea salt. The rice koji may or may not be listed.

If you are not familiar with mirin, first try some of the recipes below. As you gain experience you will find uses for mirin in all styles of cooking. It is excellent in marinades, vinaigrettes, sauces, noodle broths, simmered vegetable or fish dishes; with sauteed vegetables or fried noodles; and in dips for tempura or sushi. The process of cooking evaporates mirin's 13–14 percent alcohol content quickly, leaving only its sweet essence.

Dashi forms the foundation of Japanese cuisine. It adds subtle depth and delicate fragrance to many traditional dishes. Dashi appears simple, but it should be made carefully since the flavor and quality of the stock help to determine the taste of the finished dish.

Three Flavors of Dashi

Kombu Dashi

A mild, flavor-enhancing stock for soups, stews, sauces, simmered foods and noodle broths, kombu dashi can be quickly prepared with only kombu and water.

6-inch piece kombu
4–6 cups water

Wipe a six-inch piece of dried kombu lightly with a clean, damp cloth. (Do not rinse kombu—the whitish powder on the surface provides much of the flavor.) Place kombu and 4–6 cups water in saucepan. Bring just to a simmer, uncovered, over medium heat; then immediately remove kombu. This technique gives the most delicate and delicious results. Long boiling releases some strong, unpleasant-tasting compounds that can be overpowering in a simple vegetable soup or broth. Reserve the kombu—it can be cooked with beans or vegetables or reused to make stock. If reusing kombu to make stock, bring to a boil, then lower heat and simmer for 10–20 minutes. Lightly scoring the kombu before heating will help release the amino acid responsible for its flavor-intensifying effect.

Kombu-Shiitake Dashi

Traditionally, when a richer, heartier fla-

vor is desired, dried *shiitake* (Japanese forest mushrooms) are added.

3–5 shiitake mushrooms
6-inch piece kombu
4–6 cups water

Soak shiitake in 4–6 cups water for at least 3 hours. Then drain mushrooms, reserving the water. Cut off and discard stems. Slice caps. Place water, caps, and 6-inch piece of kombu in a saucepan and bring to a boil. Remove kombu. Add any other ingredients and continue to cook until tender.

If you do not wish to add the mushrooms themselves to the stock, but wish to utilize their flavor, the soaking time can be shortened to 15–20 minutes. Place the shiitake, the water from soaking them, and a piece of kombu in a pot and bring to a boil. Remove kombu. Simmer shiitake for 10–15 minutes, then remove them and reserve for use in another dish.

Kombu-Bonito Dashi

In Japan a rich dashi is most commonly made with kombu and dried bonito (*katsuo bushi*). Dried bonito is the product of a unique process that involves steaming, sun-drying, and woodsmoking the fish fillets, then allowing them to ferment for

about 3 months. When mature, the dried fillets look and feel like petrified wood and will maintain their quality indefinitely if kept cool and dry.

The bonito fillets are shaved into flakes on a bonito shaver (*katsuo kesuriki*). You can't beat the flavor of stock made with freshly shaved bonito. Bonito fillets and shavers are available in some Oriental supermarkets and occasionally in large natural foods stores. However, bonito flakes also come prepackaged in small, convenient cellophane envelopes that preserve their freshness well. These single-serving packets of shaved bonito are preferable to large bags or boxes, in which the flakes more rapidly lose their flavor and quality.

This versatile stock for various kinds of soups, noodle broths, dips, and simmered root vegetable dishes can be made in a matter of minutes.

6-inch piece kombu
4–6 cups water
1/4 cup bonito flakes

Follow the directions for Kombu Dashi. As soon as you remove the kombu, add about 1/4 cup freshly shaved or packaged bonito flakes and remove from heat. Let stock rest for 1–2 minutes, then strain it to remove flakes. Press all liquid from flakes into stock and discard flakes.

12. COOKING INGREDIENTS

Finding the right staples is often only the first step for the natural foods store shopper. Knowing about the wide range of high-quality cooking ingredients that are available is equally important. Some of these products, such as most of the oils and, among the sweeteners, honey, are similar to products you've probably been buying in the supermarket. Others, such as the innovative sweeteners rice syrup and amasake, and the thickeners kuzu and arrowroot, may be new and unusual to most natural foods store shoppers.

In the following pages, we'll offer some helpful hints on how to choose, use, and store cooking oils, after taking a look at the various types of oils being produced and how they differ in type and degree of processing. We'll also take a quick look at kuzu and arrowroot, those versatile vegetable starches that are the secret to smooth and creamy soups, stews, and puddings. Finally, we'll tackle the thorny issue of what exactly a "natural sweetener" is, while describing where and how we get honey, maple syrup, barley malt, rice syrup, amasake, and fruit juice sweeteners.

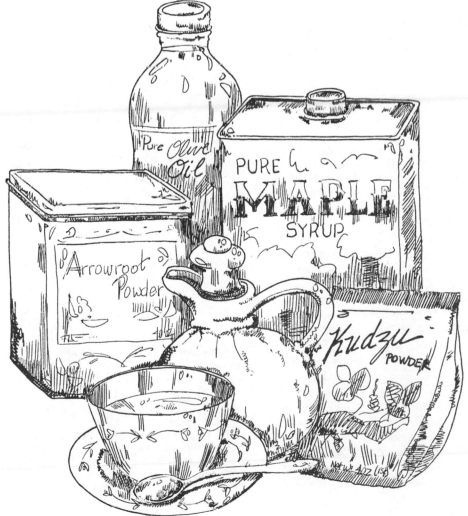

A Guide to Vegetable Oils

Vegetable oils play an important role in natural foods cuisines. Light and flavorful, they are indispensable for sauteing, baking, and frying, and are a favorite ingredient of salad dressings, spreads, and dips. Vegetable oils contribute taste, palatability, versatility, and nutrients, including essential fatty acids, vitamins A and E, and lecithin (a fat-like compound which is able to dissolve cholesterol in the body).

Vegetable oils are almost 100 percent fat, nature's most concentrated source of energy. Because fats provide over twice the caloric energy of proteins and carbohydrates, inhabitants of cold climates tend to eat more of them to generate greater warmth. They also help to create a feeling of satiety. Excess calories are stored as body fat, which holds vital organs in place, protecting them from the shocks of normal activity, and also insulates the body from external temperature changes.

The Composition of Fats and Oils

Fats and oils are composed of fatty acids, which are linear chains of carbon atoms (see illustration). Each carbon atom is attached to another carbon atom and in addition has the capacity to attract two hydrogen atoms to it. When almost all the positions for the hydrogen atoms are filled, the fatty acid is said to be "saturated." When there are many spaces that do not have hydrogen atoms, the fat is called "polyunsaturated." (Oxygen is then free to enter these spaces instead of hydrogen; this oxidation is the major cause of rancidity in vegetable oils.) "Monounsaturated" fatty acids have only a few spaces unfilled with hydrogen atoms. *Hydrogenation* is the process of bubbling hydrogen into polyunsaturated oils, so that the spaces for hydrogen atoms are filled. This makes the oils become saturated and solid at room temperature. Hydrogenation prevents separation of the oil (as in peanut butter) and extends shelf life, but it is a chemical means of altering the structure of a fatty acid. Margarines, commercial peanut butter, the palm oil in some carob candies, and shortening are all hydrogenated.

Animals store their fats in saturated chains, while plants generally contain mono- and polyunsaturated chains. The melting point of a fat is directly related to the degree of saturation as well as to the length of the chain. Highly saturated fats are solid at room temperature and are generally referred to as "fats," while unsaturated fats are liquid at room temperature and are called "oils." Coconut and palm oils are two exceptions: although considered "oils," they are highly saturated and remain solid at room temperature. Linoleic acid, the most important fatty acid, is found abundantly in plants. The percentage of linoleic acid is used as an indicator of the degree of unsaturation of a fat, with more linoleic acid generally denoting greater unsaturation.

Saturated and Unsaturated Fats

A **saturated** fatty acid is composed of a carbon (C) chain completely saturated with hydrogen (H) atoms:

Monounsaturated fatty acids are made of a carbon chain with one double bond, and thus have room for more hydrogen atoms:

Polyunsaturated fatty acids are similar, except there are two or more double bonds and therefore room for many hydrogen atoms:

Risks and Benefits

Linoleic acid and the other polyunsaturated fatty acids are essential for the maintenance of human health though the body cannot manufacture them. Essential fatty acids are found in high concentrations in whole grains, beans, seeds, and in lesser but significant quantities in some animal foods, especially fish. While polyunsaturated fatty acids are essential, there is no dietary need for saturated or monounsaturated fatty acids. Even the need for polyunsaturates is very small and may be satisfied by two or three teaspoons of unrefined oil a day.

Vegetable oils began to be heavily promoted during the mid-1970s, when it was discovered that a high blood cholesterol level was linked to heart disease. Meat and dairy foods, themselves high in both cholesterol and saturated fats, were seen as culprits. At the same time it was suggested that vegetable oils, containing mainly polyunsaturates, actually lowered blood serum cholesterol levels. A huge marketing push for polyunsaturated oils began and the most highly unsaturated, safflower, gained a reputation as the best oil. Sales soared, for here, it seemed, was a way to eat fat and get healthier at the same time.

However, studies have shown that eating a large amount of polyunsaturated safflower oil causes the blood's *triglyceride* level to rise higher and remain higher longer than does an equal amount of saturated fat. (Fatty acids are normally linked to the alcohol glycerol to form a triglyceride.) In addition, polyunsaturated oils are prone to oxidation, which can occur through high heat (as in deep-frying) as well as through exposure to air and light. It is now believed that eating oxidized oil—or obviously rancid oil—in any quantity can lead to serious health problems.

Nevertheless, there are several reasons to prefer unrefined vegetable oils over animal fats. In addition to providing essential fatty acids, vegetable oils contain fewer pesticide and pollution residues than animal fats. These residues tend to become concentrated in the fat tissues of plants and animals, becoming more concentrated further up the food chain. Thus, animal fats have more than milk and dairy fats, which have more than vegetable oils, which have more than whole fruits and vegetables.

The benefits of using vegetable oils far outweigh their dangers for those on a grain/vegetable diet. For the most part, only those persons who have had a long history of high fat consumption or whose present diet is still high in fat need to avoid vegetable oil. Used appropriately and in the correct proportion, vegetable oils are important for year-round maintenance of health.

Manufacture

All vegetable oils are derived from the seeds or fruits of flowering plants. Oils were originally obtained by roasting and crushing the seeds, allowing the oil to rise to the top of the mash. But this method does not extract all of the oil; pressing began to be utilized in order to obtain more. The oil removed by pressing is rich and cloudy, containing valuable nutrients such as chlorophyll, lecithin, vitamin E, carotenoids (provitamin A), and minerals. Oil-rich seeds such as peanuts, sesame, and sunflower yield their oils under relatively low heat and pressure and further processing is unnecessary. Olive oil does not require any heat at all.

Most commercial oils are so highly refined that their vitamin E, lecithin, and other nutrients are removed. (The amount of vitamin E the body needs is directly proportional to the amount of polyunsaturates it consumes. Eating polyunsaturated oil with its vitamin E removed creates a built-in vitamin E deficiency.) Vegetable oil production is a big business. The oils found even in natural foods stores are processed by large companies, which often crush over half a million pounds of seeds a day. But oil produced by a large company is not necessarily refined; it can be sold to the distributor after undergoing only pressing, filtering, and bottling. These rich, cloudy oils retain the color, aroma, flavor, and nutritional value which natural oils should have.

Extraction

Today, oils are extracted by two methods: pressure and chemical solvents. Pressing is normally done by an expeller press, a heavy, steel, slotted barrel with a large single screw shaft that presses the seeds against the walls. The walls retain the pulp, but allow the oil to pass through. In order to remove as much oil as possible, some manufacturers use high pressure (up to fifteen tons per square inch); this method creates an excessive heat of 300°F or more, which darkens the oil and denatures its protein. To prevent overheating, the press may be adjusted for lower pressure. Temperatures still seldom fall below 140° to 160°F (which makes the term "cold-pressed" meaningless) but the oil loses little of its flavor or nutrition. Unfortunately, the greater quantities of oil yielded by the higher pressure methods lead many producers to prefer them; lower pressure methods leave 12 to 15 percent of the oil in the seed mash.

Hexane is the most common chemical used in solvent-extraction. A highly volatile, flammable, and toxic petroleum derivative, hexane flows through toasted and flaked seed meal to dissolve and extract all but $1/2$ to 1 percent of the oil. This oil/solvent mixture reaches temperatures of about 135°F during extraction. In order to evaporate the solvent from the oil, it is heated to 250° to 300°F. Solvent-extraction is efficient, but when the solvent is removed, the natural flavors of the oil are also removed. In addition, some of the solvent residue may remain in the oil.

The prepress-solvent method is most commonly used in commercial oil extraction. Oil seeds are prepressed at lower pressure and temperature, then the remaining oil in the mash is solvent-extracted and the two oils are combined. In this way producers are able to extract over 99 percent of the oil, while still maintaining flavor components.

Refined and Unrefined Oils

To understand how unrefined oils differ from refined commercial ones, an examination of the production processes is essential.

Raw seeds arrive at the refinery and are cleaned to remove stems, stones, and other foreign material. The seeds are then shelled or hulled to make the oil-bearing part more accessible. These first two steps are accomplished by simple mechanical means—screens, blowers, vibrating tables, and rollers.

The seeds are next cooked in steam-jacketed kettles. Cooking helps to break down plant tissue, enabling the seed to yield its oil more readily. The time and temperature used depend on the type of seed, and can range from a few minutes at 110° F to several hours at over 250° F.

The cooked seeds are then sent to the expeller where they are pressed at 140° to 160° F. At this point the seed has undergone only cleaning, hulling, cooking, and pressing. This oil, called "prepressed," is the natural product we wish to obtain. It is filtered to remove any seed meal and sent to the bottlers. On the bottle it will be labelled "expeller-pressed" or "mechanically pressed," and "unrefined." Oil that is not to be sold as prepressed, together with its oil cake residue, is sent along to be solvent-extracted.

Both prepress and solvent-extracted oils or a combination of both can correctly be called "crude" or "unrefined" oil. Cleaning, cooking, pressing, and solvent-extraction are not considered part of the refining process but rather belong to the extraction process.

The words "cold-pressed," contrary to popular belief, do not mean that the oil has been processed by the low temperature and pressure method. The term does not describe how or at what temperature the oil was extracted and may be found on oils that have been chemically extracted, bleached, and deodorized. Reputable suppliers refuse to use the term on their labels. Though it is a natural product, prepressed oil is not "cold-pressed," because of the cooking and pressing temperatures it undergoes. Olive oil is the only oil that can truly be cold-pressed.

Refined Oils

Refining improves shelf life while simultaneously removing color, taste, and odor, producing the bland product many consumers have been conditioned to prefer. In contrast to the simple extraction of natural oils, this process consists of several different operations, including degumming, the removal of fatty acids, bleaching, and deodorization.

The oil is first degummed. This means it is mixed with hot water (120° F) to separate gummy substances which are then centrifuged out. The lecithin in natural oils, which causes them to smoke at high temperatures, is one of the substances removed. Degumming is the source of most commercial lecithin.

The next step—the one the term "refining" actually refers to—is the removal of fatty acids. The oil is washed in a highly alkaline caustic solution containing lye or sodium carbonate to remove the free fatty acids, which can cause rancidity. Much of the beneficial vitamin E that acts as a natural antioxidant, helping to *prevent* rancidity, is also removed by this process; synthetic antioxidants such as BHA, BHT, and propyl gallate are subsequently added. Heated to 140° to 160° F, this solution neutralizes the free fatty acids to form soaps, which are centrifuged out. These soaps are the source of the vegetable glycerines used in many natural cosmetics.

Bleaching follows refining and consists of mixing oil with bleaching clay or activated charcoal ("activated" indicates that the charcoal has been treated with sulfuric or hydrochloric acid to make it more absorbent). This mixture is then agitated under a vacuum for about twenty minutes at 180° to 220° F and filtered. Bleaching removes pigments and any soap left from the refining process.

In the deodorization process, steam is blown through the oil under a high vacuum for ten to twelve hours. Temperatures may reach 450° to 470° F. Any remaining odor, flavor, or pigment is removed, leaving a bland finished product that tastes the same no matter what source it originally came from. The defoaming agent methyl silicone is sometimes added. Since refining is pretty much an all-or-nothing process, oils that are refined are usually also degummed, bleached, and deodorized.

Additional Processes

Oils to be used in refrigerated or specialty products are further processed. "Winterization" is the process of chilling the oil for two to three days, then pressing to remove the cloudy matter that forms. This oil remains clear under refrigeration and is used for salad oils and in mayonnaise where normal oils would solidify under refrigeration and break the emulsion. Winterizing can also be done more quickly with the use of solvents.

Vegetable oil that needs to remain solid at room temperature—margarine, for instance—is hydrogenated. Hydrogen gas is bubbled through the oil as it is heated to several hundred degrees. The oil is then agitated in the presence of a catalyst, usually activated nickel, which is subsequently removed by bleaching clay and filtering aids. This process saturates the fatty acids, making the oil harder. The longer oil is hydrogenated, the more saturated it becomes, which increases its melting point. Most oils are saturated to melt at around 98° F. The margarine container that says "high in polyunsaturates" neglects to mention the oil has been hydrogenated.

Hydrogenated oil keeps margarine hard and prevents nut butters from separating. Because it spoils less quickly than unsaturated oils, it is used in fried foods such as nut mixes, chips, and puffs to increase shelf life.

Following are seven oils commonly found in the natural foods store, with information regarding their derivation, processing, and amount of saturation. A few suggestions on how to use these versatile natural oils are offered. Palm kernel oil and coconut oil, while not appropriate for natural foods cooking, do occur in products such as candies and cosmetics, and are therefore included. In addition, vegetable oil margarine is discussed. The information concerning its processing is intended to help the consumer in weighing the pros and cons of using it.

Coconut Oil

Coconut oil is colorless and almost tasteless. It contains only 3 percent linoleic acid and is 91 percent saturated. It is twice as saturated as lard (animal fat), which has only 39 to 40 percent saturated acids. This high degree of saturation keeps coconut oil hard at temperatures below 73° to 70° F but gives it extreme stability in frying and storage. However, it is used mostly in cosmetics and confections rather than in food preparation. Because of its narrow melting range it goes from solid to liquid without getting soft in-between, which adds brittleness to the confections in which it is used.

Coconut oil comes from the nut of the coconut palm, which grows wild and on plantations on the southwest coasts of North America and in the Pacific Islands. Malaysia, Indonesia, and the Philippines are the principal producers. Each palm yields 50 to 70 fruits per year. These are cracked and dried. The coconut meat, which is called copra, contains 65 to 70 percent fat. Copra can be dried in the sun, over fires, or in hot air dryers (which give the best quality). The oil is obtained by pressing; the residue is chopped up and pressed again or solvent-extracted.

Corn Oil

Corn oil, one of the most popular oils, has long been used in the United States. Natural corn oil's rich corn flavor and winey aroma add a buttery flavor to foods. Corn oil is not suitable for deep-frying since it foams easily, but it is delightful in baking, salads, sauteing and, of course, for popcorn.

Many industries use corn as a source of starch for glucose manufacturing, cornstarch, and cereal production. The oil is derived from the germ, which is separated from the kernel by steaming and mechanical action, then pressed. Most corn oil on the market is this product, but some is pressed from the whole corn kernel, and includes oil found directly under the hull. The oil under the hull, corn gluten oil, is dark red and has a strong odor like that of popcorn. Whole kernel oil is dark orange, while corn germ oil is light yellow. Although corn oil is highly unsaturated (90 percent) and high in linoleic acid (59 percent), it is very stable due to its relatively high vitamin E content, which acts to prevent oxidation.

Olive Oil

Olive oil is unique in that it is the only oil normally available that can legitimately be considered cold-pressed. The oil of the Mediterranean, it is produced almost exclusively from the fruit of olive trees grown in that area. The best oil comes from olives that are handpicked just before they are fully ripe. Other harvesting is done by shaking the trees so that the fruit falls on cloths spread out below. However, this causes bruising and as a result the flavor begins to degrade before the olives are pressed. Because olive oil comes from the soft, fleshy pulp of the fruit rather than the seed or nut, it needs no precooking or high pressure extraction.

Olives are crushed in a mill which breaks the pulp but not the pits. The first extraction is a simple, gentle pressing that doesn't heat the oil much above room temperature. The oil is then separated from the olive water either by settling (where it floats and is poured off) or by centrifuging. Oil obtained from this first pressing receives no further treatment other than filtering to remove pulp. This oil is labelled "virgin olive oil" and is the only oil that can be labelled as such.

Virgin olive oil comes in three grades: "Extra virgin" has perfect flavor and aroma; "fine virgin" has the same flavor as "extra" but a high acidity; "plain virgin" oil, the grade most often sold in the U.S., is imperfect in flavor and has the highest acidity. Olive oil labelled "pure" is still 100 percent olive oil, but not virgin. Pure grades are extracted from second pressings, which require higher temperatures, pressure, and hot water treatments or solvent-extraction. Pure grades are usually blended with virgin oil (5 to 20 percent) for better flavor. Olive oil varies according to the season of the harvest and type of olive used. The Greeks use a big, dark olive, producing a more acidic oil, rich and dark green in color. Other suppliers such as Algeria, Italy, and California use a light green olive having lower acidity, to make a pale yellow or yellow-green oil.

Pure olive oil has excellent stability and can sometimes be stored without refrigeration for over a year, but virgin oils degrade more quickly. Most of the unsaturates in olive oil are in the form of monounsaturated oleic acid, instead of the lighter polyunsaturate linoleic, which amounts to only 15 percent. This results in a heavier and more fatty oil. This fattiness allows the oil to be burned as an illuminant and lower grades to be used in fine soaps and cosmetics. Virgin olive oils are excellent uncooked to dress a salad; also, their inimitable fragrance and taste enhance any lightly pan-fried dish. Most natural foods stores sell both pure and virgin oils.

Palm Kernel Oil

Palm kernel oil is often seen as an ingredient in carob confections and other candies. This oil is produced from the kernels of the oil palm, which is grown mainly along the west coast of central Africa. The pulp and fiber around the fruit are removed to expose the kernel, which is sent to Europe for processing. The kernels are cracked to remove the nut, which is pressed and/or solvent extracted (usually both). Its oil is very similar to coconut oil, being 85 percent saturated and containing only 2 percent linoleic acid. The resulting hardness at room temperature is what makes carob candies possible. Since their main ingredient is palm kernel oil, carob candies are mostly saturated fat.

Peanut Oil

Peanut oil is a byproduct of the peanut industry, the poorer nuts being pressed or solvent-extracted for oil. Natural peanut oil is fairly high in saturated fat, about 20 percent, while containing only 30 percent linoleic acid. When used in making natural potato and corn chips, these characteristics give it better stability and longer shelf life than natural safflower oil, but not as good as the refined safflower oil. Peanut oil is suitable for use in deep-frying, sauteing, or making peanut butter cookies.

Safflower Oil

Safflower oil is the most popular vegetable oil among natural foods shoppers, although it is probably the least flavorful of the natural oils. This absence of a strong taste (it has only a slight nutty flavor) may even be one reason underlying its popularity, especially among consumers who are used to bland commercial oils.

The safflower is not known in its wild state, but is cultivated in India, Egypt, and North America, thriving in arid and semi-arid climates on land not suitable for other crops. With its spiny leaves, the plant resembles a thistle, though it belongs to the sunflower family and yields a similar oil. In the U.S. safflower is grown in California, Arizona, and other parts of the Southwest.

Safflower oil probably has the highest percentage of unsaturated fats of all the oils (94 percent) and is highest in linoleic acid (78 percent). Since unsaturated fats become rancid more quickly than saturated fats due to oxidation, one drawback of high unsaturation is short shelf life. Safflower oil is best stored in the refrigerator to retard rancidity. It can be used for deep-frying, though its flavor does not remain stable under deep-frying temperatures. Natural potato or corn chips contain up to 50 percent oil, and it is usually safflower. Because unrefined safflower oil oxidizes quickly in frying, consumers and manufacturers generally prefer refined oil (peanut oil is sometimes used as an alternative). If a processed natural food contains oil, it is usually safflower mainly because it is the least expensive.

Sesame Oil

Sesame oil is one of the oldest of oils. First used in China over 5,000 years ago, it was important for cosmetics and ink as well as for food. Two basic types of sesame oil are available: light and dark. The dark oil, made from seeds that have been roasted prior to pressing, has a toasted, smoky flavor and is commonly used in Chinese cuisine. The light oil is mild and nutty tasting, suitable for a wide variety of uses. Although it is 87 percent unsaturated, sesame oil contains only 42 percent linoleic acid. This factor and other components give sesame oil excellent stability and resistance to oxidation. It is a good choice for deep-frying, salads, and sauteing. Sesame oil production in the U.S. is not very large, since this oil does not have many commercial uses. Most of the seeds are imported from Central America and pressed in small amounts. These factors make sesame oil the most expensive of the natural oils, with the possible exception of rare brands of olive oil.

Soybean Oil

Soybean oil was almost unknown in the U.S. until the time of World War II, when the U.S. was unable to obtain vegetable oils from the Orient. The United States then began to produce them on its own and is now the largest exporter of soybean oil in the world.

Soybeans have a low oil content (16 to 18 percent), so that the commercially produced oils are usually solvent-extracted. Refined soybean oil is also usually winterized and partially hydrogenated. Unrefined, mechanically pressed soy oil is dark yellow, having a green tinge due to its chlorophyll content. As it is high in linoleic acid, which comprises about 50 percent, it is susceptible to oxidation. Soybean oil's flavor is the strongest of all the vegetable oils; thus, its main use is in baking where the taste is not so apparent.

Sunflower Oil

Sunflower oil, one of the few oils that can be produced in cold climates, is made in Canada. Its production is also of great commercial importance in Russia. In the southern United States, oil-bearing seeds such as sunflower are being planted in areas with diminishing cotton yields. Many varieties of sunflower are suitable for producing oil, the characteristics of which vary greatly with the conditions of the plant's growth. For some purposes southern sunflower oil must be winterized, while northern oils do not require this process. In degree of unsaturation sunflower oil is similar to safflower, being 92 percent unsaturated with 72 percent linoleic acid. Its flavor is a little stronger but pleasant. Sunflower oil also has better resistance to oxidation than safflower oil. As sunflower is the only oil besides corn that is indigenous to North America, it deserves attention.

Vegetable Oil Margarine

Another vegetable oil product in the health food industry is 100 percent vegetable oil margarine. Vegetable oil margarines became more popular when saturated animal fats in butter were implicated in high levels of cholesterol in the body. By using vegetable oils high in polyunsaturates, companies believe they can produce a product that will reduce the risk of heart disease or at least be suitable for vegetarians. Whether or not this is true is highly debatable. One reason is that polyunsaturated oils must be hydrogenated to remain solid at room temperature. Now research is leading many to believe that hydrogenated polyunsaturated fats are just as unhealthful as saturated animal fats and in some ways may be even more so. Hydrogenated oil has abnormal essential fatty acids from which the body derives no benefits and which in fact prevent the use of normal essential fatty acids.

By law all margarines must contain at least 80 percent fat or oil. Natural oils are not suitable for margarine production, which requires a refined, bleached, and deodor-ized oil having little color or taste. Depending on the consistency desired, 18 to 40 percent of this oil is hydrogenated. The actual polyunsaturated content of margarines can range below 35 percent. Lecithin is added to margarines for emulsification and to stop their splattering when used in cooking. Although lecithin is a natural component of vegetable oils and important for health, the commercial lecithin in margarine is a byproduct of the degumming process in refining oil. Commercial lecithin is further processed and refined, usually hexane-extracted and purified, yielding only 6 pounds of lecithin out of 2,000 pounds of soybeans. All margarines are fortified with vitamin A and almost always have coloring added, usually carotene. They also usually have salt added for taste; over 2 percent if no preservatives are used. The salt itself must be free of the trace metals copper and iron, which make fats susceptible to rancidity, so a purified salt is used.

How to Use, Choose, and Store Cooking Oils

Throughout history almost every oil-bearing seed, nut, and fruit has been used for oil production, but until recently few societies have been faced with the dilemma of which oil to choose. Most were limited to whichever one they happened to be able to produce. In Europe oil was obtained from poppy seeds, in China from cotton seeds and sesame seeds, and in Africa from the palm. India had coconut oil, Egypt radish seed oil, and the Middle East almond and sesame oils. In Central America cocoa butter was the staple. Mediterranean countries, of course, were (and are) famed for their olive oils.

A surplus of oil made the most valued oils available for commerce. Olive and sesame were traded and treasured throughout the Old World and remain popular to this day. But tastes and values change and new oils, like the highly refined ones of industrialized countries, have been developed to meet them.

The use of a natural oil is one of the most practical and efficient ways to achieve variety and dynamics in cooking. In a grain/vegetable diet based on seasonal and locally available foods, choices are sometimes limited and little can be done to make adjustments, even though weather and personal activity may vary greatly and affect the needs of the individual. But by a thoughtful use of oil, a basic diet can be adjusted to help maintain health under a wide variety of conditions and activities.

Vegetable oils are almost 100 percent fat. Since fats contain twice the calories of carbohydrates, cooking with oil imparts a strengthening quality to food, rendering a simple dish more hearty. Oil is also a source of warmth during the colder months. In the winter, stir-fried vegetables and pan-fried dishes help fuel inner fires. In the warmer seasons, raw oil has a refreshing effect. It subtly flavors salads and low-fat dishes while replenishing the body's natural stores of oil, which may be depleted as a result of exposure to sun, wind, and water.

In all seasons, simply brushing the pan with oil and sauteing over a low-to-medium flame enhances the flavors of vegetables, tempeh, tofu, noodles, and grains. This requires only a small amount of oil. To continue cooking, add water, cover the pot, and simmer until the water is absorbed and the foods are cooked.

Choosing from among the vegetable oils that are available requires decisions and judgments. The accompanying table, ranking oils and fats by their degree of saturation, can be helpful in making these choices. (See next page.)

The degree of saturation is directly related to an oil's stability. The more unsatu-rated an oil, the more it is prone to oxidation and rancidity. Polyunsaturated oils have been viewed as healthful alternatives to highly saturated animal fats, but their tendency to oxidize can be a drawback. Highly unsaturated oils are at the top of the table and the more saturated are toward the bottom. The iodine value has nothing to do with iodine in the oil but rather represents the relative degree of saturation: saturation is judged by the number of grams of iodine which can be absorbed by 100 grams of the oil; the more saturated an oil is, the more full its fatty acid chains and the less iodine it will absorb. Unsaturated oils have a lot of room in their fatty acid chains to absorb iodine and therefore have a high iodine number. Thus, a high number means light and unsaturated and a low number means heavy and saturated.

The oils are further grouped into drying and non-drying oils. Drying oils are highly unsaturated and when exposed to air absorb oxygen quickly, readily *polymerizing* to form layers of skin or film.

In polymerization, the fatty acid chains link together and the structure of the fat molecule is altered. Overheating oils—above 390° to 480° F—also results in polymerization. Since oil is heated to 375°F and above for deep-frying, it may be best to use this method of cooking infrequently.

One representative of a natural foods company stated that reusing oil for deep-frying—oil that has undergone oxidation from the high heat—"is like drinking peroxide."

The table at right shows other characteristics of oils. Semi-drying ones are food grade oils. They are light and closer to the drying oils in nature than to the non-drying oils. The non-drying oils are closer in nature to animal fats, being highly saturated and heavy. Animal fats are heavy and dense, but certain vegetable fats have a similar degree of saturation, and coconut oil is the most saturated. These heavy, highly saturated vegetable fats should be avoided. For daily use it is best to eliminate those oils at both ends of the table and concentrate on the more central oils, considering safflower as the upper limit and olive oil as the lower end of acceptability.

The table is useful only as a general guide; it would be unwise to base a choice solely on its information. The fatty acid composition of oils is as changeable as the weather. In fact, the weather and temperature during the period of seed maturation is one determinant of fat composition. The same oil will be more unsaturated in cool years and climates and more saturated in hot years and climates. Because of this tendency there is a wide range of iodine values for each oil and the table lists an average. It is possible to have a sunflower oil that is more unsaturated than a poppy seed oil.

Buy oils that say either "expeller-pressed" or "mechanically pressed" on their labels. These terms indicate that the oil has only been pressed at low temperatures and not solvent-extracted. The label should also say "unrefined." The term "cold-pressed" is meaningless as an indicator of quality; it does not mean that the oil has been extracted at low heat. (See p. 000.) An unrefined, mechanically pressed oil has a strong natural flavor and aroma which indicate the source from which it came; it will also show some sediment in the bottle.

Like the germ of the grain, seeds and nuts begin to oxidize as soon as they are pressed and exposed to air. Considerable oxidation can have taken place by the time the oil is noticeably rancid, with a discernably bitter taste and smell. Because the rate of oxidation varies with different oils as well as with how they are stored, it is advisable to follow a few general guidelines in buying and storing oils in order to maintain optimum freshness.

Purchase oil in small quantities. Four to six months is the estimated "shelf life" of unrefined oils, but it's best to use them before this if possible. Unless there is a quick turnover at the natural foods store where you purchase them, avoid buying oils that are marketed in bulk.

To prevent oxidation and retard spoilage, some distributors nitrogen-flush their bottled oil. Nitrogen, an inert gas, prevents oxygen from reacting chemically with the fatty acids. When the bottle is opened, the nitrogen exits.

Store oils in a dark container, in a cool place away from heat, preferably in the refrigerator. Keep tightly capped.

Other characteristics besides degree of saturation also determine an oil's desirability. Flavor, stability, versatility, availability, and price must be considered when choosing an oil. The satisfactory fulfillment of these considerations have made seven of the central oils the ones most commonly used. From these seven oils—safflower, soybean, sunflower, corn, sesame, peanut, and olive—we pick what best suits our needs.

Because of their high degree of unsaturation, safflower, soybean, and sunflower, although good oils, cannot be considered the best. They are fine to use when a lighter oil is called for. Safflower and sunflower have a mild taste which doesn't overpower other flavors. Soybean oil has such a strong taste—which some describe as fishy or painty—that it is hard to con-

Characteristics of Oils

Variety	Iodine Value	Uses
Drying Oils		
Linseed	175–205	paint, varnish, ink
Tung	160–175	paint, varnish
Semi-Drying Oils		
Poppy Seed	132–143	artist oil, salad oil
Safflower	130–150	salad oil, paint, resins
Soybean	125–140	food, paint, varnish
Sunflower	125–136	food, resins
Corn	115–130	food
Sesame	103–118	food, soap
Cottonseed	103–116	food, soap
Rapeseed	94–105	food, lubricant
Non-Drying Oils		
Almond	93–100	perfume, pharmacy, food
Peanut	85–100	food
Olive	75–90	food, soap, pharmacy, lubricant
Castor	80–90	medicine, lubricant, chemicals
Fats		
Palm	50–60	soap, candles, carob candy
Lard*	46–66	food, soap, pharmacy, chemicals
Cocoa Butter	32–42	chocolate, perfumery, pharmacy
Beef Tallow*	30–45	food, soap, candles, chemicals
Butter*	25–40	food
Coconut	8–10	food, soap, chemicals

*Animal Fats

sider it a light oil; as you would expect, it is not so popular. The flavor of soybean oil does not remain stable under high heat.

Safflower oil is by far the most popular oil, largely due to its mild flavor, reasonable price, and reputation for being high in polyunsaturates. This, however, means that it is more prone to oxidation and rancidity. Even though it can be used for deep-frying, its flavor does not remain stable under high heat. In addition, Dr. Rudolph Ballentine points out in *Diet and Nutrition* that in ancient India, where oils were studied and classified according to their effects, safflower oil was considered to be "excessively irritating and capable of provoking or aggravating a wide variety of disorders."

The two non-drying oils most commonly used are peanut and olive. When a heavier flavor is needed, peanut oil works very well. It is good for Chinese-type stir-fried vegetables, but many find it too heavy to use every day. In deep-frying it can flash. Olive oil is unsurpassed as a salad oil and prized for its fragrant, fruity flavor. It adds a delightful richness to cooked food, but it can also be too heavy for everyday consumption.

Two oils remain, corn and sesame. Both are fairly light but not extremely unsaturated. Both are versatile and have good stability. Corn oil has a few minor drawbacks, one of which is its tendency to foam (it cannot be used for deep-frying). The other is its flavor. Some people prefer not to have the strong taste of corn in their foods, especially if the dish is a subtle one. On the other hand, corn oil's buttery richness is just the spark that many dishes need.

The best all-around oil is probably sesame. It works well in all types of cooking. Flavorful yet subtle, sesame is available light or dark (from roasted seeds). Its natural antioxidants—sesamin, sesamolin, and sesamol—give it excellent stability. Sesame oil is relatively expensive but it is worth the price. It has a soothing, healing quality that has made it sought after throughout history and raised it to legendary status. Sesame oil's one drawback is usually due to improper storage: if it is kept in the refrigerator for long periods, moisture may condense on the inside of the bottle and react with the oil, resulting in a cheesy smell. This odor can be eliminated by gently heating the oil, but it is better to buy it in smaller quantities and store it in a cool place other than the refrigerator.

Choosing a vegetable oil is not so difficult. From all the good oils in the natural foods store, pick one that is lighter or heavier to best impart the qualities your food requires, and avoid the extremes. Don't limit yourself to only the best, for it may not be the best in all instances. Experiment and enjoy all the flavors.

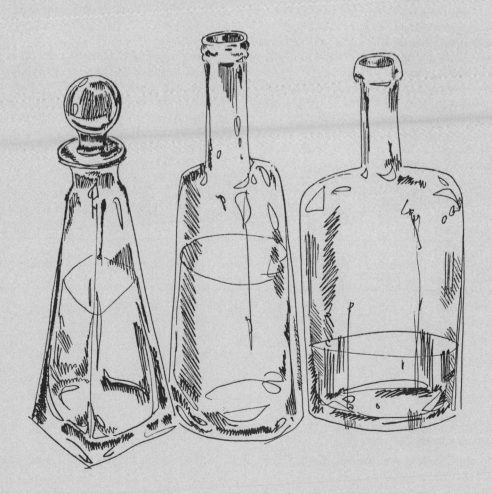

Kuzu & Arrowroot

Kuzu and arrowroot are both pure, naturally processed vegetable starches of a very high quality. Both are easy to digest and are used in traditional medicinal preparations (especially for digestive problems) as well as for culinary purposes. According to *The Book of Kudzu* by William Shurtleff and Akiko Aoyagi (Avery Publishing Group, 1985) kuzu, though more expensive, has greater alkalizing and medicinal value and is more effective as a gelling agent than arrowroot. Both starches can serve as the foundation of a delicate, glossy sauce and are effective in thickening soups, stews, and puddings. Their light, neutral flavor is prized by connoisseurs. Kuzu, a lumpy white powder, is usually diluted in cool water before it is added to other ingredients. Arrowroot, a silky white powder, can be prepared the same way but is often added dry to fruit pies to thicken them while cooking. A dusting of kuzu or arrowroot powder over vegetables gives them a crispness when they are deep-fried or tempuraed.

Kuzu grows as a wild vine in the mountains of Japan (known regionally as "kudzu," it also runs rampant over the American South, and is the subject of an exasperated,

though somewhat admiring poem, by James Dickey), and is most prized for its long (up to seven feet), thick, extremely hardy root. In Japan, kuzu is harvested in the winter, when the starch is concentrated in the root. The roots are dug up, cut, pounded, and repeatedly washed in cold running water, until the fibers disappear and the pure starch settles out.

Kuzu powder is sometimes mixed with potato starch and in this form is virtually indistinguishable (except under a microscope) from pure kuzu. Potato starch itself is sometimes sold as kuzu. Considering the rather high price of the real thing, it is best to buy brand names that you trust in the natural foods store.

Arrowroot starch comes from the rhizome (rootlike subterranean stem) of the arrowroot plant. Like kuzu, arrowroot is easily digestible. Most of the world's supply comes from St. Vincent Island in the British West Indies. This product is available in natural foods stores, supermarkets, and in Asian and Caribbean markets.

Stored in a cool, dry place, both arrowroot and kuzu keep indefinitely.

Composition of Edible Starches

Food (per 100 grams)	Calories	Moisture (%)	Protein (%)	Fat (%)	Sugars (%)	Fiber (%)	Ash (%)	Calcium (mg)	Sodium (mg)	Phosphorus (mg)	Iron (mg)
Kudzu powder	336	16.5	0.2	0.1	83.1	0	0.1	17	2	10	2.0
Kudzu root, dried	—	13.6	13.3	2.2	32.1	31.4	7.4	—	—	—	—
Sweet potato starch	336	16.5	0.1	0.1	83.2	0	0.1	35	2	18	2.0
Cornstarch	362	12.0	0.3	0.1	87.6	0.1	0.1	0	0	0	0

*Dashes indicate unknown quantities: though kudzu powder and kudzu root have been found to be rich in vitamins, exact figures have not yet been published.

Source: Shurtleff, William and Aoyagi, Akiko. *The Book of Kudzu.* Garden City Park, NY: Avery Publishing Group, 1985.

A Guide to Natural Sweeteners

Here in the foothills of the Sierra Nevada mountains of northern California on a sunny morning, it's breakfast time. Before me on the table is a slice of fresh whole wheat bread. I'd like to have something sweet with my toast.

There is a generous baker's dozen of sweeteners to choose from, arrayed before me as light, amber, and dark syrups, white and brown crystalline powders, and fruit-colored concentrates. So many choices this morning: maple syrup, barley malt, amasake, sorghum, fructose, molasses, honey, white sugar, rice malt, and others. Beyond this deployment of sweet things for my toast and palate, I envision the source of each as if also present: a maple tree, small piles of barley and rice grains, sorghum stalks, ears of corn, beet tubers, sugarcane shoots, fields of clover, baskets of fruit, a chemist's retort.

All these sweeteners come from nature, hence they all begin as "natural"—but which among them is still truthfully natural and wholesome by the time it reaches my toast? Which sweetener, after all the processing, refining, and concentrating, will I choose, and which will assuage my sweet tooth today without clobbering me with a "sugar buzz"? In the pages that follow I will recount my considerations in this search for the ideal sweetener.

The Issues

Americans today are consuming sweeteners in near-record quantities—133 pounds per person in 1984. Yet the sugar industry itself is languishing. Sugar consumption has been declining in the past decade from 89.2 pounds per person in 1975 to 67.5 pounds in 1984. The reason for white sugar's decline is the tremendous competition from artificial sweeteners (such as aspartame), cheaper ones (such as high fructose corn syrup), and a few alternative ones like honey. "The industry will just have to adjust to the reality that people want a choice of sweeteners," said a confident spokesperson for the big newcomer, NutraSweet (aspartame).

Natural foods consumers certainly are exercising their options in the sweeteners competition, but they aren't reaching with any alacrity for fructose or NutraSweet. Instead, ingredients-conscious consumers are enjoying the rise of less refined, more innovative alternatives based on whole foods—rice and barley malt syrups and fruit juice concentrates, for instance—along with the standards like maple syrup and honey. Even so, intelligent choices among the alternative sweeteners must be made with regard to several issues: origin, processing, nutritional quality, digestibility, versatility, and price.

As we search for the whole sweetener, it's useful to keep these several points in mind. First, many sweeteners are inherently natural in the sense that they are derived from nature. The obvious exceptions are the synthetics (aspartame and saccharin). White sugar comes from sugarcane or beets, fructose from corn, honey from flower nectar, maple syrup from trees, amasake from rice. It's meaningless to fault white sugar and fructose for not being "natural" in this respect.

Second, most sweeteners are processed and refined (through enzymatic or chemical hydrolysis, heating, filtration, or separation methods) and are not whole foods at all, but fractionated, isolated, and concentrated individual sugars. This distinction brings us closer to the crux of the search. Sweeteners can be ranged along a processing continuum from minimally refined (amasake) to ultra-refined (white sugar and fructose). Most sweeteners consist of individual sugars removed from of their whole food context. With white sugar and fructose, for example, little or none of the original components of the grain or vegetable are retained. Thus the degree of processing and component refinement involved should lead us to brand one as "natural" and another as "junk."

Third, sweeteners are distinguished with respect to whether their component sugars are highly concentrated simple sugars (monosaccharides, which are rapidly absorbed) or complex carbohydrates and oligosaccharides (with a range of slow-, medium-, and fast-absorbing nutrients).

The simple sugars, like glucose, fructose, and sucrose, when consumed out of their whole foods context, can cause rapid upsurges in blood sugar levels, followed soon after by dramatic plummets, commonly called "the sugar blues." It's like throwing oil-soaked soft wood on the fire rather than a slow-burning chunk of hard maple. Highly refined and concentrated simple sugars in the diet play havoc with balanced metabolism and bodily energy/fuel supplies. The more rapid the sugar absorption, the more extreme the blood sugar fluctuation, and this leads to an initial energy burst followed by depression. Sucrose (white sugar) consumption particularly has been associated with increased blood pressure, a higher likelihood of blood clotting in the veins, higher plasma triglyceride levels, and other degenerative conditions.

On the other hand, sweeteners with a high component of complex sugars, like barley and rice malt, have a gentler, slower, more balanced effect on the body's metabolism. While providing us with that periodic satisfaction for the insistent sweet tooth, their other effects are closer to those of complete whole foods than they are to the "sugar blues."

Fourth, because the simpler sugars are inexpensive, pervasive, and rapidly absorbed, people tend to consume too much of them, to the detriment of their health. The overconsumption of highly refined, simple, quickly absorbed sugars leads to an imbalanced diet and poor nutrition. It's like riding a caloric rollercoaster when what the body prefers is a smooth level train ride.

One final observation is that we must honestly assess how much sweetener—natural, unnatural, or supernatural—we are consuming every day because even the finest, most impeccably wholesome, minimally processed sweetener can still upset dietary balance when overly consumed. Too much fruit juice concentrate can be as injurious as an overdose of white sugar. Natural sweeteners are all high-calorie, low-nutrient foods, more properly regarded as food supplements or enhancements than as staples. For good dietary balance we might be better off eating a fat yam or a luscious date than using even the most complex carbohydrate-based grain syrup, with its rearranged and concentrated sugar structure.

The Nature of Sugars

Before we can look critically at the array of natural sweeteners competing for our attention on the grocer's shelf, we need to understand something about sugars.

Sugars, which are components of carbohydrates, are classified into three groups: monosaccharides, disaccharides and other oligosaccharides, and polysaccharides. Monosaccharides are the simplest sugars, and are made of a single sugar molecule (carbon, oxygen, hydrogen). They include glucose (or dextrose, or five other names), fructose (or levulose, found in fruits), and galactose (a product of lactose—milk sugar—after digestion). Monosaccharides, of which twenty occur in nature and another fifty have been synthesized, contain a chain of three to ten carbon atoms in one molecule and are very soluble in water.

Glucose is not only the most common sugar, but probably the most abundant organic compound in nature, occurring in its free state in nearly all the higher plants. It is also found in combination (a chemical linkage) with fructose in grapes, figs, other sweet fruits, and honey. Glucose is present in animal body fluids and in the human bloodstream (0.08 percent) and lymphatic system as the main energy fuel. It is absorbed through the small intestine in greater amounts than any other monosaccharide, to be later partially stored as reserve glycogen in the liver.

The second class of sugars, disaccharides, are double sugars made of two monosaccharide units joined together. Oligosaccharides are composed of two or more monosaccharide units. The disaccharides include sucrose (fructose linked with glucose), maltose (glucose with glucose), and lactose (galactose with glucose). While we see it primarily in the form of white cane or beet sugar, sucrose occurs universally throughout the plant kingdom in seeds, flowers, fruits, and plant roots (an estimated 400 billion tons are made in nature every year). Maltose derives from the malting of whole grains (such as barley or rice), a process in which grain starches are reduced to simpler forms.

Polysaccharides include gums, pectin, cellulose, starches, and many-linked monosaccharides that do not taste sweet until well-chewed and partially digested by enzymes in the saliva.

These basic sugars are distinguished by food chemists in terms of comparative sweetness. In the standard scale, in which amounts are listed as percentages of sucrose, fructose is 173, sucrose 100, glucose 74, maltose and galactose 33, lactose 16.

While consuming whole foods with their varying levels of simple, double, and complex sugars is physiologically compatible with body metabolism, when the component sugars in whole foods are isolated and concentrated, the body has an unprecedented metabolic challenge for which it may be unprepared. Fructose is 73 percent sweeter than sucrose. While the body has established glucose and glucose-fructose pathways, when fructose alone comes through at high rates, the body might experience what some nutritionists call "fructose overload," throwing everything out of balance.

We'll return to this point later, but first let's examine the individual sweeteners with respect to processing and purity standards.

Honey

Certainly honey is the most popular, best-selling, and most flavorfully varied sweetener (some thirty distinct types are recognized) on the market. Honey is available in a dazzling array of tastes, such as buckwheat, clover, orange blossom, wildflower, sage, and many others. The estimated 550,000 American beekeepers (of which perhaps 2,000 are commercial producers) derive their annual 100,000 tons (compared to 6.3 million tons for sugarcane and sugar beet) by contracting with farmers to place their hives on the edges of various clover or buckwheat acreages. Even so, about 75 percent of the honey crop is a mixture of nectars.

The only significant processing involved with honey occurs in the final filtration phase. Here the packer can either filter or strain, according to Linda Sandt of Sandt's Honey Company, Easton, Pennsylvania, a packer of "natural, unfiltered" honeys. Diatomaceous earth is a common honey filtering agent. When added to raw honey the tiny, sharp particles attract all the honey solids, but they draw out the nutritionally valuable bee pollen as well. During filtering, the honey may be heated to 175° F or higher to facilitate the process, and the high temperature can affect the honey's sugar chemistry. Mechanical straining involves a much lower heating temperature. The impurities are gathered in stainless steel mesh screens, but the bee pollen is preserved in the honey, which emerges typically a bit cloudy, indicative of the minimal heating and filtering.

Adulteration was once a significant problem with commercial honey. Honey packers sometimes added high fructose corn syrup (HFCS) to extend the honey and increase profits and failed to specify this on the labels. Technically, the FDA forbids any undeclared "economic adulterations," but detection and enforcement are time-consuming, expensive, and not a priority. The American Bee keepers Federation in Gainesville, Florida, has an informal "self-policing program," explains spokesperson Frank Robinson, whereby they independently analyze suspected honey samples submitted by consumers, then notify state and federal authorities. As recently as 1983 two major honey packers were indicted and fined for undeclared honey adulteration. Honeys adulterated by HFCS or any other ingredient are required to be labeled "artificial," while if the label states "honey" the product must be pure honey and nothing else.

Among the sweeteners (excluding the megasweet aspartame), honey has the highest caloric content, some 1031 calories per cup, compared to white sugar's 821. The total nutrient package for honey is mostly glucose-fructose and water, but some 3.5 percent of other nutrients are present. Although it is relatively unprocessed or fractionated, honey is still not a terribly well-balanced carbohydrate food. Yet it is affordable and sensible, priced about $1 to $1.50 per pound for top-grade clover, $3.50 for high-quality comb, and $4 and more for exotics.

Maple Syrup

Many regard maple syrup as the premier gourmet sweetener among the naturals. Producing maple syrup, or sugaring, as it's called in New England, was practiced by Native Americans long before the Europeans descended upon the deciduous northeast.

Initially, maple sap is only 3 percent sucrose (although this varies with weather, soil, moisture conditions, and the health of the tree) and possesses only a fraction of the characteristic maple flavor. Most of the flavor, food chemists have discovered, actually develops during the boiling phase. At evaporation temperatures reaching up to 7° F above boiling, a flavor five times as intense as that of raw sap is obtained. The final concentrated syrup, with much of the water boiled off, can be as much as 65 percent sucrose (Grade A).

Maple syrup is classified by color and light transmittance, while the actual ratio of soluble solids (sugars) to water remains fairly constant at a standard 66.5 percent solids, 33.5 percent moisture. If the solids content is higher, the sugars crystallize, while a higher moisture content invites fermentation and souring. The acceptable range (from a biological/food chemistry perspective) falls between 65.5 to 67 percent, but all maple syrups must fall within it as well to legally be called "pure maple syrup."

There is, however, a hidden potential for adulteration during the production of commercial maple syrup. This is the putting of formaldehyde pellets in tree tap holes, which is done to sterilize the opening and prevent possible fermentation of sap by unwanted microbes, and also to keep the hole open long after the tree would prefer to heal itself. Formaldehyde is toxic for humans and traces may pass from the sap into the syrup.

According to Myron Golden of Spring Tree, a Vermont-based maple syrup distributor, formaldehyde tablets were commonly used prior to 1975, but since then their use has declined dramatically. Today, says Golden, few will admit to using the tablets since producers want to protect their product's natural image.

Gary Coppola of Shady Maple Farms, St. Evariste, Quebec, a leading packer-distributor, reports that the use of formaldehyde tablets may still be "quite widespread." Nevertheless, since 1973 Shady Maple Farms has been packing and marketing maple syrup from about 3,000 Quebecois sugar bush farmers, and has been insisting that members sign affidavits describing their practices, stipulating the non-use of pellets. Moreover, the company spot checks at least 20 percent of their farmers every season for compliance. Coppola says that today about 90 percent of their syrup is "organic."

Barley Malt

Barley malt syrup or extract, although far less well-known than the standard alternatives honey and maple syrup, is unquestionably a wholesome, grain-based, complex sweetener, one which involves a natural, automatic enzymatic hydrolysis of carbohydrates. The carbohydrates in barley break down mostly into maltose. Although commercial production of malt extract by beer industry maltsters is significantly industrialized, the process is clean, simple, and free from adulteration.

The malt process begins with partially sprouted barley

Sweeteners in a Nutshell

Sweetener	Source	Sugar(s)	Degree of Refining	Cost	Calories per Cup
Refined White Sugar	sugarcane	sucrose	high	low	821
Fructose (HFCS)	corn	40–90% fructose, some glucose	high	low	736
Blackstrap Molasses	sugarcane	sucrose	high	low	699
Sorghum Molasses	sweet sorghum	sucrose	low to medium	high	848
Honey	bees	about half glucose, half fructose	low to medium	low	1031
Maple Syrup	maple trees	sucrose	low to medium	high	794
Barley Malt	barley	mostly maltose, some glucose	medium	medium	944
Rice Syrup	rice	mostly maltose, some glucose	low to medium	medium to high	752
Amasake	rice	mostly maltose, some glucose	low	high	—
Fruit Juice Concentrate	fruit	mostly sucrose, some fructose	low to medium	high	depends upon type of fruit

Dash indicates that information is not available.

grains (generally not organic), explains Tom McNealey of Malt Products in Maywood, New Jersey, a large maltster. McNealey stated that he was not aware of any unlabeled adulterations of barley malt syrup with HFCS or other cheaper extenders, but he added that the bulk of malt extract production is aimed at the mainstream food industry. Natural foods market applications are still ''relatively small'' though they seem to be ''trending upwards.''

Sometimes maltsters use additives in malting to reduce production costs and to stimulate barley's enzymatic action. Gibberellic acid, for example, may be used to shorten germination time, and potassium bromate is sometimes added to restrict rootlet formation in barley sprouts and to augment final yields. How widespread or minimal any chemical adjustments at the barley sprouting stage might be is not clear.

But there are malt extracts of whose purity we can be assured. Great Eastern Sun of Asheville, North Carolina, distributes Lima Barley Malt, produced with organically raised barley in Belgium by the well-respected European supplier, Lima. According to Bruce Sturgeon of Great Eastern Sun, the malt contains 2.8 percent protein, 0.1 percent fat, 73 percent carbohydrates (mostly maltose), ash (or minerals) 0.9 percent, moisture 22.8 percent, and about 300 calories per 100 grams. Dawn's of Philadelphia, Pennsylvania, has also recently begun bottling Lima or-

ganic barley malts under their own label.

The growing popularity of barley malt syrup and its gentle taste and slow-release complex carbohydrates have stimulated some innovative product development and marketing in America. The result has been the introduction of several varieties of whole grain rice malt, which we'll now consider.

Rice Syrup

Rice syrup's popularity first began with Chico-San's successful Yinnies. Several prominent U.S. natural foods companies, including Westbrae, Great Eastern Sun, and a newcomer, California Natural Products, have subsequently introduced Japanese-made or American-produced versions of rice syrup, which is also known as rice malt.

''Rice syrup is still pretty esoteric,'' admits Westbrae company president Gordon Bennett. But this didn't stop them from using it as the main sweetener (with raisin juice concentrate) in their popular line of whole grain cookies, Snaps. ''Actually you could do with any grain what's being done with rice today,'' say Bennett. ''Rice is expensive, something like $70 a ton compared to barley's $30, but most barley syrup is aimed at the beer makers so it's made with a strong, toasted taste and a dark color. It's not always suitable for home cooking. The ideal sugar, really, is the carbohydrate present in the whole grain. But the advantage with grain malts is that you can control the sweetness by changing fermentation conditions, whereas with honey and maple syrup, there is no such chance to make adjustments.''

Another purveyor of high-quality rice malt is Great Eastern Sun, which markets Sweet Cloud, introduced in 1984. According to Bruce Sturgeon, processing of their rice malt is simple and relatively minimal. They've found a way to obtain a wetter consistency, which means Sweet Cloud pours more easily, certainly an advantage in the kitchen.

''We were looking for a mild flavor, one that doesn't overpower foods with its own strength,'' Sturgeon recounts. ''Yet we also wanted a rice malt that was spreadable and not as sticky and hard to pour as the other malt syrups. Rice malt may be substituted for honey, but you need to use more malt for the same sweetness level. You won't get that pronounced honey flavor, however.''

Another rice malt innovation comes from California Natural Products of Mantecca, California, which has taken on the alternative grain-based sweetener category with great confidence, food chemistry expertise, and early success. In 1984 they began making Yinnies for Chico San, but since then, under the direction of the company's co-owner and resident food chemist, Cheryl Mitchell, Ph.D., they have come out with a multipurpose, modified rice malt in both liquid and powdered form. It's already finding wide applications in the marketplace, even in frozen desserts.

It's important to note, explains Mitchell, that in the corn syrup industry, the hulls and basically all the corn components except starch are removed, so that only sugars from the starch are concentrated. Rice syrup production, in contrast, begins with whole grain, only slightly polished, so that all the grain components and the complete ''nutrient package'' are retained (except some fiber from the hulls) along with the starches.

What Mitchell's process is really doing is demonstrating precision food chemistry gently applied to natural whole foods processing. Their rice syrup is in a sense a modified amasake (a fermented, blended rice beverage) which we'll consider next. Traditional amasake is high in maltose, but the modification is a combination of maltose and glucose, and has a higher proportion of glucose (10–20 percent), making it sweeter.

The advantages of rice malt in the diet are at least threefold, says Mitchell. First, rice syrup is hypoallergenic, which means few people have allergic reactions to rice (the irritant is found in the hulls, which are partially or wholly removed). Allergic reactions are more likely to occur with wheat, corn, soy, and barley. Second, rice malt has a ''light, delicate flavor that complements most foods,'' whereas honey, molasses, and maple syrup all have a strong taste. Third, rice syrup is easier on the digestive system. It has predominantly slow-digesting (one to two hours) complex carbohydrates, little free glucose, and no fructose or sucrose. According to Mitchell, rice malt provides ''a prolonged energy source without the immediate blood sugar surges'' common with other sweeteners. The maltose provides an initial energy boost, but about half of the available sugars remain in reserve and are released slowly over several hours.

Amasake

Although amasake is disappointingly expensive at about $12 per gallon, and although presently is made by only a few companies on both coasts of the U.S., it has wonderful potential as a wholesome alternative sweetener. Amasake is relatively easy to make at home, incorporates nearly all the rice, and is a mild, slowly absorbed complex carbohydrate fermented food.

Amasake takes about one day to prepare. Rice (or barley) koji consists of grain inoculated with *Aspergillus oryzae*. Prepared dry koji, which may be purchased in natural foods stores, is mixed with rice and water, allowed to ferment, then blended, filtered, or diluted to make a naturally sweet, somewhat thick, pulpy liquid. Amasake connoisseurs use this sweetener in baking, in pastries, over cereals, or in puddings as the sole basis of a kind of creamy rice ''milkshake.''

Amasake is still relatively unknown, even in the general natural foods market. According to Chris Kilham of Bread & Circus, one of the nation's leading retailers, ''Aside from the diehard macrobiotic shoppers, you'd have a hard time finding a real human out there who knows what amasake is.''

Robert Nissenbaum, president of Imagine Foods in Palo Alto, California, is one such ''real human being'' who *does* know about amasake. So well does he know that, working with California Natural Products, Nissenbaum uses a modified amasake base as the sole sweetener for his highly successful frozen dessert (non-dairy and non-soy) called Rice Dream, out since 1984.

''Highly sweetened soy desserts are harder to digest than rice,'' he explains. From the traditionalist's stance, Rice Dream's sweetener is not exactly amasake, since it's not made from whole koji, but by using specially selected koji enzymes. It does retain much of the rice fiber (beginning with only 50 percent polished grains), which, Nissenbaum says, ''gives our product a rich and creamy consistency. We don't have to add anything to improve the body of the Rice Dream mix.''

In either case Rice Dream is an ''ice cream'' sweetened with prepared brown rice and certainly that is innovative. ''We get a better balance of maltose and glucose, a subtle sweetness,'' states Nissenbaum. ''The type of sugars in this amasake make a relatively good balance for the body. We simply extract all the sugars from rice in an efficient conversion process, rather than adding more sweeteners later.''

Fruit Juice Sweeteners

One of the most promising alternatives to come along recently has been fruit juice concentrates, a simple idea but one which had apparently been overlooked. But no longer. Barbara's Bakery of Novato, California, uses a basic concentrate of pineapple, pear, and peach juice in their line of breakfast cereals, granola bars, cookies, granolas, and even in a new chocolate sauce. Company spokespeople declined to comment specifically on the products' success or their source of concentrate, but they suggested sales were more than brisk. Industry rumor has it that a retail fruit juice concentrate will soon be available.

R.W. Knudsen's, the Chico, California-based juice company, markets a line of "100% fruit juice-sweetened syrups in five flavors" (raspberry, blueberry, boysenberry, strawberry, and fruit and maple) for home use. Their composition includes "clarified" grape juice (meaning it's been passed through an ionization process), strawberry puree, strawberry juice concentrates, strawberry flavor,

and xanthan gum (a natural thickener). The product is intended as a tabletop, liquid sweet condiment, suitable for topping pancakes, cereals, ice cream, and possibly for use in baking.

Date sugar, though not widely available, is another fruit-based powdered sweetener, disarmingly simple in composition: it's all dates. The cosmetically inferior fresh dates (containing 60 percent sucrose), ones not suitable for the trade, are dehydrated to 2 percent moisture, then pulverized into a powder marketed in selected places as date sugar.

Fruit-based sweeteners have the unarguable advantage of being minimally processed, emerging in a form relatively still clearly linked with the original whole, fresh fruit. One other clear advantage with most fruit sweeteners is that orcharding is domestic. Thus, no agricultural exploitation of the Third World is involved, and commodity price manipulations do not enter into the picture (as with sugar and honey). But nutritionally, fruit-based sweeteners are heavyweight simple sugars—their punch can send the blood sugar levels reeling.

Behind the Fructose Fad

Neither white sugar nor fructose meets the standard for "natural" foods once considered by the Federal Trade Commission, which would have required that a natural food contain no artificial additives and be minimally processed. The processing for white sugar is not minimal by any standards and the same is true for fructose. In fact, Robert Shields, the marketing director of Roche Chemical (a division of Hoffman-LaRoche), which is the largest manufacturer of pure crystalline fructose, stated in a conversation that the fructose sold by his company is "definitely not natural." He went on to say that "fructose does have a natural image since it is the sugar found in fruits, but the method used to extract the pure crystalline fructose is extremely complex. This produces a very pure sugar, but one which can hardly be called natural."

Fructose generally comes in two forms, crystalline and liquid. Crystalline (granulated) fructose is produced by chemically splitting sucrose into its two component sugars (glucose and fructose) and then isolating and purifying the fructose. Liquid fructose, on the other hand, is produced

by treating corn syrup with enzymes to convert some of its starch to fructose. This product, called high fructose corn syrup (HFCS), contains 42 to 90 percent fructose and 10 to 58 percent glucose, together with small amounts of maltose, other di- and polysaccharides, and water.

Neither of these processes can be described as "minimal." Also, since refined sucrose is the "raw" product with which the production of fructose begins, manufactured fructose must be considered even more highly processed than sucrose.

Proponents of fructose claim that the fructose molecule itself is better for health than glucose or sucrose (which is composed of glucose and fructose) and has a different metabolic effect than other sugars. They reason that sucrose never actually enters the bloodstream. When it is digested it is split into fructose and glucose on the wall of the intestine and absorbed as these two sugars. The body absorbs the glucose more quickly than the fructose. The more rapid the absorption of the sugar, the more extreme the fluctuation in blood sugar level, which causes increased energy and consequent depression. Su-

crose, being half glucose, is absorbed more quickly than fructose. This swing in blood sugar level is also implicated in diabetes and hypoglycemia.

Fructose and sucrose also differ in their ability to stimulate insulin. Sucrose causes the pancreas to secrete a more immediate and larger spurt of insulin than does fructose; the glucose half of the sucrose molecule requires insulin in order to be absorbed into cells or metabolized by the liver. Fructose requires no insulin for the initial stages of metabolism by the liver. HFCS requires insulin for the portion that has been converted to glucose, but not as quickly and probably in not as large a quantity as glucose does. As a result, fructose has a less drastic effect on blood sugar levels than sucrose.

Although these effects have been observed in persons who drank 100 grams of pure fructose, glucose, or sucrose in solution, tests have not been carried out using these sugars as part of a meal. Controversy concerning the metabolic advantages of fructose over sucrose or glucose goes on and more research is necessary.

However, the high degree of refinement of fructose must still be taken into consideration. In addition, there is the question of the type of fructose that occurs in many "natural" foods. Although FDA standards require pure crystalline fructose (99.5 percent pure) in a product that carries fructose on the label as an ingredient, this is rarely the case. Because pure crystalline fructose is very expensive, most natural foods companies use high fructose corn syrup. HFCS varies in fructose concentration; most companies choose the 55 percent fructose HFCS which, as mentioned above, also contains glucose and other sugars. A solution of 55 percent fructose is only slightly better than a solution of white sugar—which is 50 percent fruc-tose—except that in the case of white sugar, the chemical bond between the fructose and glucose portion of the solution is still intact. In HFCS this bond is broken down.

Some persons believe that honey, which also contains glucose and fructose, has an effect similar to, and perhaps better than, HFCS. Honey is approximately 80 percent sugar—40 percent glucose and 40 percent fructose—which occur in the form of invert sugar. Unless the honey is heated over 180°F, this molecule does not break down and is metabolized much more slowly than refined fructose and glucose. In addition, honey contains about 16.5 percent moisture and 3.5 percent other nutrients such as minerals, enzymes, and vitamins, which help in the absorption of the sugar.

In respect to its being natural, it is hard to accuse bees of overly processing honey. Honey is relatively unrefined and whole—at least in comparison to crystalline fructose, HFCS, or white sugar.

Honey and fructose are currently the main sweeteners used in processing most natural beverages and dessert foods. Several natural foods chains, however, including Bread & Circus in Boston and Mrs. Gooch's in Los Angeles, have chosen not to carry items which list fructose as an ingredient.

The Retailers' Perspective

The sudden plethora of presumed alternative sweeteners and other sugary ingredients masking themselves as "naturals" has prompted some of the country's leading retailers, like Erewhon, Bread & Circus, and Mrs. Gooch's, to draft firm marketing policies. With such large-volume, well-known natural foods outlets as these exercising this kind of market commentary, awareness is bound to sharpen among both the public and manufacturers.

At Erewhon, with three Boston-area outlets, store manager Bruce Phlegar reports, "We don't sell any product that contains any refined sugars of any source, from beet, fruit, or cane. We do sell products with barley and rice malt."

Kilham, speaking for Bread & Circus, with four east coast stores, reiterates this view. "We absolutely do not carry any fructose, sucrose, corn syrup, dextrose, glucose, or highly refined sugar products. Fructose is an ultra-refined sweetener, an irresponsible and bogus product."

In Southern California, the four-store Mrs. Gooch's maintains a similarly restrictive policy on sweeteners. According to spokesperson Chris Kysar, "When we evaluate any product, we look not only at its dietary function but its nutritional benefit. This is why we don't allow fructose—it has no secondary benefits. We do not want sweeteners only for their sweetness, because we are a nutrition-focused store." Sandy Gooch, the store's founder and owner, notes, "We look for food value and nutrient content, which we find in the natural sweeteners like honey, maple syrup, barley, and rice malt."

The View from the Kitchen

One last consideration is a practical one. How do the alternative whole sweeteners perform in the kitchen in ordinary recipes? Not much of a cook myself (certainly not one worth quoting here), but more of a well-honed gourmand and appreciator of sweet things, I consulted two well-known natural foods chefs/writers for their professional comments.

Annemarie Colbin is the author of *The Book of Whole Meals* and director of the Natural Gourmet Cookery School in New York City. She notes that "any sweetener is concentrated out of its original context and is therefore out of balance in the ratios of carbohydrates, minerals, and moisture. At home I use very little sweetener, but when I do it's mostly fruit juice or maple syrup. Barley malt with its strong taste is good in cookies. Rice syrup, although you must use a lot, is great in tofu whipped creams. I don't use much honey, even in baking, because it's so sweet. It makes me tired and puts me to sleep."

Colbin cautions that sweeteners of any kind should play only a very minor part in a balanced diet. The sweet tooth syndrome is rampant among vegetarians, Colbin states, and often leads to bodily weakness. She says, "Our bodies expect a balance of nutrients in foods—teams of nutrients, we might say. When we eat foods fortified with extra sweeteners, the carbohydrate part is now out of balance with the protein. Thus you need more protein to correct the imbalance from using sweeteners."

Laurel Robertson, co-author of the best-selling *Laurel's Kitchen*, comments, "With sweeteners, the point is how they are served and prepared in cooking, and for what occasion, rather than the merits of individual sweeteners. We don't want to use sweeteners every day because this crowds out other foods and flattens the palate and can even become addictive. But on special occasions it feels more appropriate to indulge in a lush sweetener, to celebrate. Anyway, there really isn't a whole foods sweetener except yams or whole fruit, not one that doesn't involve some refining."

Robertson generally favors honey in bread baking because it retains moisture and keeps pastries and loaves moist longer than do other sweeteners. She recommends that fresh honey should age about three months before use, following the European baker's tradition of never using fresh honey until it has calmed down, enzymatically speaking, for about twelve months. "It's a magical, wonderful food we use with appreciation," she says. Robertson likes maple syrup, but finds the price is prohibitive. "I have an objection," she says, "to grain syrups because of all the waste of the spent grain, but I have found that barley malt is excellent for flavoring soymilk and sweetening breads. Somehow the malt imparts a rich, distinctive taste to the crust of whole grain breads and bagels. It's a strange and wonderful substance, not fully exploited to its potential yet. But it is certainly a pest to use. Viscous doesn't begin to describe its consistency. We always dissolve barley malt in hot water first, otherwise we couldn't pour it."

The Choice

The parameters for evaluating wholeness in natural sweeteners come down to, first, the amount of processing, concentrating, chemical adjustment, and overall refinement that occur in the preparation of the particular sweetener. Second, the metabolic impact of the sweetener on the human digestive and nervous system must be considered.

Third, the kind of lifestyle and eating habits the consumption of particular sweeteners tends to accentuate must be factored in. And, fourth, we mustn't overlook the various political and ecological factors at play in the production of the raw materials and their processing and distribution (negligent agricultural practices, and world commodity price/supply manipulations, for example). The most sensible course, our many commentators seem to be urging, is first intelligent, informed, discriminating choice, and second, moderate and occasional use of the more complex carbohydrate sweeteners in the context of a nutritionally rich and balanced diet.

Which brings me back to my sun-drenched breakfast table in the Sierra Nevadas with all the choices among sweeteners awaiting my decision. I won't hedge or prevaricate: I have a sweet tooth. I have enjoyed the "occasional" tofu ice cream, the almond cookie, the carrot cake, the chocolate brownie, the honeyed apple turnover. Maybe I'm even one of those improperly nourished vegetarians Colbin talks about. But on this most ruminative morning, my hand reaches for the amasake, for just a little glass of this lovely fermented rice beverage. I will allow amasake to pleasantly accompany my whole wheat toast on its long metabolic journey into the substance of my body, my blood, and the quality of my consciousness.

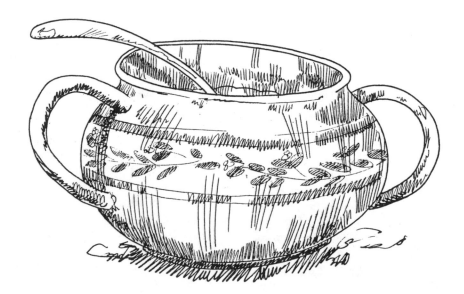

13. A GUIDE TO PRESSURE COOKERS

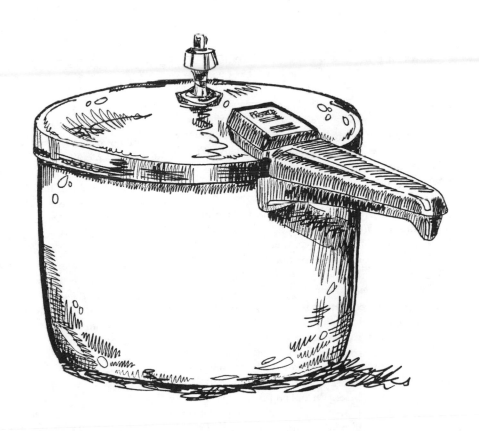

Pressure Cookers

Sweet brown rice with chestnuts. Vegetable stew and tender beans. Creamy squash pudding. These delectable wholesome dishes and an infinite variety of others are easily prepared in that invaluable and versatile pot, the pressure cooker.

If you have yet to experience for yourself the pleasures of pressure cooking—if you have thought you might like to try, but hesitated over concerns of safety and practicality—then you will be delighted to learn that today's pressure cookers are safe, economical, durable, and easy to use and care for.

What makes pressure cooking more economical than other methods of cooking? A pressure cooker cooks food more quickly, using less water and fuel, through the simple application of natural law: water under pressure can absorb more heat without boiling away. In an ordinary saucepan, the interior does not exceed 212 °F, the boiling point of water, at which time heat energy will become steam as quickly as it is created, until all the water has boiled away. On the other hand, when water boils in a sealed pressure cooker regulated at fifteen pounds per square inch of pressure, the interior temperature can reach 250 °F. This superhot water is transformed into superheated, penetrating steam that circulates through the pot and quickly and thoroughly cooks the food. A constant pressure is regulated by a metal weight or other type of regulator that will let off steam and will reduce pressure should it become too high.

A cook concerned with nutrition will find the pressure cooker economical in this respect, too. The absence of air prevents oxidation of vitamins and, because so little water is needed, soluble nutrients are not so easily dissolved. Cooking with pressure also enhances the flavors of foods rather than losing them in vapor.

Today's pressure cookers, unlike their predecessors, are lightweight, extremely dependable, easy to use, and safe. Presto, Mirro, and the Wisconsin Aluminum Foundry, which makes large-size cookers appropriate for canning, presently have the only American-made cookers on the market. The Presto model, last redesigned in 1978, is also sold under the Sears label. European pressure cookers are commonly sold through specialty stores and mail-order services. The Aeternum, SEB, and Lagostina, the best-known of the imports, are all made of mirror-finish, surgical-quality stainless steel. The Sicomatic-S, a recent import, is available in enameled carbon steel as well as stainless steel.

The European models vary a great deal. They range in size from three liters (about four quarts) to twelve liters (about fourteen quarts), and can cost anywhere from forty-five dollars to over one hundred and fifty dollars. Most of the models are available in two or more sizes. The design of the covers, pressure gauges, and safety valves also differs from one model to another.

What to Look For

If you are thinking of purchasing a pressure cooker, you will probably want to consider the following points: the material of which the pot is constructed, its shape and size, its cover, safety features, durability, availability of spare parts, and cost.

Material

Most pressure cookers are constructed of stainless steel or aluminum. The stainless steel surface is easy to clean and will not pit. Some pressure cookers are made with an extra layer of metal on the bottom to help diffuse heat and prevent scorching. (A separate heat diffuser or flame deflector, available for less than $2 in hardware stores, can be placed under a pressure cooker for the same purpose.)

Pressure cookers made entirely of aluminum, or with aluminum inner surfaces, may present serious problems from the point of view of palatability and personal health. Aluminum often leaves an unpleasant taste and may discolor food. Many studies link aluminum in the bloodstream to digestive ailments, kidney dysfunction, and brain disorders. Although the amount of aluminum transferred from the pot to the food in a single meal is probably negligible, it is also possible that over the long term these amounts could be significant.

Size

The size of the cooker is important. To cook a small amount, you'll do best with a smaller pressure cooker. Allow approximately one quart of pressure cooker for every person eating. A four-quart cooker, for example, would serve three to five people, a six-quart five to seven.

Cover

The cover is what distinguishes pressure cookers from other pots, and a variety of ingenious designs function to contain steam at a regulated pressure. To work effectively, the cover must provide an airtight seal as well as be easy to remove. The gasket is a rubber ring that fits snugly under the rim and ensures that no steam will escape. The Mirro and Presto cookers feature a twist-off cover that fits over the rim of the pot and is locked on at the handle. Several European cookers have a cover that is inserted and then lifted with a lever-like clamp to fit the sloped rim. A third type of cover is made by SEB: it fits over the rim and is secured by tightening a large screw attached to a spring mechanism.

Safety Features

Many people are hesitant to use a pressure cooker because of past bad experiences or tales they've heard. All of the modern pressure cookers discussed here, however, are self-regulating and safe. The pressure regulator keeps the steam at the correct pressure by controlling its escape through a vent. This regulator may be either a detachable weight or a fixed gauge, built into the cover. An emergency pressure escape valve will blow out to release dangerously high pressure. It can consist of a rubber plug or attached metal part. Some models, including the redesigned Presto and the T-Fal, also have a cover-blocking mechanism that makes it impossible to open the cover while there is pressure in the pot.

A cook needs only to turn up the heat at the start of cooking, lower it once full pressure is reached (indicated by the pressure regulator, which will jiggle, rock, or hiss), and turn off the heat at the end of cooking. If the heat is not turned down once pressure is reached, or if food clogs the steam valve, then the backup safety mechanism will be released and will blow off the excess steam. Food will also escape with the steam—making a mess but preventing a serious accident.

Durability

When you are looking at pressure cookers, be sure to pay attention to the following indicators of quality and durability:

- Does the cover close tightly so that no steam can escape? Is the rubber gasket flexible and well-formed?
- Are the pressure regulator and safety mechanisms functional and unobstructed?
- Are all welds, as between the body and handles, complete and strong?
- Are the edges of the metal ground smooth to prevent nicks?

- If there is a heat diffuser layer on the bottom, is it well attached?
- Hold the pot at a distance and check for any dents, bends, or other defects.
- Check also for the feeling and balance of the pot. Does it seem too heavy? Are the handles comfortable?
- Is there a lifetime guarantee against faulty workmanship? (Most good pressure cookers come with one.)

Spare Parts

Eventually, you might need to replace or repair parts of your pressure cooker, including the rubber lid gasket, safety plug, handles, and pressure regulator. Make certain that the parts will be available, affordable, and easy to install. Ask first at the store where you buy your pot whether they stock, or can obtain, spare parts. This may be your most convenient source and should indicate the store's commitment to the cooker. Beyond that, you can rely on the manufacturer or importer. (If the importer's name doesn't appear on the box, ask the sales clerk to find it for you before you make your purchase.) Spare parts are available for all the pots we reviewed. The Presto company holds ''repair clinics'' in stores throughout the United States.

Cost

Since price is an obvious consideration for most people, it pays to shop around. Most retail distributors sell for quite a bit less than the suggested price. Some stores have seasonal sales and/or offer a discount for quantity orders. There is a wide range in prices among the pressure cookers on the market. While thinking of what you want to spend, keep in mind that a well-cared-for pressure cooker is an investment that will last through many years of regular use. You will probably be happier in the long run if you get what most suits your needs.

Cookers in the Kitchen

We spoke to many cooks, distributors, and others who have had many years' experience with the daily use of pressure cookers, and asked for their comments on the different models. We found almost as many opinions as we did users. What we concluded is that each pressure cooker has its merits and disadvantages relative to the preferences and needs of each user. The ''problems'' mentioned with each cooker are minimal, occasional occurrences. Most of the models have been used daily for years without any problem.

Aeternum

This is the most widely distributed of the European cookers. Comments we heard from present users include: ''solid, compact, well-built, easy to use, good results.''

Problems included the heat diffuser bottom, which has been known to separate. Some users find the ''ear'' type handles—which necessitate holding the pot with both hands—cumbersome. The cover is an insert type, held closed by a large cam lever. Some people find that the inner-sloping rim of this model makes the food inside slightly less accessible than with other models, as well as making it difficult to use the cooker as a sauce, soup, or steaming pot. The Aeternum company was reported to be very prompt and reliable in repairing and replacing problem parts when necessary.

Aeternum–Multi

According to Aeternum, their latest design, the Multi, resulted from several years of study and experimentation by a team of engineers and cooks, and is intended to satisfy the particular requirements of ''dietetic and macrobiotic'' cooking.

The Aeternum-Multi is a strong stainless steel pot. It has a quarter-inch-thick heat diffuser bottom, and the manufacturer claims it requires no additional heat diffuser in cooking.

The Multi has a twist-off type cover. It does not get stuck, which happens occasionally with other models. Some users reported a problem with the fit of the cover, which allowed steam to escape and made the pot unusable. When we checked with an Aeternum-Multi distributor, he acknowledged the problem and told us that it was due to the pot's being knocked around during shipping. Several cooks said they fixed the lids themselves by bending the interlocking lid/body teeth into a tighter fit. Others returned their lid for a replacement.

Lagostina

The cooks who've been able to get one have high praise for the Lagostina. This stainless steel Italian cooker, which is comparable in construction and quality to the Aeternum, currently has no major importer in the United States. The super-large 12 liter (14 quart) cooker-canner is the only size available here. Many stores in Canada distribute the full line of sizes.

Mirro

The Mirro Aluminum Corporation makes only aluminum pressure cookers and cooker-canners. We don't recommend them for everyday use, unless you intend to use a ceramic pot insert at all times. Imported by the Chico-San Company of Chico, California, these ceramic pots are a Japanese invention that is meant to duplicate the heating and cooking qualities of a traditional Japanese method. Food is placed in the pot, which is covered and put into the pressure cooker, and then brought to pressure in the usual way. By this method, the food never touches the walls of the pressure cooker. The Mirro cooker, similar to Presto, is

simple and practical in design, with a twist-off cover of interlocking flanges that locks under pressure. The deluxe models have variable pressure settings.

Presto

The Presto company offers the only stainless steel pressure cooker made in the United States. You can find this cooker in hardware and department stores from coast to coast.

The Presto is lightweight, simple in its construction and use, and durable. The cooks who use it expressed a great deal of satisfaction with its cooking ability and felt it compared favorably with the European cookers. A few had occasional trouble with the twist-off cover, which can sometimes become stuck closed after cooking, and with the handles, which have been known to break. Models manufactured since 1978 have a pressure safety vent. When pressure is high, the vent rises and becomes braced against a small piece of metal attached to the interior of the pot, which locks the lid.

The Presto is available in two home-cooker sizes of both stainless steel and aluminum. Larger cooker-canner sizes are available in aluminum only. Replacement parts are readily available from Presto.

SEB

The French-made SEB has a unique cover. The lid is held firmly against the rim of the pot by means of a large screw clamp that tightens a spring mechanism. This design provides extra security, since the lid actually rises to emit steam if the pressure becomes too high. Some find the lid to be cumbersome and a bit heavy. The handles of the SEB are riveted, an advantage over welded handles, which can break off.

The SEB is of a heavy-gauge stainless steel, with a built-in heat diffuser bottom made of an aluminum sandwich wall. Many cooks appreciate the heavier weight of the pot. They feel it contributes to its durability and heating qualities.

Silit Sicomatic–S

The Silit Sicomatic-S, made in Germany, has only recently become available in the United States. The few people who have used it so far commented upon it favorably. Two types are available: an enameled carbon steel pot (in red, brown, white, or orange enamel) with stainless steel lid, and an all-stainless-steel version.

The Sicomatic cooker features two pressure settings, one for vegetables, to be used with the stainless steel steamer basket, and the other for grains, beans, and other foods that require longer cooking. The pressure regulator pops up and is non-detachable. A safety handle directs steam away from the user. The importer's brochure states that a separate heat diffuser is unnecessary.

T-Fal

The T-Fal cooker is a new model produced by the manufacturers of SEB. This pot is made of heavy-gauge steel and has a built-in heat-diffuser bottom. Its cover is a twist-off and features a unique locking system within its handle. A T-Fal representative explained that a locking pin controlled by pressure makes it impossible to raise the lid when there is more than a half pound of pressure still in the pot. A small vent on the outer rim of the cover provides additional safety.

Do's and Don'ts

It takes very little practice to become skilled in using a pressure cooker. Basic directions for operation and maintenance are outlined in the manufacturer's pamphlet that is included with purchase, and you should understand them clearly before you begin. However, we'd like to reiterate and emphasize several of the most important things to remember:

1. Always make sure all vents and pressure gauges are clear of obstruction before you fill the cooker. Make sure the rubber ring is clean and snug-fitting and that all surfaces where the cover and body of pot come in contact are clean and smooth.

2. Never fill the cooker to more than 2/3 capacity—foods swell as they cook and might plug the vent.

3. Some foods may not be suitable for cooking under pressure—oatmeal, split peas, some dried fruits, etc. They lose their integrity quickly and might plug the vent. Manufacturers will give more extensive lists of these foods in their pamphlets.

4. Never walk away and leave a cooker that is on its way up to pressure at high heat. You will need to be there to turn the heat down when the regulator starts hissing and/or rocking.

5. While the pressure is up, there should be some intermittent gentle hissing as excess steam is released, and if yours is a cooker with a detachable gauge the gauge will rock gently. If you are cooking on low heat, not enough to produce a constant hissing and rocking, you should check occasionally to make sure the contents of the pot are still under pressure. Do this by lightly tapping the pressure regulator, not by lifting it. If the pressure is still up a small burst of steam should come out. If you find that the pressure has gone down altogether, and cooking time is not yet up, turn the heat under the pot up slightly to restore pressure. Don't reheat to high unless cooking time has just commenced.

6. When cooking time is finished, remove the cooker from the heat, or simply turn off the heat under the pot. If you are in a hurry or want to stop the cooking action immediately, carry the cooker—being careful not to tilt it—to the sink and run a small stream of cold water over one edge of the top until the pressure has gone down. You will definitely know when the pressure is all the way down; the pressure regulator will not make any sound when tapped and then lifted. After the pressure is down, it is usually necessary to completely lift the regulator to release the last bit of steam before opening the cover.

7. *Never* try to remove the cover until you are sure pressure is completely down.

As intimidating as it looks at first, it will all become second nature to you, and you will soon find yourself automatically following these rules without having to think about them. Your pressure cooker is likely to become your best kitchen partner, and you'll wonder how you ever got along without one.

MAIL-ORDER NATURAL FOODS

The following companies are only some of the many sources for natural foods that can be obtained through the mail. Write or call them directly for catalogs or further information.

American Spoon Foods
411 E. Lake St.
Petoskey, MI 49770
(616) 347–9030

Diamond K Enterprises
R R 1, Box 30
St. Charles, MN 55972
(507) 932–4308

Frontier Cooperative Herbs
P.O. Box 299
Norway, IA 52318
(319) 227–7991

Garden Spot Distributors
Rte. 1, Box 729A
New Holland, PA 17557
(717) 354–4936

Jaffe Bros.
P.O. Box 636
Valley Center, CA 92082
(619) 749–1133

Kushi Foundation
P.O. Box 1100
Brookline Village, MA 02147
(617) 738–0045

Living Farms
Box 50
Tracy, MN 56175
(800) 533–5320

Mountain Ark Trading Co.
120 S. East St.
Fayetteville, AR 72701
(800) 643–8909

Neshaminy Valley Natural Foods
421 Pike Road
Huntingdon Valley, PA 19006
(215) 364–8440

Smile Herb Shop
4908 Berwyn Road
College Park, MD 20740
(301) 474–4288

Timber Crest Farms
4791 Dry Creek Road
Healdsburg, CA 95448
(707) 433–8351

Walnut Acres
Penn's Creek, PA 17862
(717) 837–0601

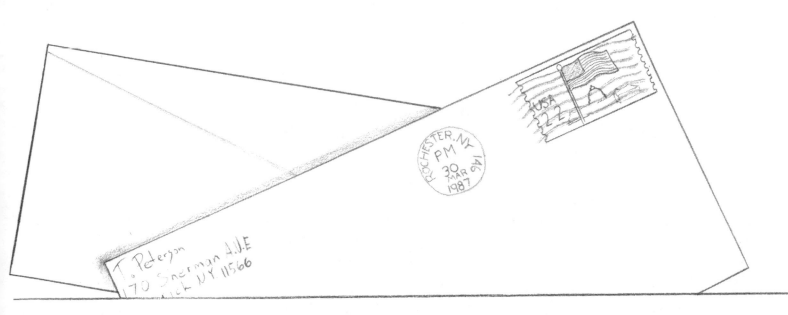

ABOUT THE AUTHORS

Jan Belleme is the co-author, with her husband John, of *Cooking with Japanese Foods: A Guide to the Traditional Natural Foods of Japan* (East West Health Books, 1986).

John Belleme, with his wife Jan, studied miso-making in Japan. He's worked for the American Miso Company, Justin Foods, the Institute of Fermented Foods, and other natural foods enterprises. John currently manages Granum East, an importer and distributor of Japanese macrobiotic foods in Saluda, North Carolina.

Ken Burns wrote frequently for *East West* about wild foods, sea vegetable foraging, and nature topics before his death in early 1987.

Steve Earle, who has lived in Japan for fifteen years, is the manager of the Overseas Section of the San-Jirushi corporation in Tokyo, the largest manufacturer of tamari in Japan.

John Fogg has been involved in various aspects of the natural foods industry for over thirteen years. A former marketing director for the natural foods company Erewhon, he now owns a consulting business, Marketing Communications, of Manomet, Massachusetts, which specializes in the advertising and packaging of natural foods.

Richard Leviton is the former editor and publisher of *Soyfoods Magazine.* He currently divides his time between Somerset, England, and Brookline, Massachusetts, where he is working on a trilogy of books on the King Arthur legend, and writing articles for *East West.*

Mark Mayell has been the editor of *East West—The Journal of Natural Health and Living* for the past four years. Previously he held a number of positions at the Center for Science in the Public Interest, including acting editor of *Nutrition Action.*

Jacqueline Ozon, a former managing editor of *East West,* is currently living and working in Hyannis, Massachusetts.

Martin Russell has been involved with natural foods baking at numerous stores and restaurants across the U.S. for the past twenty years. He is currently living in Burke, Virginia.

Meg Seaker, an associate editor for *East West,* has been on the editorial staff of *East West* for seven years, during which she has written extensively on various aspects of natural foods.

Dan Seamens worked for thirteen years in the natural foods industry both as a retailer and as a wholesale purchaser. He has written about natural foods for both consumer and trade publications and is currently the managing editor of *East West.*

Barbara Jacobs is the co-author, with her husband Leonard, of *Cooking with Seitan* (Japan Publications, 1987). She is also a fabric artist, a mother of five, and an experienced natural foods cook.

Leonard Jacobs is the publisher of *East West,* a position he has held for the past decade. He has contributed regular columns to *East West* based on his experience as a natural foods restaurant cook and manager, as well as his ten years experience teaching about natural foods, Oriental medicine, and natural healing. He lives with his family in Medfield, Massachusetts.

Kirk Johnson is an associate editor at *East West* and the co-author, with Dr. Bambi Batts Young, of *The Brain Polluters: A Consumer's Guide to Household Substances That Can Injure the Nervous System* (Random House, 1987). He holds a Master's of Science from Washington University in St. Louis, and currently lives in Jamaica Plain, Massachusetts.

Ronald E. Kotzsch is the author of *Macrobiotics: Yesterday and Today* (Japan Publications, 1986), and the forthcoming *Macrobiotics Beyond Food.* He is a longtime contributor to *East West* and holds a doctorate in comparative religion from Harvard University.

Thom Leonard has had a varied and pioneering involvement with natural foods for the past fifteen years. He was a co-founder of the first American miso company, and as a staff writer and contributing editor for *East West* has written on baking, brewing, sustainable gardening, and other topics. He recently returned to his home state of Kansas to direct The Grain Exchange, a seed preservation project of The Land Institute in Salina.

Akiko Aoyagi Shurtleff, with her husband William, is the author of *The Book of Tofu* (Ballantine, 1975) and a dozen other books on such soyfoods as miso and tempeh. Their books have sold over 600,000 copies.

William Shurtleff, with his wife Akiko Aoyagi Shurtleff, has compiled the SOYA computerized database, containing 17,500 references on soy from 1,100 B.C. to present.

The Shurtleffs are currently directors of the Soyfoods Center in Lafayette, California.

Bill Thomson is a contributing editor to *East West,* a freelance writer, and a natural foods store staffer who lives in San Francisco, California.

David Wollner has owned and operated several natural foods businesses for the past twelve years. He is currently co-owner of Columbine Market in Fort Collins, Colorado, a leading natural foods retail establishment.

Rebecca Theurer Wood is a natural foods consultant currently living in Crestone, Colorado. She is a frequent contributor to *East West, Whole Foods,* and other natural foods periodicals.

SUGGESTED READINGS

These suggested readings have been divided into the categories of health and nutrition, whole foods cooking, natural foods, chemicals in food, agriculture, and periodicals. Addresses are provided for small publishers; any reference library can provide an address for the larger publishers. Many of the following books are available through East West Book Distribution, P.O. Box 1200, 17 Station St., Brookline, MA 02147. Send a self-addressed stamped envelope for a free catalog.

Health and Nutrition

Better Health Through Natural Healing, by Dr. Ross Trattler, McGraw-Hill, 1985, 624 pp.

The Body Electric, by Robert O. Becker and Gary Selden, William Morrow and Co., 1985, 364 pp.

Bodyhealth: A Guide to Keeping Your Body Well, by the Editors of East West Journal, East West Health Books, 1985, 71 pp.

Diet and Nutrition: A Holistic Approach, by Rudolph Ballentine, M.D., Himalayan International Institute (R.R. 1, Box 400, Honesdale, PA 18431), 1978, 634 pp.

Everybody's Guide to Homeopathic Medicines, by Stephen Cummings and Dana Ullman, Jeremy P. Tarcher, Inc., 1984, 312 pp.

Fit for Life, by Harvey and Marilyn Diamond, Warner Books, 1985, 241 pp.

Food and Healing, by Annemarie Colbin, Ballantine Books, 1986, 350 pp.

Growing and Using the Healing Herbs, by Gaea and Shandor Weiss, Rodale Press, 1985, 360 pp.

Health and Healing, by Andrew Weil, M.D., Houghton Mifflin, 1983, 296 pp.

How to See Your Health: Book of Oriental Diagnosis, by Michio Kushi, Japan Publications, 1980, 160 pp.

The Hungry Self: Women, Eating and Identity, by Kim Chernin, Harper and Row, 1985, 214 pp.

Living Well Naturally, by Anthony Sattilaro, M.D., with Tom Monte, Houghton Mifflin, 1984, 228 pp.

Love, Medicine and Miracles, by Bernie Siegel, M.D., Harper and Row, 1986, 243 pp.

McDougall's Medicine: A Challenging Second Opinion, by John A. McDougall, M.D., New Century Publishers, 1985, 307 pp.

The Macrobiotic Way, by Michio Kushi with Stephen Blauer, Avery Publishing Group, 1985, 251 pp.

Making the Transition to a Macrobiotic Diet, by Carolyn Heidenry, Avery Publishing Group, 1987, 112 pp.

Natural Childcare, by the Editors of East West Journal, East West Health Books, 1984, 216 pp.

Staying Healthy with the Seasons, by Elson Haas, M.D., Celestial Arts, 1981, 242 pp.

Stretch and Relax, by Maxine Tobias and Mary Stewart, The Body Press (P.O. Box 5367, Tucson, AZ 85703), 1985, 160 pp.

The Web That Has No Weaver, by Ted Kaptchuk, O.M.D., Congdon and Weed, 1983, 402 pp.

Women's Health Care: A Guide to Alternatives, edited by Kay Weiss, Reston Publishing, 1984, 426 pp.

Whole Foods Cooking

American Macrobiotic Cuisine, by Meredith McCarty, Turning Point Publications (1122 M St., Eureka, CA 95501), 1986, 110 pp.

American Wholefoods Cuisine, by Nikki and David Goldbeck, New American Library, 1983, 580 pp.

Baking for Health, by Linda Edwards, Prism Press, 1986, 207 pp.

Basic Macrobiotic Cooking, by Julia Ferre, George Ohsawa Macrobiotic Foundation (1511 Robinson St., Oroville, CA 95965), 1987, 275 pp.

Bean Cuisine, by Janet Horsely, Prism Press, 1982, 96 pp.

The Book of Whole Meals, by Annemarie Colbin, Ballantine Books, 1979, 231 pp.

The Changing Seasons Macrobiotic Cookbook, by Aveline Kushi and Wendy Esko, Avery Publishing Group, 1985, 265 pp.

Cooking with Japanese Foods: A Guide to the Traditional Natural Foods of Japan, by Jan and John Belleme, East West Health Books, 1986, 220 pp.

Cooking with Seitan, by Barbara and Leonard Jacobs, Japan Publications, 1987, 256 pp.

The Laurel's Kitchen Bread Book, by Laurel Robertson with Carol Flinders and Bronwen Godfrey, Random House, 1984, 447 pp.

Macrobiotic Cuisine, by Lima Ohsawa, Japan Publications, 1984, 175 pp.

The Moosewood Cookbook, by Mollie Katzen, Ten Speed Press, 1977, 227 pp.

Natural Foods Cookbook, by Mary Estella, Japan Publications, 1985, 250 pp.

The New Laurel's Kitchen, by Laurel Robertson, Carol Flinders, and Brian Ruppenthal, Ten Speed Press, 1986, 512 pp.

Sweet and Natural Desserts, by the Editors of East West Journal, East West Health Books, 1986, 120 pp.

The Tassajara Recipe Book, by Edward Espe Brown, Shambhala, 1985, 225 pp.

Whole Meals, by Marcea Weber, Prism Press, 1983, 174 pp.

The Whole World Cookbook, by the Editors of East West Journal, Avery Publishing Group, 1984, 125 pp.

Natural Foods

The Book of Kudzu, by William Shurtleff and Akiko Aoyagi, Avery Publishing Group, 1986, 112 pp.

The Book of Miso, by William Shurtleff and Akiko Aoyagi, Ballantine Books, 1976, 618 pp.

The Book of Tempeh, by William Shurtleff and Akiko Aoyagi, Harper Colophon Books, 1979, 173 pp.

The Book of Tofu, by William Shurtleff and Akiko Aoyagi, Ballantine Books, 1975, 433 pp.

The Complete Book of Natural Foods, by David Carroll, Summit Books, 1985, 269 pp.

Nature's Kitchen: The Complete Guide to the New American Diet, by Fred Rohe, Garden Way Publishing, 1986, 491 pp.

A Vegetarian Sourcebook, by Keith Akers, Vegetarian Press (P.O. Box 10238, Arlington, VA 22210), 1983, 229 pp.

Chemicals in Food

Chemical Additives in Booze, by Michael Lipske and the Staff of the Center for Science in the Public Interest, CSPI Books, 1982, 133 pp.

The Complete Eater's Digest and Nutrition Scoreboard, by Michael Jacobson, Ph.D., Anchor Press/Doubleday, 1985, 392 pp.

The Food Additives Book, by Nicholas Freydberg, Ph.D. and Willis A. Gortner, Ph.D., Bantam Books, 1982, 717 pp.

Food Additives Explained, by Robert L. Berko, Consumer Education Research Center (P.O. Box 336, South Orange, NJ 07079), 1983, 79 pp.

Agriculture

Designing and Maintaining Your Edible Landscape Naturally, by Robert Kourik, Metamorphic Press (P.O. Box 1841, Santa Rosa, CA 95402), 1986, 370 pp.

A Field Guide to Your Own Back Yard, by John Hanson Mitchell, W.W. Norton, 1985, 288 pp.

The Natural Way of Farming, by Masanobu Fukuoka, Japan Publications, 1985, 273 pp.

The One-Straw Revolution, by Masanobu Fukuoka, Rodale Press, 1978, 181 pp.

Tom Brown's Guide to Wild Edible and Medicinal Plants, by Tom Brown, Jr., Berkley Books, 1985, 234 pp.

Periodicals

American Health, American Health Partners, 80 Fifth Ave., New York, NY 10011.

Delicious!, New Hope Communications, 328 South Main St., New Hope, PA 18938.

East West—The Journal of Natural Health and Living, P.O. Box 1200, 17 Station St., Brookline, MA 02147.

Everything Natural, Inverness, CA 94937.

Health Foods Business, Howmark Publishing Corp., 567 Morris Avenue, Elizabeth, NJ 07208.

Medical Self-Care, P.O. Box 1000, Point Reyes, CA 94956.

Nutrition Action Healthletter, 1501 16th St., N.W., Washington, DC 20036.

The People's Doctor, P.O. Box 982, Evanston, IL 60204.

Vegetarian Times, P.O. Box 570, Oak Park, IL 60303.

Whole Foods, WFC Inc., 195 Main St., Metuchen, NJ 08840.

Yoga Journal, 2054 University Ave., Berkeley, CA 94704.

INDEX

Twelve Important Issues that Could Change Your Life . . .

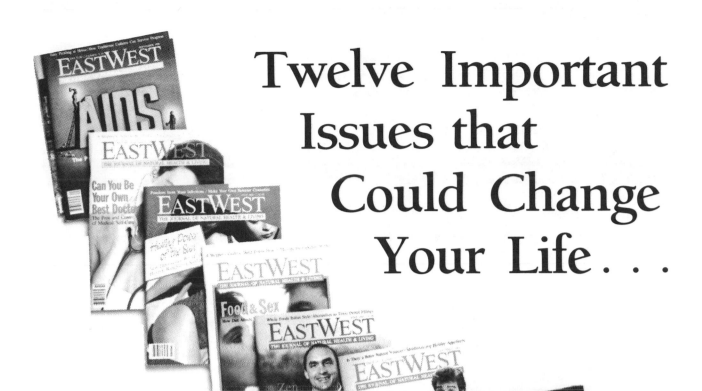

Subscribe to *East West, The Journal of Natural Health & Living*—America's leading alternative health monthly.

Each month *East West* will help you learn how to get healthy and stay healthy using natural methods such as acupuncture, diet, fasting, herbs, homeopathy, and exercise. You'll also learn about traditional healing practices from the East and West—both ancient and modern. We'll cover every aspect of health—from nutrition and diet to body and mind.

Our monthly departments feature a regular "holistic doctor" column with Christiane Northrup, M.D., plus practical and informative articles on whole foods cooking, gardening, beauty, fitness, spirituality, culture, and much more. You really can't afford to miss us—especially at the price of 12 issues for $18. That's a 25% savings off the newsstand price of $24.00. You save $6!

Naturally!

We're making this special offer because we know that our next 12 issues could change your life—naturally! Subscribe today and see for yourself. Simply fill out the coupon below and mail it back to us along with your payment. We'll both be glad you did!

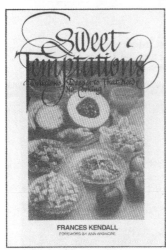
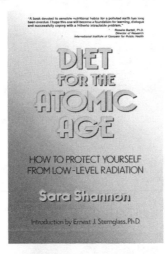
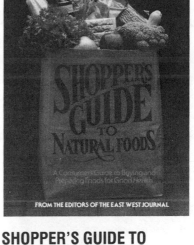
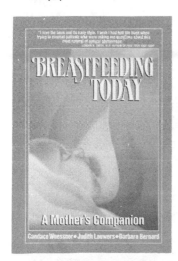
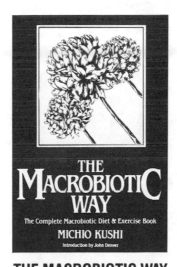
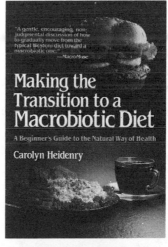
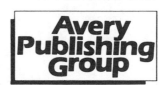

A WORLD APART

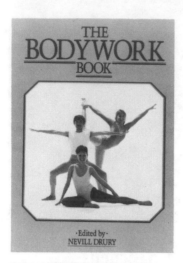

THE BODYWORK BOOK
Nevill Drury

Combines the best of Eastern and Western exercises for general fitness, including techniques for relaxing muscle spasms, correcting posture and maximizing our life-force flow.

067-2/paper/$10.95

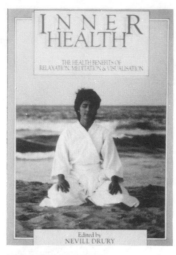

INNER HEALTH
The Health Benefits of Relaxation, Meditation & Visualization

Nevill Drury

Covers twelve major techniques—both Eastern and Western—that are designed to effectively enhance our mystical, spiritual and psychological well-being.

-73-7/paper/$10.95

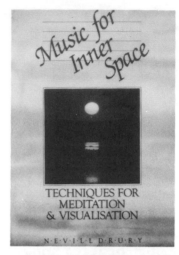

MUSIC FOR INNER SPACE
Techniques for Meditation & Visualization

Nevill Drury

Describes the use of ambient new-age music for specific types of meditation that enhance our powers of visualization and help us focus more clearly.

-74-5/paper/$9.95

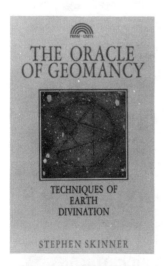

ORACLE OF GEOMANCY
Stephen Skinner

Based on Eastern wisdom, geomancy is a simple way to predict events and command success; as astrology divines by the stars, geomancy forecasts by the earth.

-82-6/paper/$12.95

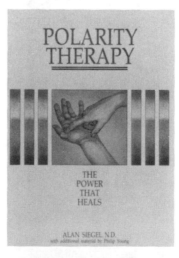

POLARITY THERAPY
The Power That Heals

Alan Siegel

This highly illustrated book provides a comprehensive, practical guide to releasing blocked energy through energy balancing, nutrition, polarity yoga and positive thinking.

-85-0/paper/$10.95

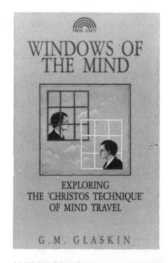

WINDOWS OF THE MIND
Consciousness Beyond the Body

G.M. Glaskin

A classic study of G.M. Glaskin's astral travels, including detailed instructions on how to achieve out-of-body experience without drugs or hypnosis.

-81-8/paper/$10.95

A HEALTHY DIFFERENCE

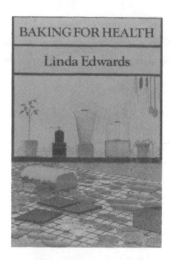

BAKING FOR HEALTH
Linda Edwards

This revolutionary cookbook creates fantastic delights from non-allergenic natural ingredients, using absolutely no refined sugar, white flour, fats, dairy products or salt.

-86-9/paper/$8.95

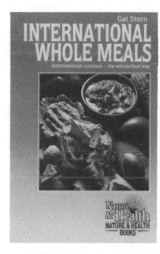

INTERNATIONAL WHOLE MEALS
Gai Stern

From France, Greece, Italy, India, the Caribbean, Scandinavia, Japan, Russia, Mexico, England and the Middle East, here are tantalizing international recipes using only whole-food ingredients.

-93-1/paper/$7.95

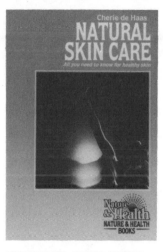

NATURAL SKIN CARE
Cherie de Haas

Shows you how to achieve healthy vibrant-looking skin using natural cosmetic treatments, tissue-toning exercises, a cleansing diet, and revitalizing nutrients.

-94-X/paper/$7.95

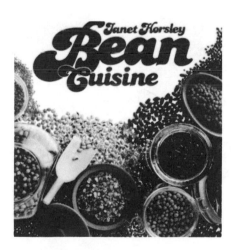

BEAN CUISINE
Janet Horsley

Finally, a complete guide to the tasty and nutritious world of beans, peas and lentils, including tips on preparation, cooking, freezing, sprouting and much more.

-33-8/paper/$6.95

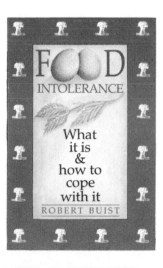

FOOD INTOLERANCE
What It Is and How to Cope With It

Dr. Robert Buist

What causes allergic congestion, stomachaches, dermatitis and migraines in millions can now be understood and overcome through Dr. Buist's effective holistic approach.

-68-0/paper/$7.95

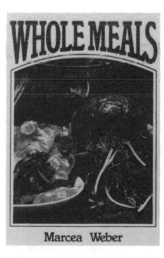

WHOLE MEALS
Marcea Weber

A well-illustrated collection of whole-food recipes that includes seasonal menus, ways to find the best ingredients, and sources of alternative proteins, vitamins and minerals.

-47-8/paper/$9.95

ORDER FORM FOR INDIVIDUALS

PLEASE PRINT:

My check for _____ is enclosed.

Charge My MasterCard _____ VISA _____

Account Number _____

Expiration Date _____

Signature _____

Ship To _____

Address _____

City _____

State _____ Zip _____

Ship Via _____

Date _____

ATT: ORDER DEPARTMENT
Avery Publishing Group, Inc.
350 Thoren Avenue
Garden City Park, NY 11040
(516) 741-2155

All prices are subject to change without prior notice and are those at which Avery sells its publications. Please specify whether cloth or paper editions are required.

Quantity	Title	Author	Price

SHIPPING	$2.00
SALES TAX FOR NY & NJ RESIDENTS.	
TOTAL	

Please make checks or money orders out in the name of Avery Publishing Group, Inc.